Getting Pregnant

What You Need to Know
Right Now

COMPLETELY REVISED AND UPDATED

Niels H. Lauersen, M.D., Ph.D.
and
Colette Bouchez

A FIRESIDE BOOK
Published by Simon & Schuster

FIRESIDE
Rockefeller Center
1230 Avenue of the Americas
New York, NY 10020

FIRESIDE and colophon are registered trademarks
of Simon & Schuster, Inc.

Designed by Pagesetters, Inc.

Manufactured in the United States of America

20

Library of Congress Cataloging-in-Publication Data

Lauersen, Niels H.
    Getting pregnant : what you need to know right now / Niels H. Lauersen and
Colette Bouchez.—Completely rev. and updated.
       p.   cm.
    Includes index.
    ISBN-13: 978-0-684-86404-4
    ISBN-10:   0-684-86404-5
    1. Conception—Popular works.   2. Reproductive health—Popular works.
3. Married people—Health and hygiene.   I. Bouchez, Colette, date.
II. Title.

RG133 .L38 2000
612.6—dc21   99-059045

No book can replace the services of a trained physician. This book is not intended to
encourage treatment of illness, disease, or other medical problems by the layman. Any
application of the recommendations set forth in the following pages is at the reader's
discretion and sole risk. If you are under a physician's care for any condition, he or she
can advise you about information described in this book.

Acknowledgments

Through the course of writing this book, many friends, colleagues, and patients have blessed us with their support, enthusiasm, insights, and knowledge. We thank each of them for every contribution, and for caring about this book.

In particular we would like to thank all the experts in the field of reproductive medicine who, through their own achievements and research, helped us to expand the boundaries of the treatment of infertility, particularly Jacques Cohen, Ph.D., Jamie Griffo, M.D., Richard Marrs, M.D., Giancarlo Palermo, M.D., J. Victor Reyniak, M.D., Zev Rosenwaks, M.D., Mark Sauer, M.D., and Richard Scott, M.D.

Special acknowledgments go to the entire Obstetrics and Gynecology Department of St. Vincent's Medical Center, particularly John Koulos, M.D., and Daniel Clements, M.D., as well as to Hugh K. Barber, M.D., former director of Obstetrics and Gynecology at Lenox Hill Hospital, for helping to establish new and higher standards of health care for women.

Our gratitude also goes to the American Society of Reproductive Medicine, to Resolve, and to the American Fertility Association, and particularly to Pamela Madsen for her support and her continued efforts to help infertile women. We'd also like to thank the March of Dimes Foundation and Nine To Five—The National Organization of Working Women, who shared their research and their insights.

Our heartfelt thanks go to the entire staff of the New York Medical Center for Reproductive Medicine for their insights and contributions, particularly Joan Affigne, Dr. Magda Binion, Donna Brummett, Rochelle Goldman, Lisa Gonzales, Anita Gutierrez, Lee Martin, Maria Perez, and Zena Rubinov.

To our friend, confidante, and colleague Yanni Antanopoulos, thank you in more ways than we can ever say. A special acknowledgment also goes to embryologists Carlos Acosta, Ph.D., and Tania Combiano, Ph.D., who shared their knowledge and their time so generously.

Many thanks to Adrian Rothenberg for her photographic contributions as well as to Ronnie Verebay, Janet Choi, and Karolina Koerna for their administrative assistance. And to Mary B. and St. Jude for always being there to pull us through—thank you.

A debt of gratitude we can never repay goes to our brilliant business and legal advisors Albert Terranova and Randy Maestro, who helped this book become a reality.

Our deepest appreciation goes to the editor and publisher of the original 1991 edition of this book, Eleanor Rawson, whose insights, wisdom, encouragement, and support remain with us always. Thank you for being there in the beginning—and in the end.

Our thanks also extends to Ballantine Books and editors Joelle DelBourgo and Judith Curr, for supporting the paperback edition of our original book.

Finally, our profound thanks goes to Simon & Schuster editor Betsy Radin Herman, who brought this book to its current updated status, and whose gentle heart and firm hand guided it to completion. She is truly an editor from heaven and we cherish her friendship and support. A special thank you also goes to assistant editor Matt Walker, who kept the wheels turning and never failed to make us smile.

And to Fireside Publisher Mark Gompertz and Editor-in-Chief Trish Todd, we are grateful that you have stayed with us to the end; we treasure your support.

—*Niels H. Lauersen, M.D., Ph.D., and Colette Bouchez*

Contents

Part I

New Discoveries: What Affects Fertility Most

Part II

The Fastest, Easiest Ways to a Safe, Natural Conception

Part III

If You Don't Get Pregnant Right Away:
How Science Can Help

Part IV

Your Personal Pregnancy Planner:
A Six-Month Guide to a Safe and Healthy Conception

Preface

Getting Pregnant in the New Millennium

Dear Mother-to-Be:

When the first edition of this book was published—in 1991—the world of reproductive medicine was, in a sense, just beginning to turn. Procedures we take for granted today, such as in vitro fertilization (IVF) and donor eggs, were in their infancy, and we had just begun to recognize the power of our individual lifestyles to influence the success and the health of the children we bring into the world.

Over the past decade, however, we have come to witness, firsthand, just how quickly that world has turned. Indeed, advances in reproductive medicine have been, at times, so astonishing that even the most enlightened visionaries could not have predicted what is commonplace today.

Equally important, much of what we have learned while solving the riddle of infertility has helped to resolve a myriad of other pregnancy puzzles as well. Today, every couple can have a faster, easier conception and, ultimately, a healthier baby than they could just a decade ago, largely due to the vast array of knowledge that research on reproductive health has provided.

Indeed, as we go forward into this new century, we can now say with some degree of certainty that nearly every couple who wants to have a baby, will have a baby—and there are few exceptions to that rule.

And this is precisely the reason we decided to write this brand-new version of *Getting Pregnant*—a book we have updated from cover to cover with what we believe is the most significant information you will need to have the family you have always dreamed of, regardless of what you think your reproductive odds may be.

- For those of you grappling with the concept of infertility right now, we offer hope *and* help, in the form of the latest, most important treatments for the most significant fertility problems affecting couples today.

- For those who have no problems conceiving but simply want to have the healthiest pregnancy possible, we give you the most significant new data on how to take charge of your reproductive health in ways that were never before possible.

- And finally, for those of you who may be trying to decide if motherhood *is* for you—whether you be a newly remarried woman over forty, or perhaps even a single woman whose biological clock is ticking louder than ever—we offer an array of new possibilities that we know can give you the confidence to pursue your dreams of motherhood.

But in many ways, we have also written this new book to say "thank you" to the countless couples who, after the publication of our first book, shared with us their trials, tribulations, and mostly their triumphs on the road to becoming parents. We are grateful that you let us be part of your journey, and we know no better way of honoring your accomplishments than to continue your legacy of hope and inspiration by inspiring yet another generation of couples to go forward with their parenting dreams as well.

So now, as we get ready to "retire" that first edition of *Getting Pregnant*, we celebrate the past and happily look to the future of our new book, and to the many new lives we hope it will help bring into our brave new world.

We look forward to hearing the good news about your pregnancy very soon. In the meantime, if we can ever be of help, please let us know. And thank you for making us a part of your parenting dreams.

Sincerely,
Dr. Niels Lauersen and Colette Bouchez
The New York Medical Center for Reproductive Medicine
784 Park Avenue
New York, NY 10021
212-744-4222

E-mail:
NLauersen@aol.com;
GettingPregnant@earthlink.net;
www.GettingPregnant.net

Introduction

The Really Good News About Getting Pregnant

When I was in medical school in the 1960s, the birth control pill was the prescription of the decade. Indeed, young men and women were far more concerned with *avoiding* pregnancy than with *getting pregnant*. Happily, this is no longer the case. Today, getting pregnant is something more and more couples view as a joyous life-expanding experience to be celebrated and cherished. And, too, we have seen the "birth" of the single mother, with many women choosing to honor the alarm on their biological clock by becoming mothers whether or not they have a suitable mate in mind.

Fortunately, along with these changes in our attitude about pregnancy came some equally important scientific advances that made it faster and easier for all women to get pregnant, and for most couples to achieve their parenting goals.

• New information about both male and female biology has given us ways to encourage not only faster but healthier conceptions, with fewer chances for miscarriage and birth defects.

• Discoveries concerning the cause of infertility have given us new ways for men and women to protect their childbearing ability as well as their sexual vitality while they safely postpone childbearing.

• Outstanding advances in nutritional therapy have given us new ways to harness the power of vitamins and minerals and in the process helped us not only reduce the risk of birth defects but also protect and even increase fertility, in both men and women.

- Stellar progress made in the treatment of infertility itself—including powerful new medications, new forms of microsurgery, and brand-new laboratory-assisted procedures—has not only allowed more previously infertile couples to get pregnant, but has given us new ways that even parents over age thirty-five can have a safer, healthier pregnancy.

In fact, thanks to what we have learned in the past several years alone, almost every woman who wants to have a baby can have one!

Why I Wrote This Book

Although the field of reproductive medicine continues to explode with new advances, my deep commitment to fertility research goes back several decades. As a member of several key scientific teams I have devoted thousands of hours to reproductive research, and my work has taken me around the world more than three times, to the capitals of Europe where the first "test tube" baby was conceived, to Russia, South America, and the Far East—anywhere I could learn the latest information on the reproductive system. Beginning in 1990, I joined forces with a team of dedicated physicians and researchers to create a medical center specifically to deal with infertility problems. As a result I have been able to see, firsthand, the exciting, almost miraculous ways in which the field of reproductive medicine has continued to grow, and how it can and does change peoples lives.

- Couples who were thought to be hopelessly infertile are now able to conceive and deliver not just one, but two and three perfect children.

- Those who previously miscarried up to fifteen times are now giving birth to healthy, full-term babies.

- Women who thought they were "too old" to have a baby are now giving birth to wonderful, beautiful children. Even those women who reach menopause prematurely—in their mid-forties, for example—have brand-new options for having a baby of their own.

Time and again my colleagues and I have witnessed a dramatic rise in the number of our fertility patients who are able to have all-natural conceptions and healthy pregnancies just by making a few simple dietary and lifestyle changes.

As astounding and important as these advances were, as I traveled the country giving lectures and making television appearances, I began to see that too many couples were still not taking advantage of all the possibilities. My colleague and coauthor Colette Bouchez, an award-winning and respected medical journalist and researcher, began to see the same thing, even among her sophisticated urban readers. While we both did our best to bring much of the good news about reproductive medicine to the public, we could see that too often, too many couples were still "in the dark" about all of their options. While some, certainly, had the basic information about such procedures as in vitro fertilization and artificial insemination, both Colette and I were continually amazed at how few people were informed about the really dramatic advances. Indeed, even many physicians were not aware of some of the great and relatively easy new fertility procedures that we knew could change people's lives.

Thus, we conceived the idea for this book—a resource and a guide to the newest, most important fertility information available today, data that has made and will continue to make a significant difference in people's lives. It is our hope that this book will make a difference in your life as well.

Part One: How the New Discoveries Can Help You

If you are planning to have a baby in the very near future or even if you haven't yet decided when motherhood will be right for you, knowing the factors that could affect your childbearing potential will enable you to take the necessary steps to protect your reproductive options and ensure that your body remains ready for pregnancy throughout your childbearing years. Part One of this book was developed to help you do just that.

It begins by exploring the very latest information on how your reproductive system functions and what biological factors can cause it to malfunction. It also explains how you can use your family history to help predict fertility problems and discusses the preventative treatments you can begin right now. It also shows how the ways in which you and your partner live, work, and play may be affecting your reproductive health, and suggests things you both can do, starting today, to make the most of your most fertile years. In Part One you will also discover:

- New information on how your immune system affects your fertility, and on the power boosters that can save your reproductive health
- How to tell if your job is harming your fertility
- The influence that alcohol, caffeine, and medication, as well as cell phones, computers, and other new technologies may be having on your reproductive health, and the steps you can immediately take to protect your childbearing options
- The kind of birth control to use to safely postpone a pregnancy without harming your fertility

Here, you'll also find a primer on the most common sexually transmitted diseases, with new information on how to keep even the most devastating infections from harming your reproductive health. You'll learn to recognize the early signs and symptoms—in both yourself and your partner—and find out the latest treatment options.

And, finally, you 'll learn important new truths about male fertility, along with vital new ways your partner can protect his virility and his potency, while decreasing your risk of miscarriage and protecting your baby from birth defects.

Part Two: Getting Pregnant Right Now — More Good News

If you are thinking about getting pregnant in the near future, and especially if you are actively trying to conceive right now, Part Two was written for you. It provides the very latest information on the factors that may influence your *immediate* ability to conceive, and to sustain a healthy pregnancy.

In this section you'll find:

- Breakthrough treatments for preventing miscarriage—and what you can do before you conceive to reduce your risks
- The links between dieting and conception—and how to find your ideal fertility weight
- How your fitness workouts may be blocking your ability to get pregnant—plus the exercises that can help you get pregnant faster
- How stress affects conception
- How to avoid major pregnancy complications
- How to get pregnant fast—including how sex affects conception
- What you can do to influence the sex of the child you conceive

Want to have a boy? Can't wait to have a girl? We'll tell you how!

In addition, you'll find an exciting new kind of nutritional guide with information on the foods that can increase your fertility and encourage your reproductive health. You will also find all the latest information on the vitamins, minerals, and herbs that can not only influence your ability to get pregnant but help reduce your baby's risk of problems from the moment of conception. You'll even learn how making love on your birthday can give your fertility a secret boost, and may help you get pregnant faster!

Finally, you'll read about the new Fertility Exam 2000, the very latest form of pre-conception counseling that can help ensure your pregnancy right from the start. Included are all the tests and treatments your doctor should be administering to help ensure that any baby you conceive will be healthy right from the start. What's more, with the information provided, you will be able to uncover any potential fertility problems you may not know you have and learn how to correct them before they seriously harm your reproductive health.

Part Three: If You Don't Get Pregnant Right Away — What to Do

In Part Three you will find the most advanced and most important new technologies developed to help you have a baby, even if you believe you are infertile. The data in Part Three not only will help you understand why you are having a problem getting pregnant, but will offer a multitude of options for solving your problem. Some of what this section offers:

- How to tell if you can have a baby long before you try to conceive — plus how to turn the pregnancy odds in your favor
- Superovulation, one of the newest ways for every woman to increase her chances for conception
- The surprising truth about fertility drugs, including new information about their safety, and how they can help you have a natural conception
- Brand-new time- and money-saving fertility surgeries that require no hospitalization and can help you get pregnant in record time

Because we now know that male fertility is a factor for nearly half of all couples who cannot conceive, this section will also offer the very latest treatments for male fertility, including the brand-new ICSI procedure.

In addition, you'll learn about the astonishing new ways that artificial insemination is helping millions of couples get pregnant, and you'll find information on the breakthroughs that can increase the success of all laboratory-aided conceptions, including in vitro fertilization, and even let you know beforehand which of the new methods is going to be best for you.

You'll also learn about the GIFT procedure and it's newest cousin, called ZIFT, both of which can help you achieve a faster, easier, healthier conception regardless of your age or how long you have been infertile.

Later in this section you will also find the latest information on donor eggs and donor sperm, as well as the new data on embryo freezing. And in a special chapter devoted to the midlife pregnancy you will find all the information you need to help you get pregnant after age thirty-five, including special dietary precautions and the treatments that will and won't help you conceive.

Part Four: Your Personal Pregnancy Planner

In Part Four of this book you'll find a Personal Pregnancy Planner—a six-month guide that takes you step-by-step through everything you need to do to have a healthy baby, whether you conceive on your own or with laboratory assistance.

Whether showing you ways to protect your fertility from current dangers or helping you restore it from dangers past, the programs in this book were developed to help you have a fast, easy, healthy conception. Not only can you be sure of your ability to get pregnant right now, but you can retain your reproductive options throughout your childbearing years. You have the power to achieve your parenting dreams. Good luck and go for it—we're on your side!

Part I

New Discoveries: What Affects Fertility Most

Chapter One

How Your Body Works:

The Latest News

From the first moment you saw him smile, you knew he was the man for you. Well, perhaps it didn't happen quite that quickly. Maybe you dated each other for months or possibly even years before that mysterious and very wonderful feeling took over and you knew you were in love.

Regardless of when in your relationship it occurred, if you are like many women, finding that special someone may have elicited another, even more powerful feeling: the desire to have a baby. While childbearing was once the farthest thing from her mind, many an obstetrical patient has told me that from almost the instant she met her mate her babylust began.

For other women, however, things can work just the opposite: The desire for motherhood may come long before a potential partner appears. In fact, some patients confide to me that it was their unrelenting desire to have a baby that prompted their search for a soulmate or at least a suitable parenting partner!

While no one is really certain what causes a woman's baby alarm to ring, the recognition that it exists was one of the elements that led researchers to a key discovery about how and why a woman gets pregnant. What was it they discovered? The vital role of reproductive hormones.

And while it was once thought that conception was strictly a physiological function of reproductive organs, today research shows that the same biochemicals that influence the desire to have a baby also play a key role in achieving conception. In fact, without your reproductive hormones, you could not get pregnant!

The New Conception Chemistry: How It Works

From the moment puberty starts and throughout your childbearing years, your body and your brain work together in a unique biological partnership to produce a series of hormones that can affect everything from your mood to your desire for sex—even your appetite for certain foods. Some new studies also suggest that some of these same hormones are what cause a woman's baby alarm to ring, stimulating a natural mothering instinct that is often perceived as a desire to get pregnant.

The strength of this feeling and when (and how often) in your childbearing years it occurs are also thought to be influenced, at least in part, by hormonal activity.

Even more important, however, is the way hormones affect your ability to get pregnant. Although the total number of eggs your ovaries can produce is predetermined before you are born (in most women, about four hundred thousand follicles exist), we now know that for you to get pregnant these follicles must be able to develop and grow, be released from your ovary into your fallopian tube, be fertilized, and implant in your uterus and grow. While it is your reproductive organs that actually perform these vital tasks, the latest research shows that it is your reproductive hormones that provide the biochemical signals necessary to put these organs into motion.

The Hormones That Help You Get Pregnant

Five reproductive hormones are necessary for conception. They send their signals to your various organs by rising and falling in a distinct and carefully timed pattern throughout the course of a single monthly menstrual cycle. The effects of all five are felt in your body, but three of these hormones are continually being manufactured and released into your bloodstream by your brain. The first two are:

- **Follicle-stimulating hormone (FSH):** Secreted by your pituitary gland (which is located at the base of your brain), it stimulates the follicles inside your ovaries to produce eggs.

- **Luteinizing hormone (LH):** Also secreted by your pituitary gland, it signals to your egg when the time is right to leave your ovary and be ovulated into your fallopian tube so that fertilization can take place.

Collectively they are called gonadotropins. Although some FSH and LH remain in your body at all times, both are secreted in greater amounts

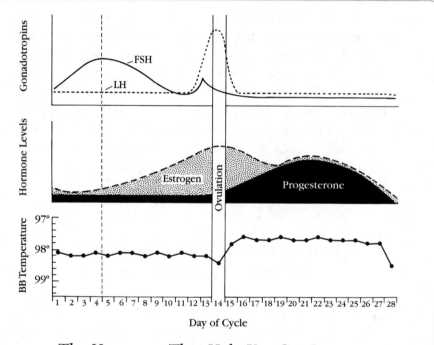

Day of Cycle

The Hormones That Help You Get Pregnant

In order for you to get pregnant, your body must maintain a fine biochemical balance among at least four of the five major reproductive hormones: FSH (follicle-stimulating hormone), LH (luteinizing hormone), estrogen, and progesterone. As their levels rise and fall, distinct patterns are formed which can be documented throughout each menstrual cycle. The changes are also reflected in corresponding changes in your body temperature. The ebb and flow of all these factors work together to create your fertility curve, the time of the month when you are most likely to conceive.

during the first half of your menstrual cycle, and levels of both drop sharply after ovulation. It was recently discovered that in order for this fluctuation to occur, another hormone must enter the fertility equation: gonadotropin-releasing hormone (GnRH). This helps release the proper amounts of gonadotropins (FSH and LH) into your bloodstream. Secreted by your hypothalamus, a tiny gland located near your pituitary, GnRH functions as a kind of biochemical radar system that pulses through your body every 90 to 120 minutes, twenty-four hours a day. It monitors your bloodstream for levels of FSH and LH and then at the proper time directs your pituitary to release more of each into your bloodstream. Finally, getting pregnant also requires estrogen and progesterone, two more fertility hormones. They are manufactured in your ovaries (and elsewhere in your body) and also rise and fall in a precisely timed pattern throughout each menstrual cycle. Their purpose is to orchestrate various steps in the egg production and release process, which you'll read more about later in this chapter. After you become pregnant estrogen and progesterone help maintain your pregnancy and protect you from miscarriage.

Getting Ready to Get Pregnant: How Your Body Works

Each month, at the start of every menstrual cycle, your body begins to prepare you for a new opportunity to get pregnant. This is a five-step process.

Step 1: Egg Production

Starting on the first day of your menstrual cycle (the day you start to bleed), your GnRH messengers sense that FSH is low. In turn your hypothalamus gland sends a signal to your pituitary to begin producing and releasing more FSH into your bloodstream. The purpose is to stimulate a new group of follicles inside your ovary to begin producing eggs.

Step 2: Getting Your Uterus Ready

As your eggs start to grow, the follicles release estrogen. In a natural anticipation of fertilization, these rising estrogen levels stimulate the tissue that lines the inside of your uterus (called the endometrium) to begin growing thicker. This helps to form a spongy nest into which your embryo (the fertilized egg) can easily implant and start to grow.

Step 3: Selecting the Egg of the Month

Within a few days after the stimulation of your egg follicles, one of them begins to surpass the others in growth and maturity. Called the Graafian follicle, it produces what is thought to be the strongest egg, the one you will eventually ovulate.

Step 4: Ovulation

As your egg of the month continues to mature, it begins to push against the top of your ovary, forming a tiny bubble on the surface. When it reaches its peak maturity, estrogen levels soar. Sensing this intense rise, your hypothalamus sends a second message to your pituitary gland to release the hormone LH, which also shoots into your bloodstream with a rapid surge. It is this fast and immediate rise in LH that stimulates your egg to leave your ovary and travel to your fallopian tube. After this occurs, your endometrium continues to grow thicker in anticipation of the arrival of a fertilized egg.

WHAT HELPS OVULATION

In addition to the push your egg receives from the hormonal surge of LH, your fimbria, the petal-like fingers of your fallopian tube, also play an important role. Using a gentle sucking action that coaxes your egg from its shell, your fimbria actually reach down and massage your ovary just before ovulation. As your egg bursts through your ovary, the fimbria act like a fertility safety net, catching and gently guiding it inside your fallopian tube so that it can meet your partner's sperm and become fertilized.

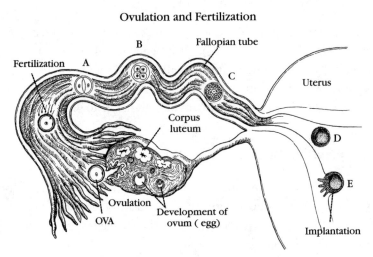

Ovulation and Fertilization

Fertilization A B Fallopian tube C

Uterus

Corpus luteum

D

E

Ovulation Development of ovum (egg)

OVA

Implantation

How a Pregnancy Occurs

At the start of each menstrual cycle, signals sent from the body to the brain help initiate the production of hormones that set your monthly egg production-and-release process in motion. When your egg is ripe and ready to be ovulated, it gently pops from your ovary and is caught by the fimbriated ends of your fallopian tubes and quickly swept inside. If you have had unprotected intercourse just prior to this event, sperm waiting in your tube will meet your egg and fertilization is likely to occur. Once this happens, the resulting embryo begins to travel down the length of your tube as it simultaneously begins to multiply and divide, first into two cells (A), then four (B), and finally eight cells (C). At this point the embryo leaves the tube and enters the uterus (D), where it implants in the lining (E) and begins to grow. You are now considered to be pregnant.

Step 5: Getting Pregnant

Once your egg is in your fallopian tube, it is ready to be fertilized. However, it only remains fertile for about twelve to twenty-four hours, after which time it begins to disintegrate. In order for conception to occur, your partner's sperm must make contact with your egg within the twelve- to twenty-four-hour time period following ovulation. You'll learn later how you can ensure that this occurs.

How Your Life Cycles Function

Whether or not you get pregnant, from the moment you ovulate, the follicle your egg leaves behind becomes a fully functioning endocrine gland. Called the corpus luteum, it continues producing estrogen (much the way your egg did) and begins producing progesterone, which helps soften the lining of your uterus and makes implantation easier, and therefore stronger. This can help you avoid miscarriage.

If you don't become pregnant (either by choice or for other reasons, discussed later in this book), your corpus luteum is programmed to pro-

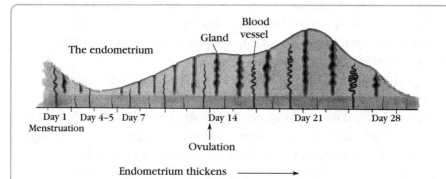

Blood
vessel
Gland

The endometrium

Day 1   Day 4-5   Day 7   Day 14   Day 21   Day 28
Menstruation

Ovulation

Endometrium thickens ⟶

The Menstrual Cycle

The purpose of the menstrual cycle is to prepare the uterus, or womb, for possible pregnancy. Beginning on the sixth day of your cycle, just after menstruation ceases, estrogen and progesterone begins to rise. This causes the lining of your uterus to thicken and grow, in anticipation of a fertilized egg.

Approximately halfway through your cycle—on about day 14—your egg is released from your ovary and whisked into your fallopian tube. If the egg is fertilized, the resulting embryo makes its way to your uterus in about 5 to 6 days, where it implants and begins to grow.

If fertilization does not take place, estrogen and progesterone levels drop sharply, and the endometrial tissue breaks down and leaves your body in the form of menstrual blood. This completes one menstrual cycle. The reproductive organs are then ready for another to begin.

duce progesterone and estrogen for just fourteen days, after which time it begins to disintegrate. As it does, estrogen and progesterone levels drop sharply. Since without high levels of these hormones your spongy uterine lining cannot exist, it begins to disintegrate as well.

Why You Get a Menstrual Period

To help cleanse your system of this now needless tissue, your body begins to produce a substance called prostaglandin, which, in turn, stimulates powerful uterine contractions. This action pulls the excess tissue from the walls of your uterus and expels it from your body. It is the combination of this tissue and the blood from the tiny vessels that rupture during the extracting process that forms the basis of your monthly menstrual flow.

Although this process should cause only minimal discomfort, some of my patients report pain ranging from mild to severe accompanying every menstrual period. Why does this happen? It was recently discovered that when, for various reasons, a woman produces extremely high levels of prostaglandin, her uterus can contract so violently during the shedding process that painful cramping occurs just before every period.

With or without pain, however, from the moment your menstrual flow begins, the entire hormonal network is reactivated, and your body begins to prepare for another twenty-eight-day cycle—and a new chance to get pregnant.

How Your Personal Biology Affects Your Fertility

In order for you to become pregnant, your body must maintain a finely balanced biochemical equilibrium. Unfortunately, current research shows this is not always possible. In fact, a woman's reproductive chemistry can be so fragile that sometimes something as simple as a cold or flu or even not getting enough sleep can throw things out of sync. As a result, you probably experience short spans of infertility far more often than you realize. This is one of the reasons you don't automatically get pregnant each time you have unprotected intercourse, even if relations take place at the time of ovulation.

Additionally, recent research has found that certain more serious personal biological factors have the power to affect your fertility in myriad ways. If left untreated, some of these factors may render you permanently infertile. In the next several chapters, you'll learn more about what these factors are. More important, however, you'll also learn how, in many instances, you have the power to prevent problems from ever occurring, as well as to reduce the effects of any problems that have affected you until now.

You Can Prevent Infertility!

With the new methods your doctor has for identifying potential problems long before they exist and a plethora of revolutionary, fast, and easy ways to treat those that do occur (all discussed in the next chapter), it's now possible to significantly reduce your risk of some of the major causes of infertility.

How can you begin to assume this new and exciting control over your reproductive fate? By becoming an active, aggressive, educated partner in your own fertility care. This is especially important if you are planning to preserve some of your childbearing options for the future. Why?

Very often the effects of reproductive damage are cumulative and silent: What is happening in your body today might not be evident for several more years. However, by remaining critically aware of what has the potential to harm you, you can catch most problems before significant damage has occurred. In this way you can have total control over your ability to get pregnant, both right now and in the future.

Chapter Two

Seven Super Fertility Threats and How to Avoid Them

Not every physiological factor that threatens reproductive health will necessarily harm *your* fertility, of course, but recent research has shown that certain conditions do routinely affect a significant number of women. Although some of these factors are obvious (for example, the much-publicized link between infertility and IUDs), some may not be so easy to see. Many of the patients who come to my fertility center are surprised, even shocked, to learn that their inability to conceive could be the result of menstrual-related conditions like endometriosis, or problems like fibroid tumors. Even simple vaginal or cervical infections that have remained undiagnosed and untreated for too long can cause fertility problems. For many women, the signs of infertility can be so subtle that problems are not even noticed until they find they cannot conceive.

How can you tell what aspects of your personal biology may be placing your fertility at risk? By listening to your body for the important signs and symptoms listed in this chapter and, when applicable, checking into your personal and family health history for factors that place you at high risk. Using this information, you and your doctor can work together to avoid or stop the most common and harmful threats to your fertility.

Threat 1: Surgical Adhesions (Scar Tissue)

One of the most devastating threats to a woman's fertility can occur as a direct result of medical treatment. I'm speaking of adhesions, also known as scar tissue. These are bands of fibrous material that develop in and

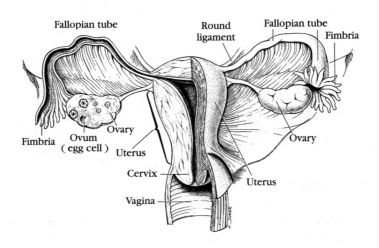

The Female Reproductive System

Enclosed in the bony structure of the pelvis are all of the organs necessary for reproduction:

- The vagina, the gateway to your reproductive tract
- The cervix, or "mouth of the womb," the entrance to the uterus
- The uterus, the layer of muscle that surrounds your endometrium, the cavity in which your baby will grow
- The fallopian tubes, the two passageways leading from the ovaries to the uterus. They provide a route allowing sperm to get to your egg and a fertilized egg subsequently to reach your womb
- The fimbria or tube ends, which help your egg to ovulate
- The ovaries, which house your lifetime supply of egg follicles

When any factor (such as disease, scar tissue, a cyst, or a tumor) blocks or restricts the function of any of these organs, or if a carelessly performed medical procedure (like an abortion or an IUD insertion) damages a portion of your system, your fertility can be placed at great risk.

around your uterus or cervix in response to any number of gynecological or obstetrical procedures, such as a Cesarean section, or a D&C (dilation and curettage) surgery. As the internal tissue is manipulated during a surgery, the body responds as if it were being wounded. In an effort to protect itself, it begins manufacturing "protective" layers of tissue in the area where it perceives inflammation. This "scar tissue" is then perceived by the body as even more inflammation, which in turn causes more protective layers to be laid down. As the vicious cycle continues, layer upon layer of adhesions can develop throughout the reproductive system.

How Scar Tissue Affects Fertility

When scar tissue forms inside the uterus it is medically known as Asherman's syndrome. Even when scarring is mild, it can block the uterus from receiving the hormonal stimulation necessary to build the soft, spongy lining necessary to maintain your pregnancy. And this can increase the risk of miscarriage. In more severe cases of Asherman's syndrome, so much scar tissue forms that the uterus is sealed shut— meaning pregnancy becomes impossible.

Scar tissue can also form in your cervix, as a result of the dilation process necessary to perform a D&C. This causes it to become rigid and narrow, a condition known as a "stenotic cervix." The dilation process can also damage the mucus-producing glands inside your cervix, which in turn can leave your internal environment so dry that it becomes very difficult for sperm to reach the fallopian tube.

Protecting Your Fertility from Adhesions

For some women, the development of scar tissue is inevitable. However, the quicker it is discovered, the easier it is to fix, and the faster pregnancy odds will improve. But how can you tell if you have scar tissue? Use your menstrual cycle as a guide: If your period does not return within three months following a D&C, scar tissue should be suspected. Although you may be ovulating, scar tissue could keep your uterus from responding to normal hormonal stimulation. As a result, no lining is building, so no shedding (in the form of menstrual blood) can take place.

It's also important to note that sometimes your surgeon can increase your risk of adhesions by being particularly aggressive when removing uterine or cervical tissue. Complications can be reduced, however, with the use of anti-inflammatory steroid medications in conjunction with your surgery.

I have found that, when given just before the start of surgery and continued for three or four days afterward, these powerful anti-inflammatory drugs can help offset the development of scar tissue by calming the body's inflammatory response in the critical forty-eight to seventy-two hours following the procedure.

Additionally, talk to your doctor about the use of laparoscopy, a minimally invasive way of performing many types of operations that dramatically reduces the incidence of scar tissue. You can read more about laparoscopy in Chapter 17.

Abnormal Pap Smear and Infertility

In the event that a Pap smear indicates the presence of abnormal cells, your doctor may recommend surgery. However, you may be able to avoid an operation and spare the formation of fertility-robbing scar tissue as well. How?

Advances in cytology are now so sophisticated that a Pap smear can detect far more abnormalities than ever before. While this can mean that cancer cells are caught at the earliest possible stage, it can also mean that sometimes a reading of "mildly atypical" or "abnormal" cells can be the result of a cervical infection or other source of inflammation—problems that can be easily remedied with medication.

As such, I strongly suggest you talk to your doctor about postponing surgery, and instead opt for a prescription of an anti-inflammatory vaginal cream or suppository, to be used daily for up to ten days. Your Pap smear can then be repeated. I have found that the second test following treatment is usually normal—meaning no surgery is necessary. If, of course, your second Pap smear still reveals abnormal cells, aggressive treatment to remove the suspect tissue is essential. To help preserve your fertility, ask your doctor about the use of a carbon dioxide laser, which gently removes the suspect tissue, or a procedure known as LEEP, a type of electrosurgical cutting that minimizes trauma to the cervix. These are the forms of surgery least likely to cause scar tissue formation.

If You Have Scar Tissue: The Treatments That Can Help

If significant adhesions have developed, and you are experiencing pain or problems conceiving, it may be necessary to surgically remove them. Unfortunately, for women who make scar tissue, the corrective surgery can cause additional adhesions to develop, with an increase in fertility problems as well.

As I mentioned earlier, one solution is to use laparoscopic surgery to remove your adhesions, which will help reduce the formation of additional scar tissue.

However, in many instances, it may be easier and more effective if you bypass the surgery altogether and proceed directly to one of the newer forms of assisted reproduction discussed in Part Three of this book. Not only will this save you the time, trouble, and trauma of a potentially unnecessary surgery, it can make the best use of your fertile time, by helping you achieve a pregnancy much more quickly.

Threat 2: Pelvic Inflammatory Disease

Although your reproductive functions are orchestrated by the hormonal activity that occurs in your brain, the conception of your child, as well as his or her growth and development, takes place within your body. The general area where this occurs is your pelvis, a bony structure that contains your uterus, as well as your fallopian tubes, ovaries, appendix, and part of your intestines. Surrounding your entire pelvic cavity is a slick, slippery membranelike material called the peritoneum. Its job is to act as a kind of semi-liquid barrier that keeps organs from sticking to each other.

However, should harmful bacteria, viruses, or other microorganisms make their way into your pelvic region, the peritoneum can become inflamed. When it does, a variety of conditions collectively known as PID, pelvic inflammatory disease, can result. Specifically, these infections include:

- Endometritis: inflammation of the uterus
- Salpingitis: infection of the fallopian tube
- Oophoritis: ovarian infection

You can also develop peritonitis, the most extreme form of PID. This results in an infection of the entire pelvic cavity and the membrane surrounding the abdomen.

Although just about anything that allows harmful micro-organisms to pass through your vagina and into your reproductive tract has the ability to cause PID, there are several factors that experts have observed (and I personally have found) to be most often responsible for these infections:

- Untreated sexually transmitted diseases (STDs) such as gonorrhea and chlamydia (see Chapter 5)
- A ruptured appendix
- An abortion performed under unsterile conditions

PID—The Signs and Symptoms

The most obvious sign of PID is extreme pelvic pain, which can either build over a period of time or be sudden and severe. Other warning signs include odorous vaginal discharge, uterine bleeding, fever and chills, painful urination, and nausea and vomiting. Sometimes, however, a woman with PID has no symptoms, or nothing more than a slight backache.

How PID Affects Your Fertility

When diagnosed and treated early on, PID will not usually cause any permanent damage to your fertility. However, as I often caution my patients, once these infections make their way inside your reproductive tract, there is always a chance for serious damage to occur.

If infections are left untreated, your organs can simply deteriorate from disease, making removal your only alternative. Fortunately, the pain leading to this drastic stage is generally so severe that most infections are caught before surgery is necessary.

Far more likely, however, is that PID will cause the formation of scar tissue within your reproductive system, particularly in and around your fallopian tubes. This makes it difficult for sperm to reach your egg, and even if it does, the resulting embryo may become stuck in the tube, increasing your risk of a life-threatening ectopic pregnancy. (You'll read more about this later in this chapter.)

In addition, if the scar tissue forms in and around the fingerlike ends of your tube (called the fimbria), the tubes may actually seal shut, in which case all chances for natural conception are lost.

In its most severe form, scar tissue can affect the peritoneum, causing organs to begin sticking together. Thus, your ovary can become "glued" to your fallopian tube, your tube to your bowel, and so on down the line. The end result here: complete infertility.

Fortunately, for most women, PID is diagnosed and treated before any of these dramatic and drastic events occur. That they can and do happen, however, underscores the need for you to see your doctor the moment you suspect you have been exposed to a sexually transmitted disease—and certainly at the very first sign of any symptoms.

Protecting Your Fertility from PID: What to Do

The best way to protect your fertility from the ravages of PID, of course, is to be on the lookout for its earliest signs and symptoms, especially vaginal discharge and pelvic pain, and to seek treatment immediately. Sometimes your doctor can see or feel the presence of PID during a pelvic exam. At other times, a procedure called culdocentesis may be needed to lock in a diagnosis. (Here, your doctor will insert a thin needle through your vagina into your abdominal cavity to aspirate fluid that is then tested for infection.) In some extreme cases, I have found that a laparoscopy—which allows me to view all the reproductive organs—is also helpful in confirming a diagnosis.

Once PID is diagnosed, an antibiotic regimen taken for two to three weeks can help. If need be, a laparoscopy can be performed later to help free the system of scar tissue that may have formed.

In addition, I have seen the following suggestions help protect many high-risk patients from contracting PID:

- Always use condoms when having sex with a high-risk partner (one who might have multiple partners or who displays any physical evidence of possible infection, especially abnormal penile discharge; see Chapter 5).
- Seek testing for STDs if you have had sex with someone you don't know well.
- Remain aware of the symptoms of all STDs (described in Chapter 5) and get tested at the first sign of infection.
- Recognize your high-risk factors: PID occurs more frequently if you are under age twenty-five, you have had a sexually transmitted disease or PID in the past, or you use an IUD.

If You Have Had PID in the Past

Don't panic now. As long as you received treatment, chances are your reproductive system did not suffer any fertility-related trauma. If you suspect you may have developed scar tissue as a result of a past infection, talk to your doctor about a simple procedure known as a hysterosalpingogram, a special X-ray of your uterus and fallopian tubes, described in Chapter 17. This can help identify scar tissue and possibly indicate whether it will affect your ability to get pregnant. There are, however, cases where the tubes will look open on the X-ray, but a laparoscopy still reveals the existence of scar tissue.

Threat 3: Fibroid Tumors

I don't think I have ever seen a patient who does not freeze with fear the moment her doctor uses the word *tumor*. As frightening as it sounds, however, I am always pleased to tell my patients that the majority of fibroid tumors are simple, *benign*, noncancerous growths that cause few, if any, life-threatening complications.

Composed of a solid mass of fibrous and muscular tissue, fibroid tumors grow in and around the uterus, and therein lies their link to fertility. Ranging in size from a tiny seedling no bigger than a pea to melon-

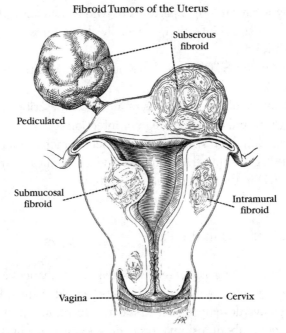

Fibroid Tumors of the Uterus

Subserous
fibroid

Pediculated

Submucosal
fibroid

Intramural
fibroid

Vagina ------   ------- Cervix

Where, Why, and How Fibroid Tumors Grow

The composition of all fibroid tumors is basically the same, and they all begin growing within the half-inch wall that surrounds your uterus. Depending on the direction in which they grow, they are categorized into three types:

- **Intramural fibroid:** The most common type of fibroid, these remain within the wall of the uterus and usually cause no symptoms.
- **Subserous fibroid:** Rooted in the outer portion of the uterine wall, they push outward into the abdominal cavity and can sometimes form a stem at their base (called a pediculated fibroid). If the stem twists (a common occurrence), it can result in severe pelvic pain. These fibroids can also cause pressure on the bladder, with pain before urination.
- **Submucus fibroid:** Pushing inward, these fibroids can grow so large they burst through the uterine lining and inflate the entire uterus. During the menstrual cycle, uterine contractions often attempt to push them out. This can cause severe pain and exceptionally heavy bleeding. If these growths also develop a stem, they can dangle down into the cervix and cause pain during intercourse as well.

sized growths, fibroids are found both individually and in clusters (one patient of mine had thirty-two growing at the same time). Primarily, they interfere with conception by causing blockages in the reproductive tract.

Where Do Fibroids Come From?

Studies show that 20 percent of all women between the ages of twenty and twenty-five and up to 30 percent of women over the age of thirty are the most susceptible to fibroids. Most often they begin growing when a woman is in her late twenties and early thirties and then continue throughout the childbearing years.

Because it is often high levels of estrogen that spark their growth, fibroids can grow especially fast during pregnancy or if a woman is very overweight (see Chapter 9 for information on weight and fertility). For this same reason, I have often seen them diminish and even disappear once a woman finishes menopause and estrogen levels drop dramatically. I have rarely seen a woman develop fibroids *after* menopause has been completed.

In addition to estrogen, these other factors can also make you more susceptible to fibroids:

• **Heredity:** If your mother or a close female relative had these growths, you may be at higher risk.

• **Predisposition:** One theory tells us that some women are born with the seedlings for fibroid tumors already in their uterus. As they reach adulthood, some biochemical event sparks an excess of estrogen, and the fibroids begin to grow. This is also why small tumors can grow like wild-fire during pregnancy, when estrogen levels are constant and high.

How Fibroids Affect Your Fertility

Although I have seen a few patients who were not able to conceive due to excessively large intramural fibroids, the submucus tumors seem to cause the most fertility-related problems by far. When left to grow large enough, submucus fibroids can:

- Interfere with the development of your uterine lining, causing implantation problems and increasing your risk of miscarriage
- Block your fallopian tube, keeping your fertilized egg from being transported to your uterus, which in turn increases your risk of ectopic (out-of-womb) pregnancy (see Threat 7: Ectopic Pregnancy)
- Alter the position of your cervix, which in turn blocks sperm from getting into your uterus, thus keeping fertilization from occurring
- Distort the shape of your uterus, making implantation impossible or difficult

In addition, because the high levels of estrogen associated with pregnancy can make even the tiniest fibroid seedlings grow extremely large, if you do conceive when these tumors are present, studies indicate you may be at a somewhat higher risk for premature labor or miscarriage.

How You Can Protect Your Fertility

The best way to protect your fertility from fibroid tumors is early diagnosis and treatment—if possible, long before you plan to conceive. I have found that one of the simplest ways to do just that is via medications that decrease estrogen levels. By creating a kind of *temporary menopause*, they encourage tumors to shrink and disintegrate, much the way they often do when you undergo menopause naturally.

Drugs in this category include danazol (Danocrine), leuprolide acetate (the same medicines used to treat endometriosis), and a promising new treatment called LHRH. This is a synthetic version of several natural hormones that suppress estrogen levels by decreasing the activity of the pituitary gland.

For most of my patients these drugs have posed no significant side effects or problems. However, in a few women, I have observed certain menopauselike symptoms, such as hot flashes and a dry vagina, as well as temporary infertility. In addition, in some patients, fibroids resume growing as soon as the drugs are withdrawn. You should also be aware that danazol can increase cholesterol levels. Therefore, I believe it should not be used for more than six consecutive months, and blood tests for liver function and cholesterol should be checked every four to six weeks during the time it is used.

Can Fibroids Disappear on Their Own?

Sometimes—most often as a result of spontaneous changes in biochemistry. For this reason I sometimes prefer a wait-and-see attitude, so long as the fibroids are not interfering with conception. If your doctor offers you this alternative, be certain *not* to use birth control pills during this time. The estrogen they contain can spark the growth of your tumors or at least discourage their disintegration.

Myomectomy: The Fibroid Surgery That Preserves Fertility

If, in fact, you do not respond well to medication, or if your fibroid tumors are so large that drugs are not an option, there is a form of fertility-sparing surgery that *can* help. The operation is called a myomectomy. It works to remove only the tumors, leaving the rest of your reproductive organs intact.

When performed by an experienced and skillful surgeon, this operation is relatively simple. Unfortunately, many gynecologists claim to have this expertise, when in fact they do not, and the consequences can affect your fertility.

Therefore, I advise you to not only get several opinions before deciding whether this operation is for you, but also speak to other women who have had this surgery and find out their doctors' success rate, particularly in terms of fertility.

If you do decide to proceed with this surgery, there are two ways in which a myomectomy can be performed. Depending on the size of your fibroid tumors and where they are located, your doctor can choose from the following operations:

- **Hysteroscopic myomectomy**: In this procedure your tumors are removed via the diagnostic procedure called hysteroscopy. Here, a periscopelike device is inserted through your vagina and cervix, allowing your doctor to visualize your uterine cavity. Once the exact location of the fibroids is noted, surgical instruments are inserted through the vagina, and the tumors are removed. No major incision is necessary. This procedure works best on submucus tumors, which are located inside the uterine cavity and are the most likely to interfere with your fertility.

- **Laparotomy myomectomy**: This more traditional form of fibroid removal uses a small but significant abdominal incision, through which your tumors will be removed. It is used primarily to excise a subserosal fibroid (on the outside of the uterus) or an intramural fibroid (located in the uterine wall). Since it is impossible to reach these growths either through the vagina or via laparoscopy, traditional open incision surgery becomes necessary. Your doctor, however, must take steps to ensure that your uterus is properly reconstructed (thus enabling you to carry a child), that your ovaries and tubes are in good condition, and that you are given special medications to prevent the formation of adhesions. You can read more about myomectomies in Chapter 17.

The New Fibroid Therapies: A Gentle Warning

Some of the very newest approaches to fibroid removal rely on a process called "embolization." Here, medications are infused into the blood vessels that feed the tumor. This helps to form tiny clots or "embolisms" that in turn choke off the tumor's nutrient supply. Without nourishment, the tumor eventually dies and disintegrates.

Although results are promising thus far, there are no long-term studies, particularly in regard to effects on future fertility. This is especially important since the procedure appears to cause a high rate of scar tissue formation, which can adversely affect your ability to conceive. If you are interested in getting pregnant in the future, it's probably a good idea to stick to more traditional forms of fibroid removal until further research verifies that these newer techniques will not interfere with conception.

Fight a Hysterectomy

If, at any time, your doctor suggests a hysterectomy for fibroids, I urge you to resist. This procedure will completely destroy your fertility, and every day evidence continues to mount that a hysterectomy for fibroid tumors is unnecessary for the majority of women in their reproductive years.

The Fake Fibroid—What You Should Know

Occasionally your sonogram or even your gyn exam may reveal a uterine growth your doctor believes is a fibroid tumor, when in fact it is not. Often it is a uterine or endometrial polyp, a growth that develops when a piece of the lining bulges away and begins to thicken. Normally benign, polyps can interfere with your fertility by disrupting your uterine lining and making implantation difficult. For this reason they should be removed before conception. The quickest and easiest way is via a D&C surgery.

Could you have a polyp and not know it? Definitely, since they often do not cause any symptoms. In some women, however, there are a few telltale signs, most notably abnormal vaginal bleeding or staining between periods, and particularly after intercourse. If your polyp becomes infected you may also experience a foul-smelling vaginal discharge.

If your doctor detects any uterine growths, ask about a saline sonogram, a new twist on the traditional ultrasound scan. (You'll learn more about how it's performed in Part Three of this book.) This test can be a big help in accessing the uterine lining and determining the exact nature of any growths or tumors seen on a normal sonogram or felt during an internal exam.

Threat 4: Ovarian Cysts and PCOD

If you have ever felt a sharp, nagging pain near your ovary, especially during ovulation or right before your period, you may already have experienced an ovarian cyst. While for most women these harmless growths come and go, with only temporary restriction of egg production or release, for others the condition can be more serious and present a more severe threat to fertility.

Different from a tumor in both structure and content, a cyst is a soft, fluid-filled sac that can appear in two different forms:

- **Functional cysts,** which are most often benign and may disappear on their own
- **Adenomas cysts,** which are solid, long-lasting, potentially cancerous growths that almost always have to be removed

Because at the onset it can be hard to distinguish between functional and adenomas, no ovarian growth should be ignored. If I discover that a patient has an ovarian cyst, I make certain to examine her again after her next menstrual cycle—and possibly again the following month—to ensure that the growth is indeed disintegrating. In order to make an accurate diagnosis, sometimes a pelvic sonogram is also used, as well as a magnetic resonance image (MRI) scanner or a computerized topography (CT) scan. For a final diagnosis, a laparoscopy is often indicated. (These methods are explained later in the book.)

How Cysts Affect Your Fertility

Regardless of the type of cyst, your fertility can be affected in a number of ways:

- If your ovary is covered by the cyst and unable to function, eggs can fail to develop. Ovulation timing and function is also disrupted and uterine preparation can be halted.

- If your cyst grows large enough, it can block your egg from leaving your ovary. This stops ovulation completely, and conception becomes impossible.

- If it turns out that your cysts are malignant (contain cancer cells), removal of part or all of your ovary may be indicated. Although you can conceive with as little as one-quarter of one ovary, whenever a reproductive organ is removed, your fertility is compromised.

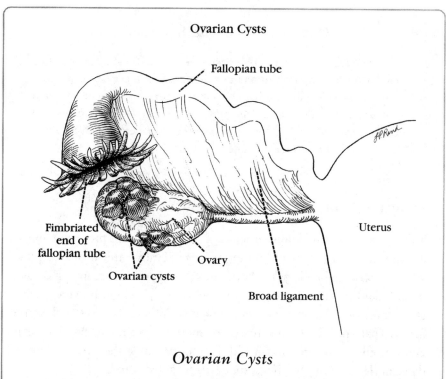

Ovarian Cysts

Fallopian tube

Fimbriated end of fallopian tube

Ovarian cysts

Ovary

Broad ligament

Uterus

Ovarian Cysts

In most women, a single cyst may form inside an ovary during any given month. It usually results when an egg fails to ovulate (leave its shell) and instead remains inside the ovary, where it fills with fluid and becomes a cyst. Sometimes the cyst can rupture on its own, usually within one or two cycles. Sometimes, however, it must be treated medically, either by draining the fluid and allowing the cyst to collapse or by surgically removing it. In a condition called PCOD—poly cystic ovarian disease—ovulation is rare or never occurs. As a result, each egg gets trapped inside the ovary, causing multiple cysts, forming the classic "chain of pearls," a series of white cysts that can be seen on the surface of the entire ovary.

> ## *Ovarian Cysts: The Symptoms*
>
> How do you know you have an ovarian cyst and not just a stomach flu? Look for these symptoms to recur each month, in a cycle that worsens when you ovulate, and right before your menstrual bleeding begins: pain localized on one side of your abdomen, pain during ovulation, menstrual irregularities, PMS, fever during ovulation or just before menstruation. Unfortunately, however, sometimes there are no symptoms.

Protecting Your Fertility: Early Treatment

To help promote the demise of cysts, I have sometimes prescribed birth control pills with a steady hormone level. Unlike the triphasic pills, which supply varying levels of hormones throughout the month and have been linked to the formation of ovarian cysts, pills that provide a constant level of hormones can encourage disintegration. When I come across a patient who, for one reason or another, does not respond to birth control pills, or when other health factors preclude their use, the drug danazol (Danocrine) has been successfully substituted.

If a cyst fails to disappear after two or three months, however, and especially if it does not respond to treatment, it may be one of three other types of solid ovarian growths, all with potentially serious fertility and health-related consequences:

- **Serous cystadenoma:** These are also known as the 50–50 cyst because they are malignant about 50 percent of the time and because they occur in both ovaries 50 percent of the time. They range from small to large and can cause various levels of discomfort.
- **Mucinous cystadenoma:** Filled with a thick fluid, these growths account for 10 to 15 percent of all malignant cysts. They are usually found on only one ovary, can grow very rapidly, and often become extremely large rather quickly. This can cause acute pain and discomfort.
- **Dermoid cysts:** Representing about 10 to 20 percent of all potentially malignant cysts, they themselves are cancerous only about 1

percent of the time. They are unique in structure in that they contain a variety of the elements of human physiology, including teeth, hair, skin, and human cells. A woman is most likely to get this type of cyst in her twenties. If they rupture, the highly toxic fluid can poison the entire system, indicating emergency treatment.

Treatment Options

If a cyst turns out to be one of the above three but is not malignant, the cyst alone—and not your ovary—may be removed. This can often be accomplished via a laparoscopic procedure or by a slightly more complex operation called an ovarian cystectomy, which removes the cyst without removing the ovary.

Another alternative is to drain the cyst by means of a needle inserted through the vagina and into the growth. Once the fluid has been removed, the cyst collapses and fertility can be restored.

To help rule out the possibility that your ovarian cyst *is* malignant, a blood test called a CA 125 can help. When used in conjunction with the pelvic sonogram, the CA 125 can rule out almost completely the possibility of malignancy. If it turns out your cyst is malignant (and I stress **already malignant and not just impending**), then and only then is organ removal necessary.

Just Say No!

At no time should you consent to a hysterectomy for a nonmalignant ovarian cyst. Some surgeons may try to frighten you into this operation, claiming that it is a preventative measure against ovarian cancer later in life. Always get a second and if necessary a third opinion.

The actual incidence of ovarian cancer among women in their forties and fifties is only between 1 and 2 percent. Even in the case of exceptionally large cysts, in most cases, your ovaries can safely remain inside your body.

Poly Cystic Ovarian Disease and Infertility

In addition to cysts, there is another type of ovarian condition that can seriously influence your reproductive health. The problem is called poly cystic ovarian disease (PCOD), or Stein-Leventhal syndrome, named after the two men who pioneered its research.

How PCOD Develops

In most women, PCOD begins between puberty and age twenty. The onset is often marked by highly irregular cycles, which continue for many years. In extreme cases, there is no menstruation at all.

First identified in the 1930s, PCOD is now considered the most common endocrine disorder among women, and a leading cause of infertility in women under age forty. Today, more than 6 percent of all women of childbearing age suffer with PCOD, accounting for some 3 million cases of infertility.

The problem itself is the result of a snafu in body chemistry, one wherein the ovaries, which normally produce tiny amounts of the male hormone testosterone, suddenly begin producing an abnormally large amount. In addition, the body also produces excess amounts of LH (luteinizing hormone) and together these two malfunctions disrupt the menstrual cycle. Although there are many theories as to why these problems occur in the first place, the most recent suggests the trouble may lie in the body's inability to properly use insulin, a hormone which, in addition to controlling blood sugar, also affects ovarian function—in this instance acting to suppress normal activity.

When the ovary can't function as it should, the developing follicles normally ovulated each month remain continually trapped inside. At some point, so many follicles collect in the ovary that cysts begin to form—often referred to as the characteristic "string of pearls" because of their white, round appearance.

Eventually, a hard shell also forms around the outside of the ovary, which further reduces any chance for ovulation to occur.

In addition to causing infertility, PCOD can also increase a woman's risk of uterine cancer. How? In all women, fat cells convert testosterone into estrogen (see Chapter 9). Since it is estrogen which stimulates the uterine lining to grow thick, the more estrogen a woman has, the thicker her lining will be.

Under normal circumstances, this presents no problem, particularly since that lining is shed each month in the form of menstrual blood.

In women with PCOD, however, not only is there more testosterone available for conversion, leading to higher-than-normal levels of estrogen and a thicker-than-normal uterine lining, but without a monthly ovulation and menstruation to help that lining shed, cells continue to build, month after month. Eventually, this results in a medical condition known as uterine hyperplasia, or cell overgrowth, which is a common precursor to uterine cancer.

Interestingly, some new research has shown that PCOD may, in fact, have a genetic component. In studies published in the British medical journal *Lancet* in 1997, researchers reported that PCOD occurred more frequently when both the baby and her mother were overweight at birth. Additional research showed that the incidence also increased when mothers were at normal weight but had a higher concentration of the hormone LH and a long gestation period of forty weeks or more.

PCOD: *The Symptoms*

- Menstrual irregularities
- Excess body hair
- Obesity, particularly in the trunk
- Inability to conceive

In addition, blood tests to verify PCOD will reflect the following:

- Elevated prolactin
- Estrogen levels that remain steady throughout a cycle
- Elevated DHEA
- Elevated testosterone
- Abnormal ratio of LH to FSH

PCOD: Treatment and Your Fertility

Traditionally, the treatment of choice for PCOD has been either surgery to reduce the size of the ovary and remove the cysts or drugs that disrupt the production of sex hormones. Medications were used to lower the level of male hormone, for example, and often birth control pills were prescribed to regulate the menstrual cycle. Women who wanted to get pregnant were sometimes treated with fertility medications, such as Clomid (see Chapter 17), and laparoscopic surgery, sometimes followed by an IVF procedure. In extreme cases of PCOD, virtually nothing could be done to increase pregnancy odds, and in those women who did conceive, the rate of miscarriage was disproportionately high.

Now, however, the focus of treatment has changed. According to such experts as Dr. Michelle Warren, medical director of the Columbia Presbyterian Center for Menopause, Hormonal Disorders and Women's Health in New York City, natural conception is not only possible for women with PCOD, but the success rate is quite impressive.

The treatment that's making the difference, says Dr. Warren, is drugs designed to help the body better utilize insulin. With less insulin available to stimulate ovarian production of testosterone, the ovaries function more normally, and eventually, ovulation kicks in.

Currently the treatment of choice for PCOD is the medication Metformin—the same drug often used by diabetes patients to help control insulin levels. However, most recently, a nutritional factor known as D-chiro-inositol has made big headlines for PCOD patients.

Specifically, in a recent study conducted at Johns Hopkins University, forty-four women diagnosed with PCOD received twelve hundred milligrams of D-chiro-inositol daily for six to eight weeks. The result: 86 percent ovulated, compared to 27 percent who were given a placebo. The women taking the nutritional supplement also showed a decrease in insulin and testosterone levels.

Perhaps most important, the new drug appears to not have any side effects. This medication is expected to be on the market in the not-too-distant future, so check with your local pharmacy as to the availability.

According to Dr. Warren, it is not surprising that D-chiro-inositol would have such positive results. The reason? This same nutrient is found in most fresh fruits and vegetables, which, says Warren, are the foods she has personally found to hold the most benefits for women with PCOD. I also believe this to be true, since many PCOD patients I have treated were able to get pregnant after I placed them on a diet that was high in these same fresh foods and when they increased their vitamin supplement intake, particularly of the B vitamins.

Diagnosing PCOD — and Protecting Your Fertility

The sooner your PCOD is diagnosed, and you receive treatment, the less likely you are to suffer any permanent fertility-related consequences. This, however, may be easier said than done, particularly since a diagnosis of PCOD can be easily overlooked, even by fertility experts. One reason is that the symptoms can be so vast, and there are a variety of conditions and problems that also affect ovulation.

And because there is no single test that points to PCOD, your doctor may not initially make the correct diagnosis.

If, however, you suspect this may be your problem, I urge you to speak to your doctor right away and discuss these possible diagnostic tests:

- An ultrasound of your ovaries, to assess their size and the presence of cysts (which, incidentally, don't always occur on every woman with PCOD)
- A laparoscopy to view and, if necessary, biopsy the ovaries
- Blood tests to check for elevations of androgens (male hormones)
- Blood tests for high levels of LH (luteinizing hormone) or an elevation in the ratio of LH to FSH (follicle-stimulating hormone)
- Monitoring ovarian response to a stimulating drug such as Lupron, or the suppressive reaction of a drug like dexamethasone

Your doctor should also seek to rule out other causes of ovulation problems, such as Cushing's syndrome (affecting the adrenal glands), or other disorders of the adrenal or pituitary glands.

If you currently suffer from PCOD and are trying to get pregnant, your doctor may suggest IVF (in vitro fertilization) as your only alterna-tive. While for some women this is a necessary procedure, studies show that for some, once insulin levels are controlled, stimulation with egg-enhancing fertility drugs (such as Clomid—see Chapter 18) is all that's necessary to bring about a natural conception. According to Dr. Warren, controlling insulin with the new medications and using a regimen of fer-tility drugs for at least one cycle gives women with PCOD a very good chance of conceiving naturally and giving birth to a healthy baby.

My precaution, however, is to make certain that you also control your weight before conceiving, and that your blood sugar is under good control as well. Women who develop diabetes during pregnancy can suf-fer some serious consequences, as can their baby, so certainly, any steps you can take beforehand to minimize these risks can be very helpful.

Threat 5: PMS

If you are like most of my patients, at some point in your life you have probably experienced PMS—premenstrual syndrome. Usually arriving about ten days before the onset of each monthly cycle, this hormone-driven condition can result in a variety of unpleasant symptoms, includ-ing bloating, anxiety, depression, achy joints, headaches, dizziness, hunger, and food cravings. The most "famous" PMS symptom is a per-sonality change that can turn an otherwise sweet-tempered woman into one who is disagreeable, argumentative, and even downright nasty, for ten days or more out of every month. The most troubling symptom of all is a feeling that your body and your mind are out of your control.

What Causes PMS?

The culprit behind nearly all PMS symptoms is a hormone imbalance, usually involving the ratio of progesterone to estrogen. While you might have the proper amount of each hormone, levels do fluctuate through-out each monthly cycle. If, for whatever reason, they do not rise and fall with the proper timing, the ratio of one hormone to another is disrupted. When this occurs, a variety of brain chemicals are also out of sync, resulting in any number of PMS symptoms.

How PMS Affects Fertility

Fortunately, for most women, PMS is a passing phase. Although strongest from age twenty to age thirty, symptoms usually abate in the later stage of your reproductive years.

For some women, however, not only do PMS symptoms continue, but more important, the underlying hormone imbalance continues as well. And this is where some serious fertility-related consequences can occur.

More specifically, in order for you to become pregnant, you must ovulate an egg, a process that requires precise coordination of the very same hormones involved in PMS—estrogen and progesterone. When your monthly hormone timing is out of sync, a variety of egg-related functions can also suffer, from growth and maturation to ovulation. Even the preparation of the pregnancy lining inside your uterus can be disrupted.

When PMS goes untreated for a significant amount of time the resulting hormone imbalances can snowball, taking you from mild fertility problems to full-fledged infertility.

Protecting Your Reproductive Health: What You Can Do

The important news here is that even if you do suffer from extreme PMS, treatment is readily available. In fact, if the hormone imbalance of PMS is behind your inability to conceive, you have one of the easiest fertility problems of all to fix. Later in this book you'll read about the fertility drugs that can help.

More important, however, you may be able to avoid fertility treatment altogether by simply getting your PMS symptoms under control before attempting conception.

Among the easiest ways to do just that is with diet, vitamins, and minerals. Specifically, research shows the B vitamin family, particularly

B_6, can be extremely helpful in rebalancing fertility hormones. I normally recommend that my patients with PMS take between two hundred and five hundred milligrams of B_6 daily, for a minimum of six weeks before conception. Because it's also important that all your B vitamin requirements are met, you should take the extra B_6 in conjunction with a high-potency B-Complex supplement.

In addition, I have found that the minerals calcium and magnesium can have a calming effect on flaring hormones, helping to alleviate some symptoms of anxiety and depression and helping you to sleep better as well. Indeed, getting adequate rest may have beneficial effects on hormone balance as well as on your fertility.

What to Eat if You Have PMS

In terms of diet, I suggest that you divide your menu into six small meals daily. Eating more frequently will help prevent a drop in blood sugar that can exacerbate PMS symptoms. Foods should be low in fat and sodium and high in protein, such as chicken, fish, turkey, and some cheeses. You may also benefit from increasing your intake of complex carbohydrates, such as whole grain breads and crackers, and cereals such as oatmeal and bran flakes, as well as fruits and vegetables.

Some of my patients have also found relief by increasing their intake of garlic, onions, and beans, all of which are rich in amino acids linked to hormonal activity.

At the same time, you should decrease your intake of high-fat foods, milk and most dairy products, and limit your intake of foods made of white flour, particularly cakes and cookies. You may also want to limit consumption of caffeine-rich foods and beverages, particularly if your PMS symptoms include breast pain and tenderness.

What Your Doctor Can Do to Help

While I always advocate natural treatments as a first line of defense, I also realize that for some women, additional help is necessary in the form of medication. Among the most helpful is progesterone therapy.

The Herbs That Can Help

In addition to vitamins and minerals, I have long been a proponent of natural herbal remedies, particularly for the treatment of hormone-related problems such as PMS. In many instances I have personally seen a number of herbal preparations play an important role in orchestrating a major change in hormone balance, and in that way, encouraging fertility.

If you find that PMS symptoms recur on a regular basis, you may want to try the following herbs, taken in either tea or supplement form:

- Ginseng
- Evening oil of primrose
- Dong Quai
- Black currant seed oil

To help reduce bloating and water retention try brewing a tea made from a combination of dandelion, nettle, and chickweed leaves.

In addition, many studies show that one of the most helpful herbs for women with PMS is Vitex. You'll find more information about how it works, and how it can help increase your fertility, in Chapter 12.

Available as a gel, vaginal suppository, or tablet, progesterone supplements are useful during the second half of your menstrual cycle, a time when your natural progesterone levels should be climbing. By supplementing your body with this hormone (you can read more about your progesterone treatment options in Chapter 15), you can not only help relieve your PMS symptoms, but also help restore the important balance between estrogen and progesterone necessary for peak fertility. I have found that in many instances a patient will need progesterone therapy only for two or three cycles before her body takes over and begins working in perfect order on its own. In any event, the sooner you correct a hormone imbalance, the less likely it is to snowball out of control.

Your doctor may also prescribe birth control pills as a way of controlling PMS symptoms. They work by shutting down your normal production of hormones, allowing only the measured amount found in the pill to circulate through your system. While this can help mediate some

PMS symptoms, I do not recommend this if you plan to get pregnant in the near future. For obvious reasons, the pill will prevent conception. But more important, very often when a woman stops birth control pills, her hormones go into a tailspin that can adversely affect fertility. Pregnancy can be difficult, even in women with no fertility problems, after stopping birth control pills. As such, you should only consider this option for controlling PMS if you do not plan to get pregnant for at least a year or more.

Reduce Your Stress — Revive Your Fertility

Finally, you should be aware that stress can play a major role in disrupting hormonal activity and can, in some women, bring on a whopping case of PMS. In fact, I can recall a number of my patients who, after undergoing personal life stresses, such as a divorce, job change, or even a change of address, began to experience severe menstrual-related problems, particularly PMS. If you are actively trying to get pregnant—and it's just not happening as quickly as you would like—the associated stress can and will affect you, sometimes turning a mild hormone imbalance into a raging case of PMS. In a round-robin effect, the PMS leads to more stress, which in turn causes more PMS, and so on down the line. Before you know it, biochemical infertility can result.

The good news: By making a conscious effort to reduce whatever stresses in your life you can control, and by making time for regular relaxation for at least fifteen minutes every day, you can keep your PMS and its resulting hormone imbalance from spinning out of control and taking your fertility with it.

Threat 6: Abortions

While no surgical procedure is totally without risk, most medical experts agree that when performed properly, in a sterile, clinical environment, by a skilled physician, an abortion is safe and poses little threat to the future of your reproductive health. However, all too often, abortions are not performed correctly, causing three main fertility-related consequences to occur:

- A damaged cervix
- A torn uterus
- A perforated bowel

In all cases, instruments involved in removing the fetus can tear open these areas, causing hemorrhaging and making future pregnancies difficult or impossible. In addition, occasionally an abscess can form inside your abdomen as a result of the abortion. If left untreated, this can lead to PID. Also, if there are bacteria or viruses present in your vagina before the abortion, the procedure can exacerbate their travel to other parts of your reproductive system, also resulting in PID.

The More Abortions, the Greater the Risk

When they are performed correctly, it is unlikely that one or even two abortions will have negative effects on your ability to conceive in the future. However, if performed repeatedly, especially at close intervals (when used as a method of birth control, for example), the operation itself can cause a number of serious problems, some of which will place your fertility in grave danger. These include:

- **Incompetent cervix:** This occurs when, as the result of too many abortions, your cervix becomes too weak to sustain a normal pregnancy. This can place you at higher risk for miscarriage or premature labor.

- **Stenotic uterus:** Because scar tissue can form after every abortion, too many operations, especially when performed at close intervals, cause potentially dangerous adhesions to develop. When they do, your uterus can become stenotic, or "too tight" to function. Eventually it can seal shut, and pregnancy becomes impossible.

- **Damaged uterine lining:** Because an abortion involves scraping the tender uterine lining in which your fertilized egg is implanted, when the procedure is performed too often, that lining can become too thin and too weak to sustain a future embryo or nourish its growth. If you do conceive, miscarriage, birth defects, or premature labor can result.

Abortion and Fertility Protection: What You Can Do

Although the majority of abortions performed today are safe, in the event that you find it necessary to have this procedure, there are some precautions you can take to ensure an extra measure of fertility protection:

- Refrain from sexual intercourse for at least four to six weeks following your abortion. Penetration that takes place too soon increases your risk of structural damage and infection.

- Remain on the lookout for signs of infection following your abortion—severe pelvic pain, prolonged abdominal cramping, fever, or hemorrhaging. Although you can expect *some* bleeding for two to four weeks, it should amount to no more than a light menstrual flow.

- Receive comprehensive follow-up care. This should include administration of antibiotics for five to seven days following the abortion to help decrease the potential for infection.

- Be tested for sexually transmitted diseases before your abortion and take prescribed antibiotics for seven to ten days if there is any chance you are harboring an infection.

Did a Past Abortion Harm Your Fertility? How to Tell

In the unfortunate event that complications do arise, they normally do so soon (hours or days) after your abortion, when immediate treatment can usually prevent any fertility damage. That means if you suffered no postoperative problems or symptoms of infection, such as heavy bleeding or excessive pain, following your last abortion, chances are your fertility was not compromised.

If, however, problems such as a torn uterus or a perforated bowel occurred, it may be wise to review your reproductive options with a fertility specialist, especially if your abortion was recent. This can help minimize damage to your reproductive organs and increase your chances for a healthy conception in the future.

Threat 7: Ectopic Pregnancy

In an ectopic pregnancy, some biological malfunction keeps your fertilized egg from reaching your uterus. Instead, it implants itself somewhere else in your body, such as in your abdomen, on your ovary, or, most commonly, in your fallopian tube, and starts to grow. When this occurs, your conception cannot survive.

In the past it was believed only one out of every two hundred pregnancies was ectopic. The American College of Obstetrics and Gynecology now suggests that the ratio is one out of every one hundred—possibly due to the concurrent rise in PID, the leading cause of ectopic pregnancy. When not treated promptly, complications stemming from ectopic pregnancy are currently the leading cause of maternal death.

How Ectopic Pregnancies Harm Your Fertility

Because most ectopic pregnancies take root in your fallopian tubes, the space in which your fetus can grow is severely limited. Not realizing it is in the incorrect location, your embryo begins to develop normally, expanding at a fairly rapid rate.

Once it starts growing, however, it isn't long before that embryo is straining against the sides of the tube. If this condition is left untreated, that tube can rupture, sometimes causing a fatal hemorrhage. In most instances, however, it is more likely to cause severe damage to the tube itself, which ultimately reduces your ability to conceive naturally in the future.

Although you *can* still get pregnant with your remaining healthy tube, ectopic pregnancies are likely to recur, so it's highly possible that both tubes can be destroyed within a relatively short period of time.

Are You at Risk?

Unfortunately, ectopic pregnancy can affect any woman who conceives. However, there are *some* factors that can place you at a higher-than-average risk:

- A history of PID
- IUD use (which leads to PID)
- Previous ectopic pregnancy
- Endometriosis
- Tubal sterilization
- Pregnancy over age thirty-five
- Two or more abortions
- Heavy smoking
- Progesterone only (minipill)
- Your mother took diethylstilbestrol (DES)

The Symptoms

One of the most devastating aspects of ectopic pregnancy is that, in the beginning, your conception appears to be normal. A pregnancy blood test will read positive, with no qualifying factors. Because, from a fertilization standpoint, your conception was successful, you will *feel* pregnant and have all the physical symptoms. However, an ectopic pregnancy is *not* normal, so as your baby begins to grow, these distinct signs will appear:

- Abdominal tenderness
- Lower abdominal pain on both sides or on the side opposite your egg's site of implantation
- Pain in your shoulder (caused by bleeding into your abdomen)
- Dizziness
- Fainting
- Urge to defecate

If your abdominal pain becomes severe or if you experience sudden and overwhelming cramping, seek emergency medical treatment **immediately.** These may be signs that your tube is starting to rupture.

Protecting Your Fertility: What You Can Do

There is no way to stop an ectopic pregnancy, but if you are at high risk for this problem, a hysterosalpingogram (an X-ray of your fallopian tube, which you will read about later in this book) can help show whether there is a blockage capable of stopping egg transport. If a blockage is discovered, a laparoscopy or other surgical procedure can be performed to help clear your tubes before you conceive again. This can substantially reduce your risk of another ectopic pregnancy and thereby increase your fertility.

Early Diagnosis: Another Way to Protect Your Fertility

Even if you are not considered high risk for ectopic pregnancy, there is no way to guarantee it will not occur. Conversely, if you are at high risk, your pregnancy could still be normal and healthy. For this reason I strongly advise every woman to have an early sonogram, which can help rule out an ectopic pregnancy. Although your doctor will rarely be able to see your baby at a very early stage, what he or she can detect is whether your pregnancy sac is inside your uterus. If it is not, and all other tests indicate a pregnancy has occurred, then there is a strong likelihood that it is in the tube. The earlier this problem is diagnosed, the better your chance of avoiding a potentially fatal tubal rupture.

In addition, the development of the ultrasensitive human chorionic gonadotropin (hCG) pregnancy blood test has also proven to be a major advancement in early diagnosis of ectopic pregnancy. Whereas it once was necessary that a pregnancy be in its eighth to tenth week for a diagnosis to be made, now, combining the results of the HCG tests and an ultrasound, correct diagnosis can sometimes be made just four to six weeks after conception. And this could very well save your fertility, or maybe even your life.

If an Ectopoic Pregnancy Is Diagnosed

Should your doctor suspect an ectopic pregnancy, the fetus must be surgically removed.

If an unruptured tubal pregnancy is diagnosed, the most common treatment is a salpingostomy (performed during a laparoscopy or laparotomy). Here, an incision is made into the wall of the fallopian tube directly over the site of the pregnancy, and the conceptus is removed. This will likely save your fallopian tube.

To help safeguard against infections that can cause PID, as well as additional ectopic pregnancies, your doctor should prescribe an antibiotic as soon as your problem is diagnosed, and add one hundred to two hundred milliliters (ml) of dextran 70 (brand name Hyskon) to your peritoneal cavity (the area surrounding your fallopian tube) as soon as the surgery is completed. If your blood type is Rh negative, you should receive a Rhogam injection immediately after the procedure (see Chapter 8).

A Final Thought About Your Fertility

Although anything that has the potential to harm your fertility is a threat that should be taken seriously, it's also important to realize that in many instances fertility problems can be prevented or damage minimized by early treatment. Use the information in this chapter to learn more about your body and your fertility and to protect against complications. Use it, too, to help find a doctor who will be your partner and treat you with the respect and care you deserve.

Chapter Three

Your Immune System and Your Fertility:

What You Need to Know About Endometriosis, Thyroid Disorder, and More

If you are like most of my patients, you are probably somewhat familiar with the workings of your immune system—a kind of biochemical "secret service," on call twenty-four hours a day, to defend your body against disease. Indeed, the moment a bacterium or virus is identified, a complex system of immunological action swings into gear. At the core of the operation lie a variety of antibodies and "killer" cells, programmed to attack the foreign "invaders" and destroy them.

How quickly, easily, and efficiently your body performs these functions is due, in large part, to the strength and the health of your immune system.

Simply put, when your immune system is in good working order, you are far more likely to avoid even catastrophic illnesses like cancer and heart disease. When your immune system weakens—due to stress, illness, even a chronic lack of sleep—you are much less able to defend yourself against not only illnesses of all kinds but also environmental assaults that can lead to disease.

There is, however, another way in which your immune system can affect your health. Instead of attacking foreign invaders, such as germs and bacteria, your body becomes biochemically "confused," turning its destructive powers on itself. As a result, you can begin producing antibodies programmed to attack your own healthy tissue. When this happens, a variety of illnesses known as "autoimmune" disorders can result—including rheumatoid arthritis, lupus, even multiple sclerosis.

Most recently, however, the idea of autoimmune malfunction has come under a new realm of investigation. Thanks to pioneers in the rapidly growing field of reproductive immunology—specifically Dr. Alan Beers of the University of Chicago Medical Center—we now have new evidence that some autoimmune reactions can and do affect a woman's fertility. Currently, much of that information is concentrated in just one area—the prevention of miscarriage (see Chapter 15).

In terms of your overall fertility, however, there are some new things we have learned about the ways in which your immune system can also affect your ability to *get* pregnant.

The Secret Immune Disorder That Destroys Fertility

If you place your fingers gently around the base of your throat, you will find your thyroid—a small, butterfly-shaped gland that quietly lies near the bottom of your windpipe.

As silent as it may be, however, the thyroid plays a very important role in not only your fertility but also your overall health. Primarily, it secretes the hormones thyroxine (T4) and triodothyronine (T3). Together, they direct many metabolic functions, including some involved in the production of fertility hormones.

When your body functions as it should, both T3 and T4 are produced on a regular basis. Stimulated by the secretion of a hormone from the pituitary gland called TSH (thyroid-stimulating hormone), it hums along without any problems.

When, however, something goes awry, causing your thyroid to produce either too much hormone (called hyperthyroidism) or too little (hypothyroidism), a variety of problems—including infertility—can result. But what causes these malfunctions to occur in the first place? The latest research reveals it may be a glitch in your immune system. For reasons we don't yet understand, some women begin producing antibodies against their own thyroid hormones.

This, in turn, causes an inflammation inside the gland itself, one that the immune system perceives as being caused by a foreign invader. In a move to eliminate what the body believes is a harmful influence (like a bacterium or virus), the immune system goes to work producing natural "killer" cells, causing further harm to the thyroid gland.

In addition, this same immune system malfunction can also cause your body to begin producing antibodies (harmful cells) against some im-

---

Thyroid Disorder: The Symptoms

Signs of an underactive thyroid include:

- A ball-like swelling in the neck (called a goiter)
- Neck or jaw pain
- Temperature changes, low fever followed by low body temperature
- Weight gain, thinning or coarse hair, puffy face
- Low energy
- Problems getting pregnant
- Recurrent miscarriage

Signs of an overactive thyroid include:

- Nervousness, anxiety, palpitations, shortness of breath
- Heat intolerance
- Fatigue
- Dry or gritty eyes, lid swelling, decreased vision
- Constant hunger
- Diarrhea
- Sweating, leg swelling, hair loss, itchy skin
- Muscular weakness
- Irregular menstrual cycle, premature menopause, inability to conceive; chronic miscarriage

portant fertility hormones, including estrogen, FSH, LH, progesterone, and hCG. This, in turn, initiates the production of even more antibodies aimed at destroying certain "neurotransmitters"—brain chemicals that are important to uterine and ovarian function. When this occurs, your ovaries may not be able to respond to normal egg-stimulating hormones, or even to those provided artificially via fertility drugs. In addition, your uterus can suffer as well, failing to produce an adequate lining for your newly created embryo to implant and grow.

Is Your Brain Chemistry Affecting Your Fertility?

When, in fact, an immune system malfunction is causing your body to manufacture antibodies against important brain neurotransmitters, some of the following problems may result:

- Fibromyalgia (an achiness in small joints and muscles, often worse upon waking)
- Depression
- Night sweats
- PMS
- Panic syndrome
- Anxiety
- Hormone imbalance
- Poor uterine lining
- Inability of ovaries to respond to fertility medications

Unfortunately, as long as this immune-mediated response continues to go undiagnosed and untreated, it's nearly impossible for a pregnancy to survive. In many instances your conception will be destroyed so soon after creation, you won't even know you *are* pregnant. Thus, what seems like an inability to conceive is really the inability to maintain a pregnancy, a problem that, ultimately, requires far different treatment than if conception were not occurring at all.

The bottom line: Unless you accurately diagnose the underlying immune problem, you could end up wasting not only thousands of dollars on worthless fertility treatments, but more important, precious time trying to conceive.

Protecting Your Fertility: What You Can Do

For many years, doctors believed that all one had to do in order to correct any thyroid-related fertility problems was to offer medication that either increased the function of a slow thyroid or decreased the function of an overactive gland. Now, however, much has changed.

The latest research shows that the key to correcting immune-related infertility lies in the treatment of the underlying autoimmune disorder that sparked the thyroid malfunction in the first place.

Indeed, before fertility problems can be corrected, treatment must first center on taming the production of natural killer cells and the antibodies being produced against the reproductive hormones. And this all must take place *before* conception and continue for at least ten weeks into the pregnancy itself. Only then will you see a reversal of fertility consequences.

Could You Have a Thyroid Problem: How to Tell

Certainly, if you experience the symptoms of a thyroid disorder noted earlier in this chapter, you should immediately bring them to the attention of your doctor. If you are already seeing a fertility specialist, he or she must be made aware of how you are feeling, particularly when the symptoms started, and begin testing you right away.

But even if you are not experiencing any significant signs of a thyroid disorder (and sometimes the symptoms can remain *very subtle*), if you are having problems conceiving, and particularly if no other significant cause of your infertility can be found, you should still speak with your doctor about the need for a complete thyroid screening.

And here is where some medical savvy on your part may really pay off. For most doctors, the typical thyroid test is a T3 and T4 evaluation. If this indicates a problem, the next step is usually medication to normalize thyroid function. But as I explained earlier, in terms of your fertility, it's imperative that your doctor identify whether an underlying immune problem is the cause of your thyroid malfunction, and if so, focus treatment in this area. Only then can you be certain that your reproductive problems will be corrected along with your thyroid disorder.

For this reason, if your thyroid tests indicate an irregularity, and you are also having problems conceiving, your doctor should perform the following additional tests, each of which is designed to measure specific immune-related factors that may be affecting not only your thyroid gland, but your entire reproductive system.

- ANA—antinuclear antibodies
- APTT—Activated partial thromboplastin time
- Lupus anticoagulant antibody
- Antithyroid antibodies
- Serum immunoglobulins
- Leukocyte antibody detection assay
- Antiphospholipid antibodies
- Anti-DNA /histone antibodies
- Natural killer cell assay

Because these tests are specialized, they may not be readily performed at all laboratories. As such, they may be costly, and many are not covered by insurance. Your doctor, however, should be able to locate at least several facilities in your area of the country that are able to conduct these analyses.

The Treatments That Can Help

The important thing to remember is that, even if your doctor diagnoses an autoimmune disorder, there are specific treatments that can help, particularly in regard to fertility-related consequences. Depending on your specific problem, normally one of two brand-new therapies may help. These are lymphocyte immune therapy, which involves injecting your body with purified white blood cells from your partner, and intravenous immunoglobulin G, involving an infusion of purified antibodies taken from donor blood. Because both of these treatments are also used to help correct immune-related pregnancy loss, you will find a detailed explanation of each in Chapter 15.

Endometriosis, Immunity, and Fertility: What You Need to Know

After more than thirty years of medical investigation and practice, there is no doubt in my mind that one of the most devastating, if not frustrating, of all gynecological ills is endometriosis. This disease develops when bits of uterine tissue and menstrual blood meant to exit the body through the cervix are instead sprayed backward into the fallopian tubes and the pelvic cavity. Once there, they can land on any organ or tissue, take root, and begin to grow. Treating the new location as a kind of "substitute uterus," they continue to be nourished each time estrogen levels climb, as they do at the start of every menstrual cycle. As a result, they continue to grow month after month, constantly being joined by new deposits left after every period. If left undiagnosed and untreated, fertility can be severely compromised—or even destroyed.

Some of the newest research on how and why endometriosis occurs involves suspected links to immune system malfunction. But before you can understand how and why, it's important to know a little more about how endometriosis develops and the ways it can affect your reproductive health.

How Endometriosis Affects Your Fertility

Among the most popular sites for renegade endometrial tissue to develop are the ovaries, a problem that can lead to the formation of blood-filled "chocolate" cysts—so called because of their color and texture. When this occurs, not only is the overall health of your ovary affected, but as you can imagine, egg growth, development, and release can be severely affected as well.

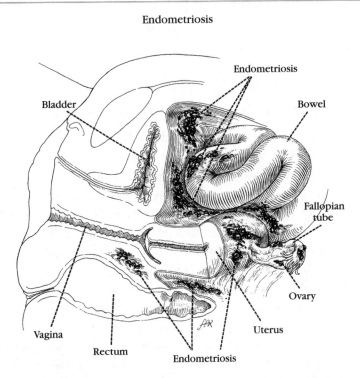

Endometriosis

Bladder

Endometriosis

Bowel

Fallopian tube

Ovary

Uterus

Vagina

Rectum

Endometriosis

Endometriosis can develop almost anywhere inside the reproductive tract, including the ovaries, uterus, and fallopian tubes. In some instances it can invade the bladder, the bowel, or even the rectum, causing great pain upon elimination. Surprisingly, pain does not always correspond to the amount of endometriosis present in your system: A small amount of deposits can sometimes cause great pain, while a lot of deposits may only cause minimal discomfort.

Another popular location is the fallopian tubes. When this occurs, scar tissue forms inside the tube causing obstructions that interfere with the ability of egg and sperm to meet, or for a fertilized egg to travel to the uterus. In some instances, so much scar tissue can develop that the ends of the tubes actually seal shut, making natural conception impossible.

In some instances, endometrial tissue can also invade the muscle wall of the uterus, causing a problem known as adenomyosis. Similar to a fibroid tumor, these growths create scar tissue within portions of the muscle wall that, if severe enough, can interfere with implantation and keep your baby from growing properly inside your uterus. The end result is a dramatic rise in the risk of very early miscarriage.

In still other instances, endometrial lesions can become so widespread that the entire pelvic cavity can become bound together, making even laboratory-assisted conception difficult.

Hormones, Endometriosis, and Infertility

In addition to the structural damage that can result from endometriosis, I have also seen this disease affect fertility on a biochemical level, with problems ranging from an increased risk of miscarriage to complete infertility. In this instance endometrial lesions emit high levels of prostaglandin, the hormonelike chemical responsible for the severe menstrual cramps that often accompany this disease.

Much the same way the production of prostaglandin causes your uterus to contract, it can also cause spasms in your fallopian tubes. If you *should* conceive, these spasms can push your fertilized egg to your uterus so quickly that it may not have the time to prepare adequately for a healthy implantation. The end result is often a miscarriage or, later in the pregnancy, premature labor. When combined with damage to the uterine lining (another effect of endometriosis), the risk of miscarriage becomes three times greater than normal.

Moreover, excessive prostaglandin in your body *before* you conceive can cause your internal environment to become so biochemically hostile that both sperm and egg are destroyed before fertilization can take place.

The Immune System Connection: The Latest News

Although no one is certain just how or why endometriosis develops, one prominent theory suggests a link to immune system malfunction. Why?

Research shows that up to 90 percent of all women experience at least some degree of the suspect "backward" flow. Yet not even half develop endometriosis. What makes the difference? Some researchers say it's the immune system. More specifically, when the body is functioning at peak levels, it is likely the immune system kicks into gear the moment the backward flow begins, destroying the renegade tissue before it has a chance to take hold and grow.

When, however, a malfunction in the immune system exists, that "blocking action" does not take place. In addition, that same malfunction also signals the release of a growth-promoting factor that actually encourages the misplaced tissue to implant on the nearest organ and begin to grow.

Further evidence of the links between endometriosis, the immune system, and infertility came when researchers discovered that the pelvic cavity and fallopian tubes of women with this disease contained higher-than-normal levels of macrophage—the immune cells that attack viruses and bacteria. These same cells were shown to have the capacity to kill sperm as it moves toward the egg, or to destroy embryos as they travel to the uterus anticipating implantation, thus creating another type of infertility.

Other Factors Linked to Endometriosis

In addition to the immune system connection, there are a number of other conditions that can contribute to the fertility-related consequences of endometriosis as well as to the severity of this disease.

Among the most prevalent is stress. Indeed, I have personally observed many patients in whom endometriosis proliferates or recurs faster and in greater quantities in times of extreme emotional stress, such as divorce, job loss, or the death of a spouse, parent, or other loved one. Since stress is also linked to a decrease in immune function, it's possible that a period of great stress may, in fact, incite the kind of biochemical imbalances that not only disrupt your immune system but, in the process, increase your risk of infertility. Later in this book you will find some impressive new evidence of the role that stress can play in keeping your body from peak reproductive health.

In addition to the factors present in your life right now, both your

Endometriosis: The Symptoms

- Severe menstrual cramps
- Ovulation pain (mittelschmerz)
- Pelvic pain that worsens before a period
- Dyspareunia (painful intercourse)
- Recurring bladder infections
- Painful pelvic cysts and tumors
- Lower back pain
- Nausea, vomiting, and dizziness during menstruation
- Difficulty conceiving

Sometimes, however, endometriosis can have no symptoms at all. In addition, you should also be aware that, ironically, there is no correlation between the degree of endometriosis and the level of infertility. Indeed, I have personally treated many women who had extremely mild endometriosis and suffered devastating fertility problems, while others who had significant lesions were still able to get pregnant on their own.

menstrual history and your family history may influence whether you develop endometriosis and whether the disease will affect your fertility.

In terms of menstruation, studies show the earlier you experienced your first period—before age twelve—the more likely you are to develop endometriosis. If your flow was also exceptionally heavy, your risk may be even greater.

In addition, this disease can be hereditary. If your mother or another close female relative had endometriosis, studies at the Baylor College of Medicine in Texas reveal that you are seven times more likely to be affected.

Protecting Your Fertility: What to Do

As devastating as endometriosis can be, there *are* things you can do to protect yourself and your fertility even if you are at high risk. One of the best ways is through diet, which can help control the growth of endometriosis that has already appeared and in some cases prevent it from occurring at all. In fact, I am continually amazed at how many of my patients are able to manage this problem, and in some cases even cure it completely, simply by eliminating certain foods.

FOODS TO AVOID IF YOU HAVE ENDOMETRIOSIS

Avoid high-fat dairy products, including cream cheese, high-fat yogurt, ice cream, whole milk, and cheese. The high fat content may stimulate an estrogen overload, which in turn may accelerate the growth of endometriosis.

Also avoid foods containing arachidonic acid, such as kidney, liver, and red meat, which can exacerbate inflammatory conditions such as endometriosis.

FOODS TO EAT IF YOU HAVE ENDOMETRIOSIS

I recommend a diet high in complex carbohydrates (grains, vegetables, and pasta). The skinless white meat of chicken and turkey and broiled fish.

There is also evidence that foods containing GLA, another essential fatty acid, may help counteract the effects of arachidonic acid. GLA can be found in cold-pressed sesame seed or walnut oil, and I recommend two tablespoons of either, once a day, if you have endometriosis.

Whenever possible eat natural foods that you cook yourself, rather than fast foods or the packaged variety, which are generally loaded with sodium and can exacerbate some of your symptoms, especially abdominal cramping.

How Your Doctor Can Help

One of the most frustrating aspects of endometriosis is that it often cannot be cured. Indeed, even when lesions are removed, eventually they usually grow back.

The good news is that treatment can *control* the development of lesions, often giving you a window of opportunity in which a healthy conception and pregnancy can occur.

Before any treatment can take place, however, your doctor should perform a laparoscopy—a minimally invasive surgery (see Chapter 17) to both confirm the diagnosis and determine the extent to which your fertility is affected. It's a good idea to select a surgeon who also has the skills to remove at least some of your endometrial lesions during this same procedure. This will save you the trauma of a second surgery, and, in fact, it may be the only treatment you'll need to get pregnant right away. Indeed, I have seen many patients who were able to conceive naturally, on their own, after a laparoscopy that removed only a minimal amount of endometrial tissue.

How Bad Is Your Endometriosis?

Once your doctor can see inside your uterine cavity, he or she will diagnose your degree of endometriosis using a four-stage system:

- **Stage one:** Small patches of endometrial lesions are found on the surface of the peritoneum—the membrane that encases the pelvis—with no resulting scar tissue formation
- **Stage two:** Endometrial lesions are found on the fallopian tubes, ovaries, and peritoneum, with or without accompanying inflammation
- **Stage three:** Larger areas of your pelvic cavity are affected, and chocolate cysts may cover your ovaries; adhesions or scar tissue may have also formed around your reproductive organs and even your intestines
- **Stage four:** Lesions are present on both ovaries, thick scarring appears on all organs, including the bladder, intestines, and all pelvic structures; one or both tubes may be partially or completely blocked

The Treatments That Can Help

If your endometriosis is classified as stage one or two, various hormonal treatments that can shrink or even eliminate the lesions may help. By reducing estrogen stimulation, these drugs keep new endometrial growths from forming, as well as causing those already formed to shrivel and die. The drugs most commonly used for this purpose include danazol (Danocrine) and leuprolide acetate (Lupron, Synarel, Zoladex).

In addition, sometimes certain birth control pills used in a particular sequence can help. Specifically, your doctor may suggest that you take one birth control pill a day for one cycle, until bleeding begins. At this point, two pills can be taken to suppress the bleeding and, in essence, stop the cycle. This two-pill-per-day regimen can be continued until bleeding begins again, at which time three pills per day are taken to once again stop the cycle. The goal here is to gradually increase the hormone dosages, thus preventing a full menstrual period from occurring. This decreases the level of estrogen in the bloodstream, which in turn allows endometrial lesions to die. Within six to eight months of this treatment, your endometriosis may improve enough to allow you to stop the contraceptives and attempt pregnancy.

Treatment for Advanced Disease

When your endometriosis is diagnosed as stage three or four, you may require surgery in order to overturn any fertility-related consequences. This usually involves the use of lasers, instruments that use a concentrated beam of light energy that rapidly heats, and then vaporizes into dust, the endometrial lesions. Normally performed via one tiny incision, the operation offers a quick recovery with virtually no scar.

In some instances, your doctor may also use microsurgical tools to physically scrape away some of the lesions and sometimes reopen your fallopian tubes.

If your endometrial lesions are particularly large and invasive, your doctor may rely on a combination of medication and surgery. In this case, the drugs mentioned earlier are used to shrink the lesions, which can then be more easily managed via surgery.

A Warning You Must Heed

Do not attempt to treat your own endometriosis by increasing your birth control pill consumption without your doctor's supervision. This treatment only works with specific *types* of birth control pills, in *certain* dosages. In addition, you must be continually monitored during this treatment to avoid adverse consequences that could ultimately cause major harm to your fertility.

When You Haven't Got Time for the Pain

Although this chapter concentrates mainly on the fertility-related consequences of endometriosis, we cannot ignore the fact that this disease can also cause a woman great pain. Although this does not directly affect her ability to get pregnant, it can certainly make the prospect of motherhood less appealing.

While not all women experience pain with this disease, if you do, a special surgical intervention may help. The procedure is called a presacral neurectomy, and it involves the cutting of nerve fibers that lead directly to your uterus and pelvis. Even if your endometriosis recurs, your pain and discomfort will be severely lessened. This surgery will also help alleviate menstrual cramps and pain with intercourse. In addition, at the time of your endometrial laparoscopy, your doctor can remove ligaments and nerve fibers that transmit pain impulses. Although this surgery can provide relief from endometrial pain as well as painful intercourse, it is an extreme procedure and should only be considered as a measure of last resort.

A Final Thought

As time marches on and we learn more about the causes not only of infertility but also of a variety of diseases affecting reproductive health, there is no question in my mind that immune system malfunctions will

Pregnancy and Endometriosis: A Warning You Can't Ignore!

If endometriosis has not blocked your reproductive organs and you can conceive, your pregnancy may temporarily halt new endometrial lesions from developing. With no menstrual cycle for nine months, no new tissue can implant in your system. However, because estrogen levels soar during pregnancy, endometrial lesions that *already exist* may grow more rapidly, with serious consequences bearing on the outcome of the pregnancy itself. For this reason, never accept pregnancy as a cure for endometriosis!

continue to be at the forefront of the research community. In fact, it's possible that, in the very near future, we may come to see that by helping to protect our immune system, we can preserve many aspects of our good health, and in the process help avoid some of the more catastrophic diseases of our time.

While no one is certain just how to ensure immune function, and in particular reproductive health, I can tell you this: Moderation is one important key. By this I mean balancing the negative factors in your life with positive actions: Eat a healthy diet, get adequate rest, use vitamin supplements, and above all, balance your stressful times with planned relaxation. Not only can all this help preserve or even restore healthy immune function, it can also influence your fertility in a very positive way.

Chapter Four

Finally! The Truth About Male Fertility

One of the most important advances in the treatment of infertility didn't happen in a laboratory. It occurred with the recognition that up to 50 percent of all conception problems were related to factors within a man's body.

Today we also recognize that a man's age, diet, lifestyle, and general state of health can also have a major impact not only on his ability to father a child but in determining how healthy that child will be.

Indeed, one of the most important discoveries made in the 1990s was that the lifestyle habits of your baby's father are as powerful as your own when it comes to not only how quickly and easily you get pregnant but also in relation to miscarriage, birth defects, even your baby's risk of catastrophic illness, such as childhood cancers, later in life.

Today, we can be certain that getting pregnant and having a healthy baby is a responsibility that must be shared by both parents.

Equally significant, we now know that, in much the same way that a woman can protect her fertility, so too can a man protect his. Not only are there things your partner can do to ensure his reproductive health, there are things he *must* do if his fertility (and his sexual vitality) are to remain at optimal levels for as long as possible. In fact, by simply learning what can influence the fate and future of his reproductive health, a man can learn to influence and control his childbearing options in ways never before possible.

Problem Within a Problem

Although new research has made it relatively easy for a man to accomplish this, in many ways, protecting and ultimately treating male fertility is far more difficult than it should be, simply because of the way many men feel about the subject. Regardless of age, race, color, occupation, location, education, or financial bracket, clear across the board I have found that most men still react with explosive sensitivity to even the slightest hint that their fertility is in question.

As a result, I have spent many hours counseling and even consoling patients after their otherwise intelligent and gentle partners left my office in a stormy fit of temper simply because they were asked to take a sperm count.

Regardless of how your partner reacts, however, it's vital that he come to understand his new and much more important role in the conception and delivery of a healthy baby and that he recognize the need to protect his fertility. I believe that your gentle understanding and love can help him accomplish all this, and in the end I'm certain he will be grateful for all the ways in which you can help him to become a healthier, happier Dad.

Understanding Male Fertility: What Every Woman Needs to Know

Before I tell you more about the ways in which you can help your partner protect his fertility, it's important that you know a little something about just how a man's reproductive system works. As is the case with your body, it all begins with hormones. Not coincidentally, the very same hormones needed to stimulate your egg production also stimulate your partner's sperm production: FSH and LH.

In both your body and your partner's, these hormones are regulated and secreted into the bloodstream by the hypothalamus and pituitary glands, both of which are located in the brain. But unlike a woman, whose hormone levels continuously rise and fall, a man has a constant level of these biochemicals surging through his body at all times, from puberty onward. This is one reason a man is considered fertile (able to conceive a child) every day of the month.

How Sperm Is Made

In a man's body, the main goal of both FSH and LH is to continually stimulate the production of testosterone, the male hormone manufactured in the tissue of the testicles. Found in a woman's body in tiny amounts but in a man's body in massive amounts, this hormone allows the testicles to manufacture sperm and must remain at constant levels in order

From Testicles to Penis: How Sperm Gets to You

Once manufactured, the sperm must be allowed to mature, travel directly from the testicles to the penis, and then be forcefully ejaculated for the male fertility cycle is to be completed. To help the sperm do that, five other equally important organs, glands, and vessels make up the remainder of a man's reproductive system:

- **The epididymis.** Two twenty-one-foot-long tubes coiled into an area just one and one-half inches wide, they sit atop each testicle inside the scrotal sac. Each sperm cell spends about twelve days passing through this structure, where it undergoes a maturing process that includes learning to swim. (This ensures that it can navigate through a woman's reproductive system and reach her egg.)
- **The vas deferens.** This consists of two thick tubelike structures that extend from the top of each epididymis through the scrotum (the loose skin sac surrounding the testicles) up into the abdomen, where they pass down into the bottom of the prostate gland and eventually empty into the urethra. Their main purpose is to transport the sperm.
- **Seminal vesicle.** These are two small glands located just below the bladder that secrete fructose, a vital component of semen, the ejaculatory fluid that helps transport the sperm into a woman's reproductive system.
- **The prostate.** This gland also secretes ejaculatory fluid and helps sperm achieve their final maturation and an increase in potency.
- **The urethra.** This is a long narrow duct that runs from just above the top of the penis down through the shaft to the tip. It transports sperm out of the body.

to keep production lags from occurring. Providing testosterone levels remain high, sperm cells are continually manufactured with production-line speed, twenty-four hours a day, from puberty onward.

How Sex Makes It All Work

Although a man generally has a constant supply of sperm ready to be ejaculated, he still needs one more signal before this process can begin. This one he receives from his partner, in the form of sexual stimulation.

Unlike a woman's body, which does not need to be sexually stimulated in order for conception to occur, a man must undergo the excitement phase, including a penile erection, to give his sperm the "go" signal. Once he is excited, the delicate nerve endings in his penis send messages throughout his reproductive system to create the power necessary to transport sperm and forcefully ejaculate it. The biological sequence of events goes something like this:

1. As sexual arousal occurs, a man's penis becomes erect. This sends a signal to the vas deferens to begin a series of rapid muscular contractions.
2. Once this movement begins, the sperm is pumped forward, from the epididymis and the ampullae (a depotlike area in which some sperm is stored) through the entire vas deferens.
3. As the sperm travels, it passes by the seminal vesicles, where a fructose solution is secreted to help push it toward the prostate gland, where more fluid is collected. Since all this seminal fluid is actually secreted behind the sperm as it passes, the first squirt of an ejaculation is always the most potent.
4. Once past the prostate, the sperm is transported into the base of the urethra, just above the top of the penis, to wait for its final release signal, the intense, rhythmic muscular contraction of orgasm.
5. The moment orgasm begins, it creates a power so strong that the sperm is pushed with shotgun force down the shaft of the penis and out the tip (ejaculation). It is this force that helps the sperm to be

deposited high in the vagina, next to the cervix, facilitating its movement through a woman's reproductive system.

Once the man ejaculates, his role in the fertility process is fulfilled, and the woman's body takes over. Nowhere in nature will you see a more complete "marriage" of the male and female anatomy than in the carefully coordinated dance of sperm and egg on their way to conception.

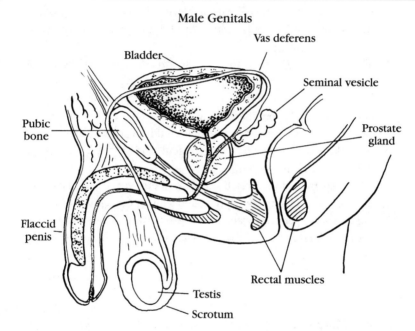

Male Genitals

The Male Reproductive System

Sperm is manufactured in the testes (or testicles) and then spends about twelve days passing through the epididymis, a twenty-one-foot coiled tube that sits inside the scrotal sac. It then passes through the vas deferens, a long, tubelike structure that winds through the abdomen past the prostate gland and eventually connects to the urethra, a long hollow tube inside the shaft of the penis. Sexual stimulation leading to orgasm is the mechanism that pumps the sperm and the fluid through the penis and out into a woman's body.

Artwork courtesy of the American Society for Reproductive Medicine

Sperm Facts You Need to Know

- Regardless of the number of times a man ejaculates, new sperm is constantly being made.
- Because making sperm is an assembly-line process with no quality control, many more imperfect sperm than perfect ones are ejaculated. That's why it's important that sperm counts remain high.
- Although it only takes one sperm to fertilize an egg, anywhere from 20 million to 200 million sperm can be ejected during an ejaculation. Because of a series of natural barriers in the female reproductive system, however, only about forty of those sperm will ever reach the vicinity of an egg.
- While semen is necessary to propel sperm into a woman's body, the size of an ejaculation in no way reflects the number of sperm a man is producing. Sterile men can produce a tablespoon or more of semen, while highly potent men may ejaculate only a few drops. However, insufficient amounts of semen could mean the sperm never reach the egg. What's the average ejaculation? From 2.5 to 5.0 cc (5.5 cc equals 1 teaspoon).
- A high sperm count (over 80 million sperm per cc of ejaculate) doesn't always ensure conception, and a low sperm count (under 10 million sperm per cc of ejaculate) doesn't always mean failure. Nature can take some surprising twists and turns, and the long shot can become the winner.

Protecting Male Fertility: What Your Partner Must Know

As you can see, sperm-making is a delicate and complex biological process. Since each step in the sperm's journey is a vital one, anything that inhibits or blocks its activity at any stage has the potential to harm male fertility. What can make a difference?

- Any activity that can injure the reproductive organs
- Bacteria, viruses, or other microorganisms that can hamper organ function or sperm manufacture or transport
- The development of scar tissue as a result of disease or infection

While there are a few villains over which he will have no control—such as congenital malformations—for the most part, most men do have at least some power over the factors that can affect them. To exert that power, a man need only become aware of *what* can harm him and then build a few basic precautions into the course of his daily living.

Fingers and Fertility

Are your partner's fingers the same length on each hand? How about the length of his ring finger versus the length of his index finger—is one longer than the other? If so, these could all be signs of how quickly and easily he can conceive a child.

Interesting new studies conducted at a fertility clinic at the University of Liverpool found that the length of a man's fingers has a surprising correlation to his ability to father a child. Specifically, if the fingers on a man's left and right hands are relatively the same size, his sperm count is probably high. If, on the other hand, the fingers on one hand differ dramatically in size from the other, sperm count may be low, and the sperm he does have may not be as active as necessary for conception. Finally, a man whose ring finger is much longer than his index finger is likely to have high levels of testosterone, so he may be more fertile.

Conversely, a woman who has a longer index finger than ring finger on either hand may have an abundance of estrogen, which in turn may mean she is more fertile.

Seven Super Male Fertility Threats and How to Avoid Them

Threat 1: The Mumps

One of the most common of all childhood diseases is the mumps, a viral infection that attacks the lymph glands, which are located throughout the body, including the groin. Contracting mumps before puberty carries no specific fertility-related danger. Once adulthood arrives, however, the virus can invade the testicles causing pain and swelling, and in the process prevent sperm from being made for several weeks. In some instances, the effects are permanent, so that the end result of adult-onset mumps is complete infertility.

MUMPS: IS HE AT RISK?

Having mumps in childhood provides a man with lifetime immunity. But because an accurate diagnosis is not always made, a man may believe he has protection from this virus when in fact he does not.

The problem stems from the fact that the symptoms of mumps (most especially swelling of the testicles) can overlap with those caused by mononucleosis and a testicle problem called torsion. Only a physician, who can rely on blood tests and a physical exam, can make an accurate diagnosis. Since, however, childhood diseases often come and go with only a parental diagnosis to confirm them, in the case of mumps, a misdiagnosis is too often made. The end result: Mumps may never have actually occurred. This is why I routinely tell each patient's husband that unless he is 100 percent certain he has had the mumps (checking with his own pediatrician if possible), he should stay away from anyone who has the disease, including his own children. This is especially important during the very early stages of the disease, when transmission factors are the highest. If exposure does occur, a man should seek immediate medical attention.

Threat 2: Sports Traumas

More than ever, fitness is a part of everyone's life. However, as important as being physically active is, it can harm fertility. How? Through sports-related genital trauma—accidents that can damage or even permanently impair a man's reproductive system.

Adult Mumps: A New Warning!

Even though a highly effective mumps vaccine has been available since 1967, the U.S. Food and Drug Administration (FDA) recently announced that more and more young (unvaccinated) adults are coming down with the disease. The FDA advises that both men and women born after 1956 make a point of discovering if they had mumps, and if they have not had it, they should ask their doctor about a vaccine. A man exposed to the mumps virus should seek medical treatment immediately, especially if the following symptoms appear:

- Low-grade fever
- Swelling in neck, underarm, or groin glands
- Mild sore throat
- Achy, flulike feeling

If mumps is diagnosed, he should seek immediate treatment from a urologist or a fertility specialist and keep a close check on his sperm count until levels return to normal.

WHAT CAN HARM HIM THE MOST

Although a genital trauma can come from almost any activity, the most common problems occur during team sports, particularly:

- Football
- Basketball
- Soccer
- Hockey
- Baseball

However, a man can also get hurt during one-on-one competitions, for example in tennis or racquetball, where the speed and impact of the ball itself can completely shatter a testicle, or even when engaged in solo activities. Accidents occurring during bicycling and horseback riding, for example, have been responsible for some of the most traumatic of all genital injuries.

WHAT HAPPENS WHEN A MAN GETS HURT

Although the type of sport a man is playing largely determines the type of injury he can sustain, certain types of traumas tend to be more common than others:

- *Ruptured epididymis:* Damage here can keep sperm from maturing enough to fertilize an egg.
- A *split or torn vas deferens:* Damage can act much like a vasectomy and stop sperm transport.
- *Shattered testicles:* This not only destroys sperm production but also ends the ability to manufacture the important male hormone testosterone.
- *Injured seminal vesicles or prostate gland:* Since both these organs supply seminal fluid, damage can lead to ejaculatory problems that could keep sperm from leaving the body.
- *Bladder damage:* This could harm the delicate muscle structure that keeps sperm from mixing with urine and urine from leaking into the urethra and damaging sperm.
- *Back trauma:* In the cast of a slipped disk or a spinal cord injury, for example, nerves controlling erection or other actions of the male reproductive system may be severed or damaged.

BIKER'S IMPOTENCE: A NEW DISCOVERY

Studies from the University of Southern California School of Medicine shows that a serious cyclist might be placing his fertility in extreme danger. According to Harin Padma-Nathan, assistant professor of urology at USC and a specialist in sexual disorders, many of his male patients suffering from impotence had one important factor in common: They all rode their bicycles at least one hundred miles a week. The problem? Repeated thrusting on the pedals was causing a banging of the groin against the bicycle seat, damaging critical arteries and nerves. The danger was increased when riders used a hard, narrow seat and maintained an ag-

---

Can a Penis Break?

Although every part of a man's reproductive system is subject to destruction from injury or disease, one of the most resilient organs, as well as one least likely to be affected, is the penis. Composed of exceptionally strong muscle and tissue, it can't break and usually rebounds from injury quite rapidly, due primarily to a surplus of blood vessels, which encourage speedy healing.

---

gressive riding style for long periods of time. A lean body also seemed to contribute to the problem.

To help ensure his fertility, every man who regularly rides a bicycle should remain critically aware of the following warning signs of biker's impotence:

- Numbness in the backside
- Difficulty in getting an erection after biking, or for one or two days that follow
- Pain in the genital area

If any of these symptoms appear after biking and last longer than two days, a man should see a doctor immediately.

To help keep problems from occurring, Professor Padma-Nathan recommends the following precautions:

- Periodically pull your body up from the bike seat when riding long distances.
- Position the bike seat so that body weight does not shift on the downstroke.

It is also important to note that damage from biker's impotence is cumulative. Without treatment, this temporary problem could become permanent.

PROTECTION AGAINST ALL SPORTING INJURIES

Because nearly every sporting activity has the potential for genital harm, any man who is athletically active must use adequate protective equipment, even when the possibilities for problems are slim. In fact, so important is the concept of adequate protection that in professional sports today team physicians, managers, and even the players themselves are actively campaigning for more stringent regulations regarding the mandatory use of protective gear during all types of sporting games.

What are the most important forms of protection?

- Penile cups
- Jock straps
- Padded genital protectors
- Sturdy protective clothing

Since injuries most often occur in players who are young and inexperienced, it's extremely vital that young men always use protection for every single sporting activity.

WHAT TO DO IF AN INJURY OCCURS

Even when protection is used, the risk of sports-related genital injury still exists. Should an injury be sustained, it's vital that a man take the following steps to ensure that his reproductive organs remain in good health:

- Seek *immediate* emergency medical treatment. It is not smart to suffer in silence, and forgoing treatment, or waiting too long, can be disastrous. When genital traumas are treated early enough, damage to reproductive health can be greatly minimized.

- Seek follow-up care. Even if emergency treatment is received, follow-up visits with a urologist, a physician who generally specializes in male fertility, can help minimize damage and monitor the healing process.

- Ask your doctor to check your sperm count. Although sperm count can remain low for several weeks or even months following an injury, it should rise again if the damage was not permanent. Checking sperm count periodically until that rise occurs can facilitate getting additional medical care if needed.

Threat 3: Fitness Workouts

Although a man seldom experiences genital injury while jogging or doing aerobic exercise, there is some evidence that certain fitness activities can affect fertility by altering the temperature of the testicles. How does this cause problems? In order for a man's testicles to function at peak efficiency, their temperature must remain between 94 and 96 degrees Fahrenheit, approximately two to four degrees cooler than normal body temperature. To help ensure that it does, nature placed the testicles outside the body and equipped them with a special set of muscles that draw the testicles close when they get too cold and drop them loose when the temperature rises too high. In this way a constant, healthy temperature is maintained, regardless of most environmental influences.

Sometimes, however, certain activities temporarily override this natural reaction, allowing the testicles to overheat. When this occurs, sperm production stops or significantly decreases. In addition, there is some evidence that prolonged exposure to high body heat may also affect the epididymis, the organ where sperm mature and learn to swim. This can affect a man's immediate ability to conceive a child and sometimes results in permanent sterility. A defective epididymis can also increase the risk of miscarriage or birth defects by allowing greater numbers of abnormal sperm to be produced.

Since certain fitness activities can, and usually do, increase overall body temperature, sometimes they can affect fertility as well. Fortunately, for most men, once the body cools, any sperm production that *was* disrupted returns to normal. However, for those who have a borderline low sperm count or testicles that are already too hot due to certain vascular problems (discussed later in this book), fertility can be affected by fitness activities.

Hot Baths, Hot Sex, and Infertility

If you're thinking that a romantic candlelight "bubble bath for two" might get you and your partner in that baby-making state of mind, think again. While the atmosphere might be conducive to romance, unless your bubble bath is in cold water, you could be harming your chances for making a baby. Why?

Studies show that very hot baths can harm a man's fertility—primarily by reducing sperm count. And the more times he takes a dip in the steamy waters, the more likely he is to experience problems.

If you are trying to get pregnant, and particularly if your partner has been diagnosed with a low-normal to low sperm count, be certain he refrains from taking very hot baths for at least six weeks before attempting conception. Although men continually manufacture new sperm daily, the complete process takes from three to six weeks. So, avoiding the hot baths for at least that amount of time can help give sperm a healthy start.

If your partner has already been taking hot baths regularly, don't despair. Research shows that a sperm-related problem caused by the steamy baths will usually resolve itself within a few weeks.

THE WORKOUTS THAT CAN AFFECT HIS FERTILITY

While any activity that substantially raises body heat has the potential to affect sperm count and motility, the following fitness workouts are thought to bring about the most temperature-related problems in the least amount of time:

- Rowing machines
- Simulated cross-country ski machines
- Treadmills
- Duration aerobics
- Repetitive calisthenics or aerobics
- Jogging

In addition, *any* exercise can be made more hazardous when certain workout clothes are worn, primarily those that hold in body heat. These can include:

- Exceptionally tight, spandex shorts
- Synthetic fabrics that don't breathe
- Tight-fitting spandex jeans (worn right after working out)
- Tight spandex bikini underwear

Boxers Versus Briefs: The Latest News

You've probably already heard the long-running rumor about the effects of tight briefs on male fertility. As the myth goes, men who wear very tight-fitting underwear are more likely to suffer fertility problems than those who wear loose-fitting boxer-style garments, ostensibly because the briefs hold in body heat, which in turn causes the temperature in the testicles to rise too high. While the theory makes perfect sense, the studies don't bear out the results, at least not according to the latest research published by the *Journal of Urology*. Here, research on ninety-seven men with fertility problems found that those who wore boxers were no more likely to be fertile than their brief-wearing counterparts.

However, I believe that if your partner has a moderate to low sperm count, continually wearing tight underwear still could make a difference. If he really hates the boxer style, then simply encourage him to take off all underwear and put on a robe for several hours every evening. Indeed, studies also show that men who frequently allow their genitals to move freely may have fewer problems trying to conceive.

THE GOOD NEWS

Fortunately, the solution to most fitness-related fertility problems is simple. A man doesn't have to stop working out, as long as he makes sure his testicles remain free enough to pull away from his body when temperatures get too hot. The avoidance of tight underwear when working out and tight jeans afterward could be all his body needs to ensure a high sperm count and steady production.

In addition, he should try to spend time aerating his genitals, by removing all clothing from his lower body and covering himself with just a light robe or a towel wrap after exercising. This can go a long way toward helping his genitals recover from heat buildup and constriction.

HEALTH CLUB FERTILITY HAZARDS

In addition to the workout, some of the perks provided by health clubs can affect male fertility by further increasing the temperature of testicles. If you are trying to conceive, your partner should stay away from the following "luxuries" for at least three to six weeks before the time you want to get pregnant:

- Sauna
- Steam baths
- Hot tubs
- Extra hot showers

These can be especially hazardous directly after vigorous exercise, when body heat can rise to a point that is dangerous to sperm.

Threat 4: Stress

Interesting new research has shown that stress affects not only a woman's ability to get pregnant, but also a man's ability to father a child. While we previously believed the only link between stress and male fertility occurred when tension prevented an erection, we now know a man's reproductive system can be affected in a variety of ways.

In recent studies by the Department of Physiology at the Medical College of Ohio in Toledo, the following facts were learned:

- Both a man's autonomic nervous system and his adrenal hormones actively participate in the stress response, which in turn can impede sperm production and release.

- Emotional stress can depress testosterone levels and thus interfere with sperm production.

- In animal studies it was learned that stress can affect testosterone levels and mating behavior, with varying effects on the testicles.

- Extreme tension and fatigue for prolonged periods of time can lead to psychological impotence. This in turn often leads to more worry (about the impotence itself), which can add enough stress to affect the hypothalamus gland, alter levels of FSH and LH, and ultimately lower both testosterone levels and sperm count.

In addition, many independent studies have confirmed that even minimal stress has the ability to cause a man's sperm count to drop. The greater and more prolonged the stress becomes, however, the more serious the damage that can occur.

Stress, Loss, and Infertility

Has your partner recently suffered the loss of a loved one? If so, his sperm count may suffer. New studies show that sperm motility can decrease by as much as 10 percent following an emotional loss, such as a death, job loss, or even a divorce.

THE GOOD NEWS

The good news is that the effects of stress on male fertility are usually only temporary, lessening or even disappearing entirely when the stressful situation is resolved. In addition, experts say that by keeping stress levels under control (especially *not worrying* about temporary bouts with impotence), a man can give himself a good measure of fertility protection as well as a boost to his sex life.

Threat 5: Colds, the Flu, and Other Diseases

In much the same way that a woman's menstrual cycle can be affected by changes in her body chemistry, so can a man's sperm-making abilities be jeopardized particularly if an illness causes his white blood cell count to rise. When it does, the result can be a bout of infertility lasting anywhere from several days to several months or even longer.

What kinds of health problems can cause this temporary effect on a man's fertility?

- The flu
- Diarrhea
- A bacterial infection
- A virus
- An acne flare-up
- An abscessed tooth
- Mononucleosis
- Epstein-Barr virus

Naturally, this doesn't mean that a man with a cold can't make you pregnant. Of course he can! But depending on the strength of his immune system, a man's fertility is at least somewhat compromised every time he gets sick.

High Cholesterol and Infertility

There may be a new reason for your partner to cut down on those cheeseburgers and T-bone steaks: Their ties to high cholesterol may affect more than his heart. In a study of some thirteen hundred men, doctors found low levels of high-density lipoproteins (the "good" cholesterol) were directly linked with the ability to have an erection—an obvious cause of infertility. The cholesterol-related sexual problems are thought to occur when circulation to the penis is compromised.

The Infections That Can Harm His Fertility

In addition to those problems that can temporarily cause a man's sperm count to suffer, there are some diseases, as well as some infections of the reproductive tract itself, that can have a more powerful and long-lasting effect on his fertility. They include:

- *Urethritis,* an inflammation of the tube that carries sperm from his body
- *Epididymitis,* an infection of the epididymis, which can affect sperm maturation and transport
- *Prostatitis,* an infection of the prostate gland, which can affect sperm motility and cause impotence and ejaculatory problems

When left untreated, any of these infections can partially or even completely destroy a man's reproductive organs, rendering him permanently infertile.

The Good News

Although almost any bacterium or virus that invades a man's body can settle in his reproductive tract and cause one or more of these problems, the culprits are most often the microorganisms associated with STDs (sexually transmitted diseases). You'll learn how and why they occur (and what you and your partner can do to protect your fertility) in Chapter 5. Right now, the good news to remember is that, when diagnosed early, nearly all of these infections can be easily cured using a simple antibiotic regimen for just seven to ten days.

To help ensure that he does receive that all-important early treatment, a man should remain critically aware of any of the following symptoms and report them to his doctor immediately:

- Infection, especially in the penis
- Pain, anywhere in the genital area
- Genital swelling
- Difficulty in urinating, including a burning sensation

- General genital sensitivity or discomfort
- Fatigue
- Low-grade fever
- General feeling of malaise

Diabetes and a Man's Fertility

One of the most physically threatening conditions is diabetes, a disease in which the biochemistry needed for the proper metabolism of sugars and simple carbohydrates is somehow disrupted. Since diabetes affects both nerve impulses and circulation, a diabetic man can suffer ejaculatory and impotency problems. Because these difficulties can usually be controlled when the diabetes is treated, it's imperative that your partner be checked for this disease if he has any of the following symptoms:

- Excessive thirst
- Craving for sweets
- Excessive urination
- Unexplained impotence

Because diabetes can be hereditary, he should also be checked regularly (via a simple urine or blood test, or both) if any close family members have had this disease.

Threat 6: Poor Nutrition

By now I'm sure both you and your partner are aware of the power of antioxidant vitamins (such as C, E, and beta-carotene) to protect against both heart disease and cancer. But did you know that these same powerful nutrients can also have a significant impact on male fertility? It's true. Studies now show that when a man is deficient in certain key nutrients, particularly antioxidants, his sperm production can suffer.

One of the most interesting of these new studies involved the effects of vitamin C. While researching the overall health effects of a vitamin-deficient diet on men, one researcher at the U.S. Department of Agriculture decided to see if, in fact, sperm was one of the factors affected by nutrition. He collected sperm samples from the men in the study—both the group with a low vitamin intake and the control group, which were getting an adequate vitamin supply.

What he found: The sperm samples from men whose intake of vitamin C was low (about ten milligrams a day, or one-sixth of the RDA) were two and half times more likely to be damaged than the sperm from men who were getting adequate vitamin C.

When you look at the role of this nutrient in a man's body, however, this finding isn't hard to understand. Semen naturally contains about eight times the amount of vitamin C found in blood. Since this is the fluid in which sperm resides, as well as the vehicle that carries it into a woman's body, it's easy to see how a decrease in vitamin C may alter the natural environment necessary for optimum reproductive health.

ANTIOXIDANT PROTECTION FOR SPERM

Perhaps more important are the new studies showing the effects of antioxidant nutrients, such as vitamins C, E, and beta-carotene, on sperm cells.

Research conducted at Tulane University discovered that an imbalance in antioxidants makes sperm more susceptible to harm from environmental factors, while doctors at the Cleveland Clinic found that antioxidants can keep sperm DNA from becoming damaged. For this reason, antioxidant nutrients appear to have an important protective effect on male fertility, and can also help when added *directly* to sperm during preparation for laboratory conception. (You'll read more about this in Part Three of this book.)

THE "MANHOOD" MINERAL

Although it's an important nutritional component for both sexes, it is men who appear to garner the most benefit from zinc, a mineral that is secreted naturally by the prostate gland and found in great abundance in semen. Plentiful in nuts and whole grains, and readily available as a supplement, zinc has been shown to be particularly beneficial to fertility in men suffering a deficiency, increasing sperm production by a significant margin. One caveat: Too much zinc—going vastly over the RDA—could be toxic to sperm and yield a negative effect on fertility.

Male Fertility Nutrients: What He Needs to Protect His Sperm

- Beta-carotene: 10,000 units daily
- Vitamin D: 400 mg daily
- Vitamin E: 800 IU daily
- Vitamin C: 1,500 mg daily
- Vitamin B complex: 100 mg daily
- Vitamin B_6: 500 mg daily, total
- Calcium: 800 mg daily
- Zinc: 100 mg daily

VITAMINS AND MALE FERTILITY: A WARNING

While it's important that your partner maintain a high nutrient intake, particularly when you are trying to conceive, make certain he does not give in to the temptation of megadosing—taking extraordinarily large doses of any single nutrient, or even more than one potent multivitamin daily. Studies show that, in some instances, too many vitamins can have a negative effect and actually reduce a man's fertility. This, however, is not the case with nutrients you get naturally from food. Indeed, you should encourage your partner to eat as much of the healthy foods listed below as possible throughout his childbearing years.

FOODS THAT PROTECT SPERM

One of the best ways your partner has of ensuring the health of his sperm is eating a healthy diet. While supplements can help him meet at least basic nutritional needs, I believe that nothing can replace the power of the nutrients that you receive from eating fresh whole foods. In fact, later in this book you will find an entire chapter devoted to the foods that I believe will increase a woman's fertility.

Likewise, here are some of the dietary components that research shows, and I personally have seen, help men protect *their* fertility. While it's important that he eat these foods every day, his diet becomes critically important in the weeks before you plan to conceive.

- Eat three to five servings of vegetables and at least three servings of vitamin-rich fruits every day—particularly those high in vitamin C, including oranges, grapefruits, and lemons. If eating these many fruits is a problem, encourage him to drink more fresh juices.

- When possible, choose whole wheat grains (including bread and pasta) over white flour products to increase his intake of the B vitamin folic acid. Other sources include green vegetables, such as broccoli, collard greens, kale, romaine lettuce, and Swiss chard—all high in folic acid.

- If your partner loves chili, you can satisfy his appetite and meet some of his fertility needs in a single meal, particularly if you reduce the amount of beef and increase the amount of beans, which are a powerful source of folic acid. Meanwhile, the tomatoes can supply a heavy dose of vitamin C. Serve it up with some whole wheat garlic bread and you've got a super fertility meal. If that doesn't appeal to him, perhaps munching a bowl of peanuts and sunflower seeds will be more to his liking— both are also high in folic acid and vitamin E, another powerful antioxidant food.

In Part Two of this book you will find detailed information on the herbs and other natural ways to protect and increase his fertility.

FATTY FOODS AND MALE FERTILITY

Avoiding certain fats may not only help your partner protect his heart, but recent research shows it may also help to ensure his fertility. As with heart disease, saturated fats, hydrogenated oils, trans-fatty acids, and coconut and palm oils should be avoided. Also on the "no" list is cottonseed oil, which has been shown to retain pesticide residues, and has high levels of *gossypol,* a substance known to inhibit sperm function.

In addition, when saturated fat intake is high and essential fatty acid intake is low, the fatty acid composition of sperm membranes undergoes changes that ultimately interfere with motility.

Meanwhile, increasing his intake of polyunsaturated oils, such as olive or canola, can help increase not only your partner's sperm development and motility, but also his sexual virility.

Threat 7: Rough Sex

While the male genitalia are built to endure both the friction and thrusting of even the most active intercourse, there are times when sex can get too rough:

- If testicles are squeezed too hard or subjected to weighted pressure for a prolonged period of time, damage to the epididymis as well as the testicles can occur.

- Oral sex performed too vigorously can cause some trauma and bruising that could have residual effects on a man's ability to make sperm for up to several weeks.

- The sharp plastic edges or the "tails" of certain IUDs can make contact with the penis during heavy or deep thrusting and cause some inflammation or localized trauma or bleeding. This is even more likely if a man is uncircumcised: His foreskin can be ripped or torn during especially deep intercourse.

Although no permanent damage usually ensues from any of these activities, if bleeding occurs or persists even after pressure is applied or if localized infection sets in, a man should seek medical treatment as soon as possible to ensure that no harmful bacteria invade the urethra.

In addition, if a man experiences any unusual pain or discomfort in his penis, testicles, or general genital area during sex, he should seek medical treatment immediately. As is the case with women, painful intercourse for men is a sign that medical attention is needed.

Sex Toys and Male Fertility

In addition to rough sex, some sex toys or aids, such as penile rings and vibrators, can, when used in a rough or vigorous manner, produce trauma to the male genitals and have some effects on fertility. I heard about a couple in France who, during a particularly vigorous sexual encounter, were worked into such a frenzy that they didn't notice that the electric massager the woman was using had begun to short out. When she reached down to touch her partner's genitals, he received a shock of enough impact to destroy his epididymis and all future sperm production. That was, of course, an uncommon injury (most vibrators today are battery operated and shockproof); still, it shows that whenever the genitals are involved, precautions must be taken to protect them.

The Male Fertility Protection Exam

While it is immeasurably important for a man to continually monitor his own health for the signs and symptoms of the fertility-robbing conditions already discussed, self-care alone is not enough. Although there is no equivalent of the gyn exam for men, every man should undergo at least one yearly physical. For optimum fertility protection and care, the examination should include the following areas:

The **testicles,** the most vital of the male reproductive organs, should be carefully examined regularly by the man himself, as well as by his physician, for:

- Lumps
- Tenderness
- Discoloration
- Swelling
- Rigidity of the testicles themselves or in the surrounding scrotal sac or genital area

Not only can these be signs of genital infections, they can also signal testicular cancer, a growing concern for men of all ages.

The **penis** should be checked for these signs:

- Discoloration
- Growths
- Lesions
- Blisters
- Warts
- Abnormal discharge

The doctor should gently squeeze the tip of the penis to see if any abnormal discharge is emitted. If there is, a urethra culture might help track down the presence of harmful bacteria or viruses.

Current Sexual Health History

Every physical should also include a detailed history of any sexual malfunctions, including:

- Inability to have an erection
- Loss of sexual desire
- Inability to maintain an erection
- Premature or no ejaculation
- Pain during intercourse or any sex-related activity

Any or all of these situations could be symptoms of underlying physical problems, many of which can be related to fertility-robbing diseases or conditions.

A Check for Hernias and Undescended Testicles

Although a hernia itself is not a direct cause of infertility, tearing of the abdominal tissue can cause a decrease in the blood supply to the vas deferens, possibly with long-term effects on the functioning of this organ.

Because surgery to repair a hernia and the procedure to correct the congenital malformation known as undescended testicles are both done very close to the spermatic cord, the blood supply to the testicles can be endangered during these operations. If the blood supply is inadvertently cut off the testicle will atrophy and die, destroying any chance for future sperm production. Only a sperm count immediately following hernia repair surgery can alert the physician to this mishap. If the count is low and does not return to normal within a few weeks' time, a second surgical procedure might be needed to restore blood flow to the testicles. This can sometimes keep permanent damage from occurring.

The Prostate Exam

Although prostate disease was once thought to be only a concern of "older" men, the latest statistics show that even those who are forty years of age, and sometimes younger, can also be affected. Divided into two basic categories—benign (nonmalignant) prostate disease and prostate cancer—this condition can affect fertility in a number of ways.

First, the prostate secretes a good portion of the ejaculatory fluid necessary to move sperm out of a man's reproductive system and propel it with enough force to navigate through a woman's reproductive tract. This can only occur when the prostate gland is healthy.

If prostate disease should develop, particularly cancer, the gland must be removed. This will affect his ability to conceive naturally, not only because of the decrease in ejaculatory fluid but because the surgery to remove the prostate also severs the vas deferens, the result of which is similar to that of a vasectomy.

If a man diagnosed with prostate cancer wants to preserve his child-bearing ability, he can opt to freeze his sperm before receiving any treatments. His partner can then later be treated with one of the new reproductive technologies featured in Part Three of this book.

To ensure a healthy prostate gland, your partner should receive a rectal exam (which checks for prostate size and consistency) once a year. After age forty, he should also receive a PSA (prostate-specific antigen) blood test every two years. After age fifty (or age forty-five if there is a family history of prostate disease), he should receive the PSA every year.

High Blood Pressure and Diabetes

Although high blood pressure will affect neither sperm production nor movement, it can affect blood flow to the penis, and that in turn may cause impotency. Additionally, some of the medications used to treat hypertension can have a negative effect on fertility. Catching and treating high blood pressure early has obvious benefits, including fertility protection.

As previously noted, diabetes can have direct and devastating effects on a man's reproductive system, so early diagnosis and treatment can help preserve fertility, as well as general health.

A Final Word About Male Fertility

As medical science continues to learn about the male reproductive system, one point becomes increasingly clear: A man's fertility *cannot* be taken for granted.

The shocking truth: In the past twenty years alone, the average sperm count for healthy college men has dropped from 60 million to below 40 million per cc of ejaculate.

Researchers speculate that increasing levels of stress, the proliferation of sexually transmitted diseases, wider use of alcohol, drugs, and tobacco, and exposure to radiation and toxic substances have all contributed to this statistic. And later in this book you and your partner will learn how these factors can damage reproductive health and what you each can do to protect your fertility.

In fact, unless men, like women, begin taking steps to protect their reproductive health, sperm counts may drop even further, and the incidence of male infertility can climb to an all-time high. If we are to alter these statistics significantly in the next generation, the men of today must set an example for the men of tomorrow. Young boys need to be taught fertility protection at an early age—in school, on the radio and TV, in books, and most important, by the examples set by both parents. Seeing us taking care of our reproductive health, our children will learn to do the same.

Chapter Five

Sex and Infertility:

What Every Couple Needs to Know Right Now

"It can't be—I'm married. How could this happen?" (Kiersten, lawyer).

"There must be a mistake. I don't hang around with 'those' kind of men" (Jennifer, health club instructor).

"What? No way! My partner and I are completely faithful" (Roger, computer programmer).

What are these men and women so surprised about? They've learned they have a sexually transmitted disease (STD), an infection caused by any number of rapidly spreading bacteria or viruses that are usually passed on during sexual intercourse. This year alone it is estimated that more than 3 million people will contract one or more STDs. Many won't even know it. What is most alarming: The latest studies show that, when left untreated, STDs are the leading cause of infertility in the United States today, for men as well as for women.

The Good News

As frustrating and damaging as STDs can be, there is good news. Once they are diagnosed, especially in their early stages, treatment is fast, painless, and easy, via a regimen of antibiotics. In most cases, a complete cure is possible in a matter of days, eliminating nearly all threats to fertility. To accomplish this, however, you must learn the important signs and symptoms of these diseases, as well as the lifestyles and other health factors that may place you at high risk. With this information, you and your partner can protect your fertility and your sex life throughout your childbearing years.

STDs: What Are They? Who's at Risk?

Medically speaking, a sexually transmitted disease is any one of a number of infections that develop in your body primarily as the result of a sexual encounter with an infected partner. Currently, more than twenty sexually transmitted diseases have been identified. Among the most common, however, are the following:

- Chlamydia
- Gonorrhea
- Syphilis
- T-mycoplasma
- Herpes
- HIV/AIDs
- human papilloma virus (HPV), which causes condyloma acuminata, or venereal warts

Because they can be transmitted during sex, some physicians now also classify three forms of vaginitis as STDs:

- Candidiasis (yeast infection)
- Trichomoniasis
- Bacterial Vaginosis (BV)

While not all of these organisms can lead to infertility, if left untreated they can compromise the delivery of a healthy child and impair your sex life. For this reason it's imperative that you don't overlook any of the symptoms of these diseases or underestimate your chances for infection.

How STDs Are Spread

Contrary to popular belief, STDs are not confined to those who have a wildly active sex life. However, they are mainly transmitted via sexual contact, so naturally, the number of sexual partners you have increases your risk. It's also important to remember that you can easily catch an STD having sex with only one person, if that person has an infection.

Over the past several decades, government reports indicate, the incidence of STDs has risen, particularly among young adults—men and women from eighteen to twenty-five years of age. Part of the reason has to do with changes in our culture, particularly sexual experiences beginning at a younger age. This, combined with marrying at a much older age than previous generations and a rising incidence of divorce, means that most men and women today will have more sex partners in their lives than in generations past. And that means a greater risk of sexually transmitted disease.

Another problem, however, is that many of today's most prevalent STDs can be harbored in the body for years without a visible trace. And that means transmission is more likely. In fact, just because you don't see or feel the symptoms of an STD doesn't mean that the disease itself cannot be transmitted—in essence, silently passed from one partner to the next. In fact, some diseases can remain silent in the body for so long that even those of you who are in a five-, ten-, or even fifteen-year monogamous relationship have no guarantees that you and your partner are disease-free.

Hot Tubs, Health Clubs, and STDs

Although all STDs can be transmitted during sex, under certain conditions some can also be contracted in other ways. That is another reason why these bacteria and viruses have spread so rapidly. The most risky environments include:

- Hot tubs
- Steam rooms

- Saunas
- Bathrooms
- The showers and dressing areas of some health clubs

Because their atmosphere is similar to the moist, warm conditions found in your genital area, these environments can make excellent breeding grounds for certain bacteria and viruses. In fact, touching your genital area with a contaminated towel can sometimes provide enough of a transmission factor to allow you to become infected. Because your body is often unprotected when you are using these facilities, your risk of infection via casual contact increases even further.

What Can You Catch Through Casual Contact?

Venereal warts, BV, yeast infections, and herpes can all be contracted in nonsexual as well as sexual circumstances. Contact with active syphilis lesions or gonorrheal discharge could allow for nonsexual transmission as well.

Increasing your risk of all STDs are the following factors:

- **A previous infection:** If you have had an STD in the past, studies show your chances for contracting one again are increased.

- **Age:** The younger a woman is the higher her risk of contracting an STD, primarily because the uterus remains partially open until early to mid-twenties, allowing for easier passage of any number of bacteria into the body.

- **Choice of birth control:** Using a barrier method of birth control—a condom or a diaphragm—will decrease your risk. The pill offers no protection, and an IUD may actually increase your risk by allowing for easier passage of bacteria into your uterus.

How STDs Can Affect a Woman's Fertility

Although complications associated with STDs affect both sexes, it is women, by far, who risk the greatest reproductive consequences. When left untreated, even a mild infection can upset many aspects of your reproductive system. Indeed, once an STD microorganism is allowed to pass from your vagina into your reproductive tract, an acute inflammation of your cervix (a condition called cervicitis) can result almost immediately. If left untreated, that infection can easily pass into your uterus and from there into your fallopian tubes and your ovaries. As these organs become infected, PID results. As you read earlier in the book, depending on the organ involved, once PID occurs, your entire reproductive system may be placed in jeopardy.

How STDs Can Affect a Man's Fertility

Because the bacteria and viruses associated with STDs first make contact with the male body via the penis, it is also relatively easy for these microorganisms to enter a man's system. They do so by moving up through the urethra (the narrow shaft inside the penis), causing an infection called urethritis. Then, by working through the vas deferens (the hollow tubes that lead from the penis), they can attack the prostate gland, causing prostatitis. If they continue traveling to the epididymis (the small gland located on top of each testicle), an infection called epididymitis results. Finally, an STD can invade the testicle.

Infections that go on indefinitely without treatment can not only impair the organs themselves (resulting in defective or no sperm), but also cause an abundance of scar tissue. This can result in blockages that inhibit both sperm maturity and travel.

Finally, if an STD invades the testicles, permanent sterility can result.

An STD Primer: The Most Common Sexually Transmitted Diseases and How to Treat Them

The most essential part of STD protection is the care you give yourself in the form of body awareness. To help you and your partner get a head start on the protection you *both* need, use the following STD primer to learn what to look for in each of your bodies, along with the fast, easy treatments that can help you avoid future problems.

Disease: Gonorrhea

Signs and symptoms:
Female body:
- Mild genital burning or itching, or both
- Slight vaginal discharge
- Frequent urge to urinate or urinary discomfort, or both

Male body:
- Yellow, puslike penile discharge that rapidly increases in volume and is much thicker than the normal mucus secretions of arousal
- Penile discomfort (primarily at tip) two to five days after being infected
- Painful or burning urination

Incubation period: Forty-eight to seventy-two hours.

Potential reproductive damage: Most commonly affects fallopian tubes in women; constriction and closure of all sperm passageways in men.

Test: A urine test or a swab culture taken from the inside of the cervix and then examined for the genes of the bacteria itself is the newest and possibly most accurate form of diagnosis. An alternative method examines the vaginal or ejaculatory fluids under a microscope.

High-risk factors: Multiple partners; an infected partner.

Treatment: Broad-spectrum antibiotics, including tetracycline; an injectable drug, spectinomycin hydrochloride; and some penicillin-related drugs such as ampicillin. In certain individuals an untreated infection may cure itself in anywhere from a few weeks (in men) to a year (in women). However, chances of reproductive and other bodily damage increase when no treatment is provided.

For your information:
- Early symptoms are not always present, particularly in women. When they do occur, look for signs from two to ten days after you suspect exposure.
- Gonorrhea can be spread to the eyes and lead to irreversible blindness.
- Oral sex with an infected partner can result in gonorrhea of the throat, the most common symptom of which is a sore throat. This form is less contagious.
- Condoms dramatically cut the risk of infection and should always be used if the activities of your partner or his or her physical symptoms are in question.

Warning for Men

Two out of every ten men who contract gonorrhea do not have symptoms. They must rely on the honesty of their partner to inform them that they have been exposed. Any man who is told of gonorrheal contact should be tested and treated immediately, even if no symptoms are present.

In addition, often right after infection and sometimes before any symptoms appear, a slight irritation stimulates the nerve endings in the penis, causing a man to feel an increased desire for sex. This is one of the reasons the disease can be so easily spread.

Disease: Chlamydia Trachomatis Infection

Signs and symptoms:
Female body:
- Slight discharge and some vaginal burning beginning anywhere from three days to three weeks after infection begins
- Very often, there are no signs or symptoms. Two out of every three women and two out of four men have no symptoms.

Male body:
- White discharge from penis
- Frequent urge to urinate or some burning

Incubation period: Five to seven days.

Potential reproductive damage:
- Experts estimate that fully one-third of all women with chlamydia go on to develop PID and subsequent fertility problems.
- In some women, chlamydia causes a hostile vaginal environment capable of killing or damaging sperm.
- Undiagnosed chlamydia can affect the lining of the womb, leading to premature birth, stillbirth, or neonatal death. It may also lead to salpingitis, an inflammation of the fallopian tubes.
- In men, chlamydia is the leading cause of nongonococcal urethritis (NGU), an infection that attacks the prostate gland and the epididymis. In severe cases it can cause so much scar tissue that complete infertility results.

Tests: Traditional testing analyzes vaginal and seminal fluid for the chlamydia bacteria, with results in about a week. There are also several new rapid tests that can be done in your doctor's office, with answers in several minutes. Using a system of bacteria identification known as DNA amplification, the tests are quick and easy, but may not be as accurate as the more traditional fluid analysis. Finally, a third method uses a urine sample to detect bacteria. Although slightly less accurate than the traditional culture, it can be used effectively when other testing is not possible or practical, as in a college infirmary.

High-risk factors:
- For women: IUD use; youth
- For both sexes: Multiple partners or an infected partner

Treatment:
- Broad-spectrum antibiotics, such as tetracycline or doxycycline (Vibramycin), taken orally for seven to twenty days.
- Occasionally the body's own immune system can overpower the chlamydia microorganism and stop the infection on its own. This, however, is rare and should never be relied upon for a cure.

On the horizon: A vaccine for the prevention of chlamydia as well as a topical preparation that works much like a spermicide to kill the bacteria on contact may soon be widely available.

For your information:
- If you are sexually active, with multiple partners, or if the activities of your current partner are in question, you should have a chlamydia test every six months.
- Tests for chlamydia are not 100 percent accurate, especially if the disease has progressed from your cervix into your fallopian tubes. For this reason, always seek treatment if your sex partner is diagnosed as having this disease, even if you do not test positive.
- Use of condoms containing the spermicide nonoxynol-9 during sex can offer an extra measure of protection against transmission of the chlamydia bacteria.

Disease: Condyloma Acuminata (Genital Warts)

Signs and symptoms:
Female body:
- Firm, light or dark pink or red growths that usually appear in clusters on the vulva, or outer vagina, and can cause itching, irritation, or bleeding
- Warts can also appear on the side walls of the vagina or even on the cervix itself, in which case they can be seen only during a gyn exam.

- Warts can spread from the vagina into the anal area, with or without anal sex, if you simply touch the infected area, or if you do not practice good bathroom hygiene (wiping front to back).

Male body:
- Warts may appear on the penis or anywhere in the genital area.
- Warts may also appear in the anal region if transmission took place during a homosexual encounter, or if this area of a male's body came in contact with a toilet seat, towel, or any moist, warm environment in which the virus was living.

Incubation period: Seven to fourteen days.

Potential reproductive damage:
- Venereal warts in the vagina may contribute to a hostile environment, inhibiting or disrupting conception.
- Since pregnancy stimulates the development of almost any growth, venereal warts present after conception can grow so large that they can block the vagina or the birth canal and increase the risk of Cesarean delivery.
- The potential for reproductive damage in men is not completely known.

Tests: For both sexes, diagnosis is usually made by on-site observation. For women, the ViraPap test or a Pap smear can also indicate the presence of the infection linked to genital warts. On rare occasions, a biopsy may be necessary to confirm the finding. In 1999 the FDA approved a brand-new test called Hybrid Capture II, which uses sophisticated DNA technology to diagnose and classify strains of HPV.

High-risk factors:
- Youth: Young women in their teens and early twenties are at highest risk, especially if they have more than one sexual partner.
- Smoking
- Birth control pills
- History of genital herpes

Treatment: Since there is no cure for a virus, genital warts cannot be totally eradicated. Treatment, however, can remove the symptoms, which is the warts themselves.

Primarily that treatment falls into two categories. The first is prescription drugs that you can topically apply at home, on your own. These include podofilox and imiquimod. The other option is to use more potent medications that your doctor must apply. These include podophyllin, trichloracetic acid (TCA), bichloracetic acid (BCA), and interferon.

Additional treatment options include chemically "freezing" the warts into disintegration (called cryotherapy) or surgically removing them. The size of each wart, the number of warts, the cost, convenience, and adverse effects of treatments help determine which procedure may work best for you.

For your information:
- More than 70 different strains of HPV exist, some of which dramatically increase the risk of cervical cancer. However, genital warts are generally caused by just two strains—HPV 6 and 11, which are not generally associated with cervical cancer.
- If warts have not improved substantially within three treatments, or cleared completely within six treatments, you and your doctor need to discuss an alternative approach.
- Because venereal warts can be transmitted via casual contact as well as sexually, remain acutely aware of any symptoms and be tested immediately if signs of this disease appear.
- Since moist, warm towels, public showers, saunas, and steam rooms make excellent breeding grounds for this virus, be tested regularly with the new ViraPap smear if you normally find yourself in these environments.
- Because this disease is highly contagious, regular testing is advised if your partner or any close family member has been diagnosed as having venereal warts.

Disease: T-Mycoplasma Infection

Signs and symptoms: **Male and female body**
Generally none, although some individuals may experience a slight burning during urination and a light, odorless discharge.

Incubation period: Seven to fourteen days.

Potential reproductive damage:
- Although no link has been found between the T-mycoplasma organism and infertility, when the organism is present in either the male or the female body at the time of conception, there may be an increased risk of miscarriage.
- In men, T-mycoplasma is responsible for up to 25 percent of all occurrences of nongonococcal urethritis.

Tests: A vaginal culture or a sperm check for the specific T-mycoplasma bacterium.

High-risk factors: Multiple partners.

Treatment: Ampicillin or tetracycline taken orally for seven to fourteen days, or other antibiotics, depending on culture sensitivity.

For your information: T-mycoplasma is still a relatively new disease, discovered in Europe in the 1970s and found in significant numbers in the United States beginning in the 1980s. To date, its main link to infertility in women is an increased risk of miscarriage. Recent evidence also shows that men who harbor this bacteria may increase their wives' chance of miscarriage. Since this disease is usually totally silent, if you are having a problem carrying a pregnancy to term, be certain both you and your partner are checked for this bacteria.

Disease: Syphilis

Signs and symptoms (general—male and female body):

First sign: Chancre:
- The chancre (pronounced "shanker") is a sore that appears anywhere from two weeks to two months following initial contact with an infected partner.
- It is usually brownish in color and hard in texture, and often resembles a large pimple. There can be one chancre or a cluster, and they are usually painless.
- Chancres can appear almost anywhere on the body where contact has been made with the infection: fingers, mouth, breasts, rectum. Most often they occur in the genital area. In women they can be internal or hidden in the folds of the vagina, or both.
- While chancres are the usual sign, they don't appear in every case, and they usually disappear on their own, even when not treated. The disease, however, remains in the body and produces what is called secondary syphilis.

Secondary syphilis:
- From a few weeks to a few months after the chancre disappears a brownish rash resembling German measles may result. The most common sites are the palms of the hands, soles of the feet, mouth, and nose.
- There are also flulike symptoms, swollen lymph nodes, and fatigue, lasting about two weeks.
- Untreated, these symptoms disappear, and the disease seems to be gone, sometimes for many years. The microorganism responsible for syphilis lives on, however, continuously multiplying in your body. In time it causes extensive damage, including heart disease, paralysis, mental illness, blindness, and eventually death.

Incubation period: Two to eight weeks.

Potential reproductive damage: Although the first symptoms of syphilis are ulcerated sores, the bacteria eventually travel through the entire body, damaging many organs in the process, including those in the reproductive system. During the "silent" period, the years when no symptoms are present, syphilis can easily be passed on to any fetus that is conceived, and any baby born to a mother who is infected will likely have the disease as well.

If a syphilis infection is active during the first trimester of pregnancy, there is also an increased risk of miscarriage, premature labor, and birth defects.

In men the syphilis virus causes no direct, specific reproductive damage. However, by infecting his partner, a man with syphilis can indirectly cause severe damage to the pregnancy.

Tests:

Early stage: The "darkfield examination," a method of examining the chancres through a microscope for an on-site diagnosis.

Later stages: There are four basic blood tests:
- Venereal disease research laboratory (VDRL) test
- Fluorescent treponemal antibody absorption (FTA-ABS) test
- Rapid plasma regain (RPR) test
- Treponemal hemagglutination assay (TPHA)

The VDRL and RPR are fast, inexpensive, and easy, but they can show a "false positive," indicating syphilis where none exists. Oftentimes a doctor likes to confirm the results of these tests with the FTA and TPHA. These tests detect syphilis antibodies (proteins made by the immune system in response to infection).

High-risk factors: Sex with an infected partner, multiple partners.

Treatment:
- An injection of long-acting penicillin works the best. If, for whatever reason, a person cannot tolerate penicillin, then other antibiotics can be used.
- In advanced or stubborn cases, a second or even third injection may be needed at one-week intervals.

For your information:
- Fortunately, just twenty-four hours after a penicillin injection, syphilis can no longer be transmitted.
- While relegated to a medical backseat for quite a number of years, syphilis has been making a comeback of late, with an alarming number of new cases developing each year. For this reason, don't assume this disease belongs to another generation.
- Of continuing concern is the fact that syphilis appears to increase the risk of transmission of HIV, the virus that causes AIDS.
- Because it can attack any tissue or organ, syphilis often causes destruction throughout the entire body. It is not only a painful disease, but a deadly one that you cannot afford to dismiss.

Disease: Genital Herpes

Signs and symptoms:
Female body:
- Clusters of small blisters on a reddened area of skin that eventually break and form small scabs and sores. They can be painful and usually itch.
- Most often they appear in and around the outside of the vagina, the most common site being the labia, or outer lips.
- Signs and symptoms appear anywhere from two to ten days after contact with the disease.
- During the initial outbreak there can be swollen glands, particularly in the groin, with a slight fever and flulike symptoms.
- Before any outbreak, the vagina may appear red and feel sore, swollen, and itchy.

Male body:
- Symptoms are the same as in the female body, with lesions appearing mostly on the tip or the shaft of the penis.

Incubation period: Two to four days.

Potential reproductive damage:
- An active herpes infection at the time of delivery can cause your newborn to contract the disease. Since infants have little or no immunity to infection, the virus can ravage their tiny, defenseless bodies. As many as 25 percent of all newborns who contract herpes die. If the virus attacks their eyes, they can be permanently blinded.
- In men a herpes infection can cause nongonococcal urethritis (NGU) in up to 10 percent of all cases.

Test: Although the sores are usually diagnosed on-site, to help distinguish them from other infections, your doctor may use a viral culture. Here, he will swab the active lesions and send the sample to a laboratory. A newer, more rapid, but slightly less effective test involves detecting signs of the virus directly in the lesions.

Although a blood test cannot determine if you have an active genital herpes infection, it can detect antibodies to the virus, which were made during a previous herpes infection. Unlike other viruses, where the formation of antibodies protects against subsequent attacks, herpes can still recur. Once you have the virus in your system, contact with an infected person is not necessary in order for new lesions to develop.

High-risk factors: Sex with an infected partner; lowered immune system due to stress, illness, or fatigue.

Treatment: The drug Acyclovir, available as both an internal and an external medication, has been shown to provide some relief of symptoms and may be able to decrease the length of an episode. In addition, the FDA has recently approved two new medications for herpes treatment. They are valacyclovir and famcyclovir, the latter of which has also been approved for use in suppressing viral activity and preventing recurrences.

Since no antibiotic has been found to be effective in treating viruses, there is no cure for herpes.

For your information:
- Once in your system, the herpes virus continues to reactivate at in-

tervals, the length of time between outbreaks varying for each individual.

- Herpes cannot be spread during a remission period. However, there is evidence that once the virus becomes active in the body (as it does several days before the appearance of symptoms), it can be transmitted.
- Because at certain stages herpes lesions can resemble syphilis, it's important that all cases be verified by a physician as soon as symptoms appear.
- Herpes outbreaks may be exacerbated by stress, which lowers the functioning of the immune system and allows the virus to go from its dormant state to an active one.
- No related diseases (including herpes simplex, which causes cold sores; herpes zoster, which causes shingles; chickenpox; Epstein-Barr syndrome; and cytomegalovirus) provide an immunity against genital herpes.

Disease: Vaginitis

While many forms of vaginitis can be self-generated (that is, they develop within the body, without the invasion of any outside bacteria or viruses), they are generally not communicable. However, there *are* three types that can be sexually transmitted and are found both in the male and in the female body:

- Yeast infection (candidiasis)
- Trichomoniasis
- Bacterial vaginosis (BV)

For this reason many doctors choose to categorize them as STDs.

YEAST INFECTION

Medically known as moniliasis or candidiasis, a yeast infection results when the delicate alkaline-acid balance of the mouth, vagina, or rectum is biochemically disrupted, allowing the healthy flora that normally live in these areas to start growing out of control. The result is a fungus infection that can spread rapidly throughout the body. When the genitals are involved, this infection can be transmitted during sexual activity.

Signs and symptoms:
Female body:
- Discharge (thick and white, similar to cottage cheese, with a "yeasty" odor)
- Itching
- Burning (particularly on the labia or lips of the vagina)
- Sometimes painful intercourse
- Reddening of the vagina, the irritation and subsequent pain spreading into the rectum, making sitting or even walking very painful

Male body:
- Genital itching
- Genital rash
- Penile discharge

Incubation period: One to two days.

Potential reproductive damage:
- A yeast infection in the vagina may interfere with sperm transport to the egg. It can also alter vaginal environment, making it difficult for sperm to survive.
- In men, yeast infections can cause an inflammation of both the urethra and the prostate gland and thus affect sperm transport. There is also some evidence that the yeast fungus can attach to sperm, weighing it down and causing motility problems.

High-risk factors:
- Stress
- Antibiotics
- Allergies
- Hormone imbalance
- Sex with an infected partner

Treatment: Current treatment for yeast infections in women include antifungal suppositories and creams such as Nystatin, Monistat, Femstat, Gyne-Lotrimin, plus the oral medications Diflucan (tablets) and Nystatin (tablets). For men, Nystatin taken orally in tablet or powder form is most often prescribed. In addition, some studies show that diet modification may have some positive effects on rebalancing normal flora levels and eliminating the yeast fungus.

Foods that may inhibit a yeast infection:
- Yogurt
- Cranberry juice
- Garlic

Foods to avoid:
- All yeast products
- Refined sugars and carbohydrates
- Fermented foods (including miso soup, soy sauce, vinegar)
- Dried fruits
- Peanuts (dry-roasted)

For your information: While oral monilia infections are usually caused by antibiotic medication, they can also be transmitted via oral sex. When this occurs,the mouth becomes red and inflamed with cheesy white patches that bleed when scraped.

TRICHOMONIASIS

Trichomoniasis is caused by a parasite known as *Trichomonas vaginalis,* which can live in the vagina, and in the male, in the urethra or prostate gland, and is passed on during sexual intercourse. Capable of causing a chronic infection that is often symptomless, it can live silently inside the body for many years. When it is finally activated (due to changes in the genital environment brought about by stress or other illnesses, for example), it is often difficult or even impossible to ascertain when or from whom the parasite was contracted.

Signs and symptoms: Once this parasite becomes active in a woman's body, the following symptoms can appear.

- Yellow-green vaginal discharge
- Foul vaginal odor
- Severe itching
- Irritated genital membranes
- Painful urination
- Painful intercourse

Should the infection spread to the uterus, pelvic pain can also result.

In the man's body the primary symptom is a yellow-green penile discharge and genital itching.

Incubation period: Three to five days.

Potential reproductive damage: While studies linking trichomoniasis and reproductive health are still inconclusive, I believe that because this parasite is associated with changes in the vaginal environment, it can contribute to conception difficulties or increase the risk of miscarriage. In men it may interfere with fertility by attaching to sperm and affecting transport. Once diagnosed and treated, however, trichomoniasis should have no residual effects on your ability to conceive.

Perhaps most important, however, is that new research shows trichomonas is associated with an increased risk of transmission of HIV. Additionally, when present during pregnancy, trichomonas may also cause you to deliver a low-birth-weight baby, or to develop premature labor.

Treatment:
- The standard treatment in women is a 250-milligram tablet of metronidazole (Flagyl) taken orally three times a day: This usually brings about a full cure in about ten days. Alternative treatment can include a megadose of two grams of metronidazole taken in twenty-four hours.
- In men the general treatment is 250 milligrams of metronidazole

taken twice daily for ten days or one megadose of two grams taken in twenty-four hours.

- Intercourse should be avoided during treatment, and both partners must be treated simultaneously (even if only one has symptoms) in order to avoid reinfection. In addition, do not drink any alcohol while taking this treatment. Combining the two has been shown to cause severe nausea and vomiting.

Warning: The Misdiagnosis You Must Avoid

The most accurate diagnostic measure for detecting trichomoniasis in women is a Pap smear or a direct examination of the discharge itself under a microscope. The latter is also the method used to detect this condition in men. Some doctors believe correct diagnosis can be made after a pelvic exam alone, but I must caution you against this. I have often seen monilia infections mistaken for trichomoniasis and consequently mistreated with metronidazole. Since that medication can exacerbate monilia symptoms and actually worsen this infection, treatment for trichomoniasis should never be accepted without proper documentation that the disease does indeed exist in your system.

BACTERIAL VAGINOSIS INFECTION

Formerly known as nonspecific vaginitis, or Gardnerella, the name of this disease was changed to bacterial vaginosis (BV) when researchers discovered how many different strains of bacteria were capable of causing essentially the same type of vaginal infection. It occurs when the physiological environment inside of the vagina changes, allowing different types of bacteria that normally reside in small amounts to begin growing out of control. The end result is an overload of nasty germs that cause a variety of symptoms.

While BV can be transmitted on clothing or towels and is considered highly contagious, it can also be passed on during sexual intercourse when a BV-related virus that silently rests in a man's body is passed to the woman, causing the changes in the vaginal environment that allow the various bacteria to proliferate.

Signs and Symptoms:
- The most significant female symptom produced by this bacteria is a grayish-white discharge with an extremely unpleasant odor. It does not cause any local irritation, swelling, or itching. Over half the women diagnosed with this infection, however, have no symptoms.
- In men there usually are no symptoms.

Incubation Period: Three to five days.

Potential reproductive damage: Because the presence of BV in your reproductive system can create a hostile vaginal environment, it may affect the ability of sperm to reach or fertilize an egg.

In men, some of the bacterium associated with BV can affect the reproductive glands, as well as the quality of sperm that is produced.

Special warning: Should conception occur while a woman is harboring a BV infection, her chances for preterm birth, or even miscarriage, may increase. For this reason many doctors now routinely prescribe certain antibiotics, namely erythromycin or penicillin, for any woman who gets pregnant and has a history of repeated miscarriage.

Diagnosis and treatment: This infection can be verified by testing the pH (acid level) of the vagina, and then examining a sample of vaginal fluid under a microscope to detect the presence of certain organisms. Diagnosis is also made based on the absence of certain other organisms, and by the presence of "clue cells," which are bits of vaginal tissue coated with the bacteria. A fishy odor and decreased acidity in the vaginal fluid are also signs.

The most common treatment for BV is oral metronidazole. Topical treatment is also possible using metronidazole cream or gel, or clindamycin cream. Clinical trials have shown that oral versions of clindamycin are also effective, but widespread use is still limited. Metronidazole should not, however, be used if there is even a chance you might be pregnant, since it has been linked to increased incidence of birth defects. Although clindamycin has not been shown to cause any birth defects, testing is still considered inconclusive. If you contract BV while you are pregnant, oral antibiotics can help.

HIV, AIDS, and Your Fertility

As recently as the 1990s, a diagnosis of HIV—the virus that causes AIDS (acquired immune deficiency syndrome)—was, more or less, a hopeless situation. With little or no knowledge of how and why this disease occurs, doctors were at a loss for how to treat it. Most people diagnosed with HIV died, often within a relatively short time after being diagnosed.

Not so anymore. While HIV is still considered the most deadly of all STDs—currently there is no cure—there are important new ways to manage this disease, and in the process, greatly extend the life expectancy of its victims. For many diagnosed with HIV today, the progression to full-blown AIDS may not come for twenty or thirty years. In some, it may never come at all.

How HIV Is Contracted

Because HIV is most easily transmitted through bodily fluids, it can be easily passed between partners during sex. This includes anal, vaginal, and oral sex, all of which involve the transmission of semen as well as vaginal fluids, and sometimes small amounts of blood.

Sharing needles or other injection equipment with an HIV-infected person is another key method of disease transmission, as well as being accidentally stuck with a needle that contains infected blood. In addition, many cases of AIDS have occurred as a result of a transfusion with HIV-tainted blood. While today we have sophisticated screening methods that make nearly all transfusions 100 percent safe, this was not the case as recently as the mid-1990s, when tainted blood did slip through the system on more than one occasion.

Once inside the body, the virus heads straight for the immune system cells—primarily the T-cells, which work to defend the body against diseases. Once inside the cell, the virus instructs it to begin replicating copies of itself and release them into the bloodstream. As more T-cells continue to be attacked, they are forced into making more copies of the virus and releasing it as well.

Eventually, so many cells are affected that the body can no longer defend itself from even minor infections. When the "viral load" (the amount of HIV cells in the blood) becomes high enough, virtually all immunity to disease is lost and the diagnosis of AIDS is made.

Contrary to myth, HIV is not a disease limited to the homosexual community. Although it has devastated this segment of the population, there are hundreds of thousands of heterosexual HIV victims around the world.

Although it only takes one encounter with an infected person to contract HIV, oddly enough, not everyone who is exposed will contract this disease. While doctors aren't certain why this is so, many believe the strength of a person's individual immune system and general state of health may protect him or her them from infection. That said, you should never risk exposure to HIV, no matter how healthy you think you are. You can, in fact, greatly reduce your risk of infection by always using a latex condom during sex with any partner whose health may be in question (and that includes anyone who has not been tested for AIDS within six months, or who has had more than one sexual partner within six months).

HIV Transmission and Testing: What You Should Know

The incubation period for HIV is almost immediate, although the infection does not appear in blood tests for anywhere from twenty-five days to six months. Rarely does the virus show up after this time, so a negative test six months after exposure usually means you did not contract HIV.

Currently, there are two types of tests available. Both use blood to test for antibodies to HIV, which is what your body begins making after you contract the virus. The first test, which is available only in limited areas, is called the rapid HIV screen. It produces results in five to thirty minutes. The second test, known as the EIA (enzyme immunoassay), takes from one to two weeks, and is usually the test found in most home kits. The rapid test and the EIA are equally accurate.

STDs and HIV: The Risk Factors

Some STDs can also increase your risk of contracting HIV when you have sex with an infected person. Any disease that causes open sores or breaks in the skin (such as syphilis or herpes) can allow for easier passage of infected bodily fluids. In addition, any STD may increase the risk of contracting HIV by stimulating an immune response in the genital area.

HIV Treatment

As I explained earlier, in the not-so-distant past there were virtually no medications to treat HIV. Today, there are many. Most, however, are a form of antiviral drugs, medications that stop the replication of the virus at some point along the way. The stage of the disease when you are diagnosed often determines the type of antiviral medication that works best for you.

Currently, there are some fifteen different antiviral drugs available, and many times they are given in what is called a "cocktail"—meaning more than one drug is given at the same time in order to improve results. Among the most common antiviral medications are zidovudine (AZT), didanosine (ddI), saquinovir, ritonavir, nevirapine, and the newest, amprenavir.

In some individuals, these medications can not only stop the virus from replicating, they may even reduce the viral load in the blood to a negligible amount. Unfortunately, there is no way of telling who will respond to which medications, and which combinations may work best for any one individual. Still, results continue to be promising, so much so that many experts contend that in the not-too-distant future HIV will be as manageable a disease as high blood pressure or diabetes.

Fertility and HIV: What You Need to Know

When the first edition of this book was written, I could not offer any hope, and certainly no encouragement, to any couple diagnosed with HIV, particularly in regard to their reproductive future. In fact, it almost seemed cruel and insensitive to discuss HIV and infertility in the same book, let alone the same breath.

Again, this is no longer true. Because many HIV patients can live a nearly normal life for years, often in a relatively healthy state, there are some couples for whom having a baby is a reality that can be achieved. Many experts believe the healthiest way to have that child is via assisted reproductive technology.

Although the criteria for both medical success and ethical treatment is specific—the mother must be disease-free and the father must be diagnosed with HIV that has not progressed to full-blown AIDS— still, remarkable advances in the treatment of infertility have now made it possible for these couples to have a disease-free child.

Among the world's leading experts on this subject is Dr. Mark V. Sauer, chief of reproductive endocrinology at Columbia Presbyterian– New York Medical Center in New York City. According to Dr. Sauer, the key to success with HIV patients is a brand-new technology known as ICSI (intracytoplasmic sperm injection). This laboratory procedure (which you will read about in great detail in Chapter 22) injects a single sperm into an egg, which is then cultured in the laboratory. After fertilization occurs, the resulting embryo is transferred into the mother's body, allowing a normal pregnancy to then develop.

Because the sperm is subjected to treatment before injection (including a washing process that separates it from semen and white blood cells that are thought to carry the infection), so far, Sauer's studies show that the resulting embryo will be disease-free. Additionally, the mothers do not appear to develop HIV, even after the fertilized egg is transferred into their bodies.

Dr. Sauer's studies are still considered preliminary: He has so far treated thirteen HIV couples, resulting in three healthy pregnancies. Although only one child has been born thus far, that baby is healthy and disease-free. As small as this sample is, however, the results are incredibly promising, and seem likely to yield an important breakthrough for couples who are living with HIV.

Certainly, there are ethical questions here—most involving whether the infected father will have any chance to see his child grow up. The answer is that we don't know. What we do know is that bringing a healthy child into a world in which he or she is loved and desperately wanted, and where we are sure that there will be one healthy parent able to care for that child, tempers our ethical concerns with a compassion and an understanding that we must extend to these couples.

Indeed, as Dr. Sauer often states, it is far better for such couples to undergo fertility treatments and to create a baby in the healthiest of environments than to risk creating an unhealthy child on their own, which studies show many of these couples eventually attempt to do.

If Your Partner Has HIV: What to Do

Not every doctor who treats infertility will agree to treat a couple who has HIV. In fact, I would venture to say that most will not. However, there are centers around the country and experts like Dr. Sauer who do have expertise in this area and can help you. In most instances, a local medical school or teaching hospital will help you find such a doctor in your area.

Be aware, however, that of those fertility specialists who do treat HIV couples, most will require a long and extensive battery of both physical and psychological tests and usually several interviews with physicians before determining if you and your partner are good candidates for assisted reproduction.

And, in case you are wondering whether a center that treats HIV couples is safe for all couples to use for their fertility treatments, usually the answer is yes. In Dr. Sauer's center, for example, both the equipment used to treat HIV couples and the medical professionals who work with them are kept very separate from that used to treat healthy couples. In fact, health regulations concerning any form of medical treatment of persons with HIV are so strict that for the most part you have no risk of contracting an infection if you are treated in a center that also treats HIV-infected couples.

STDs: Are You at Risk?

To help round out your knowledge not only of STDs but of the ways in which they can affect your life, here are some of the most commonly asked questions about these diseases, along with the answers that can help you relax and enjoy your sexuality for years to come.

Q: **Can I get an STD from kissing?**

A: Generally, no. However, since gonorrhea is capable of living in the throat, it may possibly be transmitted this way. In addition, any open sores in your mouth, such as fever blisters or dental lesions, could increase your chances of infection of oral gonorrhea. While the AIDS virus is not generally transmitted via saliva, there are still some conflicting reports about the role that deep mouth kissing may play in transmitting this disease.

Q: **I had PID in the past. Does this mean I won't ever get pregnant?**

A: No. It is the extent and severity of your PID, and whether you were treated promptly, that determine whether your fertility was affected. If no scar tissue formed and there was no damage to your fallopian tubes, your chances of achieving a natural conception are good. In addition, even if damage has been done, a laser laparoscopy or some form of microsurgery could help reverse any problems that did occur, allowing you to conceive. If, however, your tubes underwent severe damage, you might need some laboratory assistance, such as in vitro fertilization, to help you get pregnant. (Review the discussion of PID and its link to infertility in Chapter 2.)

Q: **My husband and I both had gonorrhea in college and were treated with penicillin. Could we be sterile now?**

A: Most likely not, if you were treated immediately and PID was not diagnosed.

Q: **Can I get an STD from oral sex?**

A: Yes. During oral sex, gonorrhea, herpes, syphilis, yeast infections, and possibly AIDS (if an open sore is present in the mouth), as well as a few lesser-known STDs, *can* be transmitted. If sores appear in your mouth or a sore throat develops a few days after oral sex, report these symptoms to your doctor and request cultures and tests for these diseases.

Q: **Is it true you can't get an STD from just one encounter?**

A: No. You can catch an STD any time you have sex with an infected partner. Your chances for catching any disease increase the more times you are exposed, but you are at great risk even after one encounter with a person carrying an STD.

Q: **Can I have an STD and not know it?**

A: Yes. Chlamydia, venereal warts, T-mycoplasma, and gonorrhea can all be symptom-free or have signs that appear only for a short period of time and then disappear. That the symptoms are gone, however, doesn't mean the disease has been cured. Chlamydia can linger for years, with a slow, silent means of destroying your organs, while gonorrhea can wreak havoc in the few days before symptoms become apparent.

Q: **Can an STD disappear by itself?**

A: Yes. Several, like gonorrhea, can burn out on their own, after causing destruction. Syphilis can also disappear for ten or twenty years and then reappear. In addition, there is evidence that venereal warts disappear on their own. However, since it is almost impossible for you to tell if a disease has disappeared or is merely "hiding" silently in your body, never take a lack of symptoms as a sign that all is well. Be cultured and tested any and every time a possibility for infection exists and begin treatment immediately if any of these diseases are discovered in your body.

Q: **I was a virgin when I got married and never slept with any man but my husband. Could I get an STD?**

A: Yes. If your husband was sexually active before marriage, he could have been harboring a silent infection that was ultimately passed on to you. The most common are T-mycoplasma and chlamydia.

Q: **Can an STD get into my reproductive system during anal sex?**
A: Certainly HIV can be transmitted this way via tiny breaks in the skin during anal sex. In addition, many bacteria that are deposited in the rectum during anal sex can work their way into the vagina later on and then penetrate your pelvic region. Chances of this increase during exceptionally vigorous vaginal penetration, which can drive any bacteria or viruses present in your vagina deeper into your system. Your partner *must* cleanse his penis thoroughly before attempting vaginal sex after anal penetration. You can also increase your risks via improper wiping or cleansing after a bowel movement. To help protect yourself, always wipe front to back, away from the vagina.

Q: **I just found out my husband has an STD. Does this mean he had sex outside our marriage?**
A: It could, of course, mean that. However, it could also mean he was harboring the disease in his body long before he met you or that his infection came from an infection you may be unknowingly harboring in *your* body. In addition, since some STDs are spread nonsexually as well as through intercourse, it's possible your husband contracted his disease in a totally innocent encounter with a wet towel or unsanitary sauna or steam room.

Q: **Can I get an STD from a toilet?**
A: Yes, but not all STDs are equally contagious in this manner. Some bacteria and viruses, such as those responsible for herpes, yeast infections, and venereal warts, live outside the body longer than others, so transmission via toilet seats, vibrators, or any other object that comes in contact with your genital area can more easily occur. Other microorganisms, such as chlamydia, T-mycoplasma, and those causing gonorrhea, usually don't live outside the body very long, so your genitals would have to come in contact with an ob-

ject, say, a toilet seat, almost immediately after vaginal or penile fluids of an infected person had been deposited. While this time factor significantly reduces the risk of transmitting many STDs in this manner, transmission can still happen. To be safe, always use a paper toilet seat cover when using any public facility or the bathroom of any person you suspect may be infected.

A Final Word: Safe Sex, Not Fearful Sex

While the perils of a sexually active life cannot be denied, this chapter was not meant to scare or inhibit you or to decrease your ability to enjoy sex in any way. It was written to help you demystify some of the physical problems that can arise in the course of a sexual relationship and help you keep those problems from affecting your health and your fertility, now and in the future. It was also meant to help you understand your own body better and thus spot trouble signs before the problem arises. My intention has been to reassure you that, whatever the ways you have enjoyed sex in the past or will enjoy it in the future, you can protect yourself from *any* and *all* problems.

Chapter Six

Your Fertility from Nine to Five:

Reproductive Hazards of the Workplace and How to Avoid Them

Mary Ellen lies quietly in her bed, her hands resting atop her now-rounded tummy. Five months pregnant and just beginning to feel life, she senses a rush of anxiety each time her baby moves inside her. Although she is healthy and strong (and a sonogram shows her baby is fine as well), Mary Ellen lives in constant fear of miscarriage. Why? She just found out that seven out of every ten women in her office complex have miscarried in the past eight months. The health department is looking into the matter, but by the time any answers arrive, Mary Ellen's fate—and that of her unborn child—will already have been decided.

"If only I had known what was going on," she told me, "maybe I could have done something to try and avoid the problems."

The Workplace and Your Fertility

Astonishingly, studies show that reproductive disorders are among the top ten work-related illnesses for *both sexes*. Currently, there are more than 14 million men and women exposed to potential reproductive hazards on the job every day. In fact, a report issued by the U.S. Office of Technology Assessment in the 1980s revealed that out of the sixty thousand chemicals in widespread use in U.S. industries, only a handful are regulated, in part, on considerations of human reproductive health. Unfortunately, matters are not much different today. In short, no matter what you do for a living, the workplace and its potential for affecting both male and female fertility is now a major issue, and one that no couple in their childbearing years can afford to ignore.

The Reproductive Hazards: Who Is at Risk?

Because each workplace has its own specific hazards, it's often difficult to generalize the risk factors. However, when problems do occur they are usually linked to one of the following factors:

- Exposure to radiation, including that which comes from office equipment such as fax machines and computer terminals
- Contaminated or low-oxygenated air due to poor ventilation, dirty heating or air-conditioning systems, or chemical pollutants
- Direct contact with toxic chemicals, including those used for copy machines and printers, as well as those used in various manufacturing processes
- Dangerously high temperatures—especially hazardous for male fertility (over one hundred degrees—often seen in bakeries, restaurant kitchens, and many factories)
- Atmospheric pressure, which can contribute to premature labor or miscarriage

These factors could be present in the specific job tasks that you or your mate perform, or they could be fundamental to the nature of your company's business. Moreover, toxic elements used in the workplace can pollute the general atomosphere.

Depending on the substance, how long you have been exposed, and most important, the level to which you are exposed on a regular basis, a variety of reproductive problems can occur, such as:

- Fertilization difficulties
- Implantation problems
- Interference with ovulation
- Menstrual irregularities
- Increased risk of miscarriage
- Increased risk of birth defects
- Decrease in libido (sex drive)

In addition, there can be problems even after your baby is born. Studies show that workplace contaminants (such as lead, pesticides, cadmium, carbonyl, and other manufacturing chemicals) can show up in breast milk, leading to an increased risk of cancer, respiratory problems, or immune system deficiencies for your baby (check specific risks for many types of jobs later in this chapter).

You and Your Partner: At Equal Risk

Although much of the attention on the workplace–fertility link has been focused on women, the problems are by no means limited to the female population. A man's fertility is equally vulnerable. Indeed, men sometimes experience more damage in less time and with less exposure than women. Making matters worse, many employers continue to ignore the dangers to male reproductive health. According to studies conducted as early as the 1980s by the Massachusetts Occupational Health Program, out of 198 chemical and electronic firms queried on reproductive hazards, only one took the importance of male fertility into consideration by restricting hazardous jobs for those men whose partners were trying to conceive. Many experts estimate that number is even lower today.

How can reproductive hazards threaten your mate's fertility? When exposed to certain harmful factors, he can experience one or more of the following problems on a temporary or even long-term basis:

- Lowered sperm count
- Higher rate of abnormal sperm
- Increased risk of birth defects

- Sperm motility defects
- Testicle damage
- Impotence
- Loss of sex drive

The effects on him can also increase *your* risk of miscarriage.

The Good News: The Workplace Can Be a Safe Place

The good news is that there are many ways your workplace can be made safer, for general good health and to protect your fertility. Laws have already been passed to ensure valuable reproductive rights; you'll read about them later in this chapter. In addition, you and your partner can both take steps to eliminate many work-related fertility hazards. A good place to start is by identifying potential problems.

Computers and Your Fertility: What You Need to Know Right Now

Although much of what has been alleged about computers and fertility was based on rumor and not fact, there are some links that have proven true. These include:

- Increased risk of miscarriage
- Increased risk of birth defects
- Decreased fertility overall for men and women

For a long time these problems seemed to appear in clusters—isolated groups of computer workers in various industries and in different geographical locations reported increases in reproductive problems, particularly miscarriages and birth defects. Because, however, the effects were not universal, many skeptics doubted the existence of what I like to call "high-tech" infertility. Over the past decade, however, studies have been emerging to show that these concerns may, indeed, be real.

In 1997, for example, research published by the Department of Preventative Medicine and Environmental Health at the University of Iowa College of Medicine revealed an important link between women who worked on video display terminals and an increased incidence of endometriosis, as well as a greater incidence of cervical-factor infertility, although currently there is no adequate explanation of why this is so.

These findings back up studies conducted as early as the 1990s of some fifteen hundred women by the Kaiser-Permanente Medical Group in northern California. They exploded the cluster theory by following the pregnancies of 1,583 women. What they learned:

- Those women who spent more than twenty hours per week working at video display terminals (VDTs) had twice as many miscarriages in the first three months of their pregnancy as did workers who did not use computers.

- When compared to nonusers, women who were exposed to just five hours per day of VDT use had a 40 percent increase in the number of babies born with congenital malformations.

- Whether problems result from exposure *before* or *after* conception is still not known. Still, the potential dangers of computers for fertility are hard to ignore.

How Computers Can Harm Your Fertility

According to the most recent research, the link between computers and reproductive health is not the machine itself, but the monitor used to display the information. Most emit one or both of the following types of radiation:

- Extra low frequency (ELF)
- Very low frequency (VLF)

Some experts report that continued exposure to either one damages the reproductive system as well as a developing baby. The end result can be miscarriage, birth defects, or difficulty in conceiving. In addition, the effects of low-level radiation are thought to be synergistic—made worse by outside factors. An important study conducted on the reproductive risks of nurses found that multiple workplace factors, including VDTs, other sources of radiation, and exposure to chemotherapeutic drugs, all work together to bring out the worst in each other. So, even minimal exposure to a single factor can sometimes cause problems.

VDTs and Your Menstrual Cycle

Early in the technology revolution, studies conducted in the 1980s by the School of Management at UMIST (University of Manchester, Institute of Science and Technology, in Manchester, England) found prolonged exposure to VLF radiation of VDTs leads to a variety of menstrual irregularities, leading to yet another possible cause of infertility. Problems included:

- Cramps
- Anxiety
- Irritability
- Stress
- Amenorrhea (loss of menstrual cycle)

Since that time, smaller but significant studies continue to report that prolonged regular exposure to either VLF or ELF radiation can cause biological stress that manifests itself in improper brain metabolism and malfunctioning of the endocrine system, which produces the hormones responsible for reproduction. I believe this research may provide another connection between menstrual problems, VDTs, and infertility.

VDTs and Male Fertility

Since a man's reproductive system is even more sensitive to the effects of radiation than a woman's, when regularly exposed to even minimal levels he can experience:

- Decreased sperm count
- Testicle damage
- Hormonal upsets
- Chromosomal damage within the sperm, leading to birth defects and miscarriage

Because the effects of radiation are cumulative, simply spending time in an environment where many VDTs are regularly used can take its toll on his reproductive health, and on the health of your baby.

Working on Computers: The Good News

Whether your job entails regular, daily work at a computer terminal or just occasional exposure or use, there *are* things you can do to help reduce the reproductive hazards:

- Whenever possible use laptop computers or the new flat-style digital display monitors, particularly if you are pregnant. Both offer significantly reduced levels of radiation exposure.

- Several companies are now manufacturing accessories to help cut exposure to VDT radiation, including shielded cables, specially designed work stations, and portable radiation monitors to measure dangerous leakages.

- Finally, there are steps you can take to minimize any harmful effects of the computer equipment you are working on right now—at home or in your office.

Nine to Five—the National Organization of Working Women—did a tremendous job in helping to research the VDT-infertility link, and in educating women and men about computer safety. The following is a sample of their suggested guidelines for making your computer safer for you and your baby.

How to Protect Your Fertility

- Since one source of VLF radiation is the flyback transformer located at the rear of your monitor, stay clear of this area when doing other work tasks.

- Push the screen back as far as your work station will allow, so long as you can read your screen without straining. Most VDT radiation projects only about ten feet from the front or back of the monitor.

- Avoid doing noncomputer tasks or taking breaks near the side of your terminal, or turn your monitor off if you do.

- Arrange your office so that you are not sitting close to the back or the side of a coworker's terminal.

- Insist that your employer provide periodic, thorough testing of VDTs for excessive radiation leaks, as well as regular maintenance to prevent problems from occurring. Systematic testing can prevent X-ray emissions due to design flaws or a malfunction in your system.

Can a Lead Apron Protect Your Baby?

Because a lead apron can shield one from the harmful effects of *some* radiation, many of my patients ask whether it can also protect against the harmful effects of VDTs. It cannot. A lead shield protects one *only* from the effects of ionizing radiation, which is negligible in VDTs. It offers no protection against nonionizing VLF or ELF radiation, which are thought to be the most significant sources of VDT-related fertility damage. Moreover, continual, long-term use of a lead apron when you are pregnant adds a weight on your stomach that may be more harmful to your baby than any radiation.

Another Important Warning

Don't be fooled by clever packaging or unsubstantiated advertising claims about screens, monitors, and other computer accessories. A random sampling found that many "radiation-reduced" and "radiation-free" products reduced only one type of frequency, leaving the others barely changed or untouched. To be sure that the product you purchase gives you all the protection it advertises, write to the manufacturer for specifics—if possible, for *written* guarantees about the type and amount of radiation reduction provided.

Workplace Cautions:
What Else You Need to Know

In addition to computers, there are a variety of other workplace factors that can have equally troubling effects on your ability to conceive. For women, these include:

- Organic chemical solvents and glues
- Pesticides used in and around the work environment
- Industrial dusts

In addition, physical stressors (particularly shift work), long hours standing on one's feet, and heavy lifting have all been associated with increased risk of miscarriage and premature labor. If you are actively trying to get pregnant, pay attention to these factors at work as well as at home and you may soon discover that you can conceive—and maintain your pregnancy—much more easily than you thought.

For your partner, the list of dangers is even longer. Indeed, a wide variety of published studies have shown that a man's reproductive system is extremely sensitive to even limited exposures to many toxic chemicals regularly found in many workplaces, often the result of poor ventilation.

What are the chemicals most toxic to male fertility?

- Alkylmercury
- Antimonide
- Anesthetic gases
- Boron
- Carbon disulfide
- Chloroprene
- Inorganic lead
- Manganese
- Methyl chloride
- Organic solvents
- Synthetic estrogen and progestin
- Combined exposure to styrene and acetone

(For a complete listing of the occupations where these chemicals are most often found, see the Workplace Fertility Guide below.)

Both heat and excessive vibration may also affect male fertility. Fortunately, reducing exposure whenever possible, particularly in the months before you want to conceive, can go a long way in ensuring that your conception is not only fast but also healthy.

Workplace Fertility Protection Guide

Although it's difficult to ascertain which potentially dangerous factors will be present in your particular work environment, the following guide should help you determine if your job might be harming your fertility. Although every attempt has been made to provide the most accurate, up-to-date information, please note this guide is by no means complete.

- Some substances that test as safe today may prove to be hazardous later on.

- Some things that are suspect today may be proved safe when further studies are made.

- Some factors medical science simply has not yet explored. That a substance doesn't appear on this list, or any list published anywhere, does not automatically mean it is safe.

This guide also does not suggest that everyone who works at these occupations or in these industries is exposed to these substances, nor does it imply that everyone who is exposed is in definite danger. It simply represents guidelines to help you investigate how your job might affect your ability to conceive and deliver a healthy baby, now or in the future. Occupations are listed alphabetically. Their order suggests no ranking as to danger or intensity of harm.

Airline Personnel (pilot, navigator, flight attendant)

RISK: OVEREXPOSURE TO HIGH-ALTITUDE RADIATION

Male: Decreased sperm count, increased risk of birth defects, decreased fertility, impotence

Female: Increased risk of miscarriage, premature labor, menstrual irregularities

Artist (fine)

RISK: MANGANESE DIOXIDE

Male: Impotence, reduced sex drive, decreased fertility
Female: No data available

RISK: FORMALDEHYDE

Male: No data available
Female: Menstrual irregularities

RISK: GLYCOL ETHERS

Male: Abnormal or reduced sperm count, decreased fertility
Female: Increased risk of birth defects

RISK: LEAD

Male: Impotence, reduced sex drive, abnormal or reduced sperm count, decreased fertility, miscarriage in wife

Female: Menstrual irregularities, decreased fertility, increased risk of miscarriage, birth defects, stillbirths, infant mortality, contaminated breast milk

Baker

RISK: ELEVATED TEMPERATURES

Male: Reduced sperm count
Female: No data available

Ceramic and Craft Workers

RISK: LEAD

Male: Impotence, abnormal or decreased sperm count, decreased fertility, miscarriage in wife

Female: Menstrual irregularities, decreased fertility, increased risk of miscarriage, stillbirths, infant mortality, contaminated breast milk

RISK: GLYCOL ETHERS

Male: Abnormal or reduced sperm count, decreased fertility
Female: Increased risk of birth defects

RISK: MANGANESE DIOXIDE

Male: Impotence or reduced sex drive, decreased fertility
Female: No data available

Chemical Laboratory Worker

RISK: CARBON TETRACHLORIDE

Male: Change in personality
Female: No data available

RISK: BENZENE

Male: No data available

Female: Menstrual irregularities, increased risk of stillbirths, low-birth-weight babies

Clothing and Textile Workers

RISK: TRIS (FLAME RETARDANT)

Male: Decreased fertility
Female: No data available

RISK: FORMALDEHYDE

Male: No data available
Female: Irregular menstrual cycles

Computer Personnel (programmers, keyboard operators, technicians)

RISK: RADIATION

Male and Female: See section on VDTs earlier in this chapter

Cosmetics Manufacturer or Worker

RISK: MERCURY COMPOUNDS

Male: Impotence, reduced sex drive, reduced sperm count, increase in abnormal sperm, decreased fertility

Female: Menstrual irregularities, increased risk of miscarriage, stillbirth, infant mortality, birth defects

RISK: FORMALDEHYDE

Male: No data available
Female: Irregular menstrual cycles

RISK: NITROSAMINE

Male: Chromosomal abnormalities and mutations
Female: Chromosomal abnormalities and mutations

RISK: ESTROGEN

Male: Decreased fertility
Female: Ovulation upsets, hormonal imbalances

Dental Care Personnel (dentist, nurse, hygienist)

RISK: ANESTHETIC GASES, NITROUS OXIDE

Male: Abnormal or reduced sperm count, miscarriage in wife, decreased fertility
Female: Decreased fertility

RISK: X-RADIATION

Male: Abnormal or reduced sperm count, decreased fertility, chromosomal or genetic damage
Female: Menstrual irregularities, decreased fertility, increased risk of birth defects, possible increased risk of miscarriage and stillbirth

RISK: MERCURY

Male: Impotence or reduced sex drive, low sperm count, increase in abnormal sperm
Female: Menstrual irregularities, increased risk of miscarriage, stillbirth, infant mortality, birth defects

DES Manufacturers and Workers

RISK: DIETHYLSTILBESTROL

Male: Abnormal or reduced sperm count, decreased fertility
Female: Increased risk of birth defects, contaminated breast milk

Dry-cleaners

RISK: CARBON TETRACHLORIDE

Male: Reduced fertility
Female: No data available
Note: For more information on the effects of dry-cleaning chemicals on fertility, see the chapter on miscarriage later in this book.

Exterminator

RISK: PESTICIDES (DIBROMOCHLOROPROPANE, KEPONE, DDT, DBCP CARBARYL, DDVP, MALATHION)

Male: Decreased sperm count, decreased fertility
Female: Menstrual irregularities, decreased fertility, contaminated breast milk
Note: For more information on the effects of pesticides see the next chapter on lifestyle factors that affect fertility.

Farm and Agricultural Worker

RISK: PESTICIDES (SEE EXTERMINATOR)

Male: Decreased sperm count, decreased fertility
Female: Menstrual irregularities, decreased fertility, contaminated breast milk

RISK: ARSENIC

Male: Reduced sperm count, decreased fertility
Female: Increased risk of miscarriage, stillbirth, infant mortality, low-birth-weight babies, birth defects

Foundry or Oven Workers

RISK: ELEVATED TEMPERATURES

Male: Reduced sperm count
Female: No data available

Hairdresser, Cosmetologist, Barber

RISK: LEAD IN HAIR DYES

Male: Reduced fertility
Female: Reduced fertility

RISK: HAIR SPRAY RESINS

Male: Decreased fertility, increased risk of miscarriage in wife, impotence
Female: Increased risk of miscarriage, stillbirth, infant mortality

RISK: NAIL POLISH SOLVENTS

Male: Decreased fertility
Female: Menstrual irregularities, decreased fertility

Hazardous Waste Disposal Worker

RISK: LEAD, PBBs

Male: Impotence or reduced sex drive, increase in abnormal sperm, reduced sperm count, decreased fertility, increased risk of miscarriage in wife
Female: Menstrual irregularities, decreased fertility, increased risk of miscarriage, stillbirth, or infant mortality, contaminated breast milk

Health Care Worker

RISK: ETHYLENE OXIDE (DISINFECTANT), X-RADIATION

Male: Decreased fertility
Female: Increased risk of miscarriage and birth defects, decreased fertility

House Painter

RISK: BORON

Male: Impotence, reduced sex drive, low sperm count, abnormal sperm

Female: Increased risk of miscarriage, stillbirth, infant mortality, birth defects

RISK: CADMIUM

Male: Impotence, abnormal or reduced sperm count, decreased fertility

Female: Menstrual irregularities, low-birth-weight babies, contaminated breast milk

RISK: PCBs

Male: No data available
Female: Menstrual irregularities

RISK: FORMALDEHYDE

Male: No data available
Female: Menstrual irregularities

RISK: AROMATIC HYDROCARBONS

Male: Decreased fertility
Female: Decreased fertility

RISK: GLYCOL ETHERS

Male: Abnormal or reduced sperm count, decreased fertility
Female: Increased risk of birth defects

Lawyer, Paralegal, Legal Secretary

RISK: COMPUTERS, ELECTRIC OFFICE EQUIPMENT, STRESS

Male: Reduced sperm count, decreased fertility
Female: Increased risk of miscarriage and birth defects, menstrual irregularities
Note: See section on VDTs earlier in this chapter.

Medical Personnel (doctor, nurse, aide, technician)

RISK: ANESTHETIC GASES, NITROUS OXIDE

Male: Low sperm count, increase in abnormal sperm, increased risk of miscarriage in wife
Female: Increased risk of miscarriage

RISK: ANTICANCER DRUGS

Male: Impotence, reduced sex drive, low sperm count, abnormal sperm, decreased fertility
Female: Increased risk of miscarriage, contaminated breast milk

Perfume Industry

RISK: BENZENE, OTHER ORGANIC SOLVENTS

Male: No data available
Female: Menstrual irregularities, increased risk of low-birth-weight baby, infant mortality, birth defects

Pesticide Workers and Farmers

RISK: JOB-RELATED CHEMICALS

Male and Female: See Exterminator; see next chapter on lifestyle factors and infertility

Photographic Processor

RISK: FORMALDEHYDE

Male: No data available
Female: Menstrual irregularities

RISK: GLYCOL ETHERS

Male: Decreased fertility
Female: Increased risk of birth defects

Police Officer

RISK: STRESS

Male: Impotence or decreased sex drive, abnormal or reduced sperm count, decreased fertility, increased risk of miscarriage in wife

Female: Menstrual irregularities, decreased fertility, increased risk of miscarriage and stillbirth, contaminated breast milk

Printer or Graphics Designer

RISK: ETHYLENE GLYCOL PD

Male: Testicular atrophy, decreased sperm count, increase in birth defects

Female: Increased risk of birth defects

PVC Manufacturer or Processor

RISK: POLYVINYL CHLORIDE

Male: Decreased fertility, increased risk of miscarriage in wife, possible impotence and reduced sex drive

Female: Increased risk of miscarriage, stillbirth, infant mortality

Radar Operators

RISK: MICROWAVES

Male and Female: Decreased fertility

Rubber Worker

RISK: CHLOROPRENE

Male: Impotence, reduced sex drive, low sperm count, abnormal sperm, increased risk of miscarriage in wife

Female: Menstrual irregularities

RISK: VINYL CHLORIDE

Male: See PVC Manufacturer or Processor
Female: Increased risk of miscarriage, stillbirths, and infant mortality

Smelters

RISK: CADMIUM

Male: See Storage Battery Worker
Female: See Storage Battery Worker

RISK: NICKEL

Male: Reduced fertility
Female: No data available

RISK: MANGANESE DIOXIDE

Male: Impotence, reduced sex drive, decreased fertility
Female: No data available

Soil Treater

RISK: CARBON DISULFIDE

Male: Impotence, abnormal or low sperm count, increased risk of miscarriage in wife
Female: Menstrual irregularities, increased risk of miscarriage

Stockbroker

RISK: COMPUTER TERMINALS, LOW-VOLTAGE APPLIANCES (FAX MACHINES, TOTE BOARDS, ETC.), STRESS, CARBON MONOXIDE (CIGARETTE SMOKE)

Male: Reduced sperm count, abnormal sperm
Female: Menstrual irregularities, increased risk of miscarriage and birth defects

Storage Battery Worker

RISK: CADMIUM

Male: Impotence, reduced sex drive, low sperm count, increase in abnormal sperm, decreased fertility
Female: Increased risk of miscarriage and stillbirth, decreased fertility

Utility Worker

RISK: EPICHLORODRIN

Male: Decreased fertility
Female: No data available

RISK: ETHYLENE OXIDE

Male: Decreased fertility
Female: Increased risk of miscarriage, birth defects

RISK: BUTADIENE

Male: Decreased fertility
Female: Decreased fertility, increased risk of miscarriage and birth defects

Viscose Rayon Worker

RISK: CARBON DISULFIDE

Male: Impotence, abnormal or low sperm count, increased risk of miscarriage in wife
Female: Menstrual irregularities, increased risk of miscarriage

Welder

RISK: MANGANESE, NICKEL

Male: Impotence or reduced sex drive, decreased fertility
Female: No data available

X-Ray Inspector, Technician

RISK: IONIZING RADIATION, MICROWAVES

Male: Abnormal or reduced sperm count, decreased fertility
Female: Menstrual irregularities, decreased fertility, increased risk of
birth defects

The Workplace Chemicals That Can Affect Your Pregnancy

A wide variety of toxic substances found in the workplace not only affect
your ability to *get* pregnant, but can harm your baby after conception occurs. If you are pregnant, take special precautions to avoid overexposure
to these substances.

- Anesthetic gases
- Dibromochloropropane
- Ethylene oxide
- Lead
- Methyl Mercury
- Organic solvents
- Vinyl chloride

How to Make Your Workplace a Safe Place

Regardless of your occupation, the federal Hazard Communication Standard guarantees your right to obtain information about potential health
hazards in your working environment, including those that can threaten
your unborn baby, without fear of employer retribution. In many cities
across the United States, the Occupational Health and Safety Administration (OSHA) or the National Institute for Occupational Safety and
Health (NIOSH), both found in the government listings of your phone
book, can provide you with information about your employer's *obligations
for protecting you.* Here are just a few things federal law requires your
employer to disclose:

- Any hazardous chemicals present in your work environment (all such material must be clearly marked with the name and address of the supplier)
- Complete health and safety information about all hazardous chemicals, including product name, possible health effects, symptoms resulting from exposure, and handling procedures
- Precautions to take when working with these chemicals, including any need for protective clothing or equipment, and emergency treatment in the event of an accident
- The results of any company studies, exposure records, or air monitoring that could affect the health and safety of workers

You Can Make a Difference!

In addition to taking advantage of federal and state regulations, don't overlook your own power to initiate even more laws in your behalf. Remember, some of the most important changes in labor standards and practices have been brought about by employees who took an active, even aggressive role in job safety.

For example, in 1977 a group of male workers at a California plant manufacturing the chemical DCPB discovered over lunchtime conversation that none had been able to father a child since they'd begun their jobs. A subsequent semen analysis showed a marked decrease in the sperm counts of the men working with this chemical, many of them so low that they were completely sterile. The workers joined forces and fought for important changes. What started as a casual lunchtime chat turned into a major issue that eventually led to the government ban on the manufacture of DCPB.

Seven Steps to a Safer Workplace

If you do believe your working environment may be a threat to your fertility, I strongly urge you to take some kind of action right away. The following guidelines for a safer workplace were issued by Nine to Five, the

National Organization of Working Women, and the Southeast Michigan Coalition on Occupational Safety and Health (SEMCOSH). They can help you obtain a safer, healthier environment for everyone.

1. Share your reproductive health concerns with other workers. Discover how many female coworkers, as well as how many wives of male coworkers are having problems conceiving or have been plagued with an unusual number of miscarriages, premature labors, or babies born with birth defects. This may shed light on whether your workplace is suspect.

2. Document problems you can clearly identify, then organize an employee task force to investigate specifics. Share your discoveries with your coworkers and encourage them to do the same. Pooling information can help everyone determine where specific problems might lie.

3. Discuss your concerns with your employer. You cannot be fired, punished, or discriminated against for inquiring or complaining about health and safety concerns of your job.

4. Request copies of all company studies concerning reproductive or other health hazards of your workplace. Your employer is required by law to share with you any significant health or safety information about your job.

5. If you have reason to believe that the air in your workplace may be contaminated, request that air samples be taken. If your employer refuses, contact your local Coalition on Occupational Safety and Health (listed in your phone directory under government agencies).

6. File grievances with your employer and encourage coworkers to do the same. If possible, organize petitions specifying clear demands to improve health and safety, including reducing exposure to dangerous chemicals, substitution of safer chemicals wherever possible, and improving ventilation. In addition, work to have reproductive safety concerns included in union negotiations or other employee contracts.

7. Learn what information your employer is legally required to give you in regard to the reproductive hazards of your workplace. Your local department of labor, your union, NIOSH (National Institute for Occupational Safety and Health), plus your local state and city

coalitions or occupational safety and health can provide the specific
regulations your employer must adhere to in regard to your welfare.

You Are Not Alone: Where to Get Help

If you believe your working environment may be harmful to your fertility—or to any aspect of your health—or if you would like further information on the reproductive hazards of the workplace, the following
organizations can help you:

Computer Databases:

- Medline: National Library of Medicine, Bethesda, Maryland. References from over three thousand biomedical journals can help you
  zero in on the specific health hazards of your job. To find Medline
  on the Internet: Http://www.Medscape.com.
- Toxline and Toxnet: National Library of Medicine, Bethesda, Maryland. Four hundred thousand references on human and animal toxicology: On the Internet: Http://www.toxline.com.
- Reprotox: Reproductive Toxicology Center, Washington, D.C. Ref-
  erenced summaries of more than seven hundred reproductive toxins. On the Internet: Http://www.reprotox.com.

Hotline Organizations

For additional written material and/or references to help you in your area
or occupation, contact the following organizations:

Nine to Five
National Organization of Working Women
614 Superior Avenue, N.W.
Cleveland, Ohio 44113
216-566-9308

National Network to Prevent Birth Defects
Box 15309 SE Station
Washington, DC 20003
202-543-5450

Occupational Safety and Health Administration (OSHA)
U.S. Department of Labor
200 Constitution Avenue NW
Washington, DC 20210
There are also regional and state offices. OSHA will perform work-place inspections at the request of an employee, a union, or a physician.

National Institute for Occupational Safety and Health (NIOSH)
101 Marietta Tower
Atlanta, GA 30323
There are also local state offices. NIOSH investigates health and safety hazards in the workplace upon request.

Office of Technology Assessment
U.S. Congress, Washington, DC 20510
Provides literature on reproductive hazards of the workplace.

Chapter Seven

Fertility Protection 2000:

A Couple's Guide to a Healthy Lifestyle

Every day, it seems, we discover not only new fertility threats, but new dangers in things that have been present in our lives for a long time. From alcohol to diet pills, tranquilizers to caffeine, pesticides, tobacco, computers—you name it—sometimes the list seems almost endless.

The good news is that the same research that has helped us to identify new risks to our reproductive health has also helped to shed light on what we can do to protect our fertility—actions that often require little more than a few modifications in our daily living.

To help you and your partner get started in the right direction, I have prepared a short Lifestyle Fertility Quiz. Based on information from worldwide studies on reproductive health, these questions—and their provocative answers—can provide important insights on what you and your partner can do to begin protecting your fertility right now.

The Lifestyle Fertility Quiz

Each of the following twenty-four statements was designed to help you and your partner learn something about a particular aspect of your lives. The connection between the questions and the subject of fertility is sometimes obvious; at other times the significance of your responses will be more subtle. For this reason, I ask that you both answer each question spontaneously, and then go on to the next, without stopping to wonder what your answers mean. The Fertility Scorecard at the end of the test will help you understand the meanings of your responses, as well as provide some important information on the current status of your reproductive health.

To take the test, simply read each statement and then record how true it is for you, indicating A for always, S for sometimes, and N for never. Keep a numbered list of your answers. The same format is applied throughout the quiz.

	ALWAYS	SOMETIMES	NEVER
1. I drink more than four cups of coffee a day.			
2. I drink more than two cans of cola a day.			
3. I take pain relievers regularly–more than twenty tablets monthly.			
4. I smoke at least twenty cigarettes a day.			
5. I need at least two alcohol drinks a day to relax and unwind.			
6. I drink more than ten beers or ten glasses of wine a month.			
7. I use marijuana more than once a month.			
8. I use cocaine/crack more than once a month.			
9. I have trouble falling asleep at night.			
10. I have trouble remaining asleep, or wake frequently during the night.			
11. I regularly use a variety of over-the-counter medications.			
12. I spend more than twenty hours per week at a desktop computer terminal.			
13. I hate my boss.			
14. I watch twenty plus hours of TV weekly.			
15. My job requires exposure to radiation or chemicals on a regular basis.			

	ALWAYS	SOMETIMES	NEVER
16. I fly more than eight hours a month.			
17. I spend most of my time outdoors in a major city.			
18. For women only: My menstrual cycle is regular. For men only: My sex drive seems to be decreasing.			
19. I exercise more than five hours a week.			
20. For women only: I use an IUD for birth control. For men only: I take medication for high blood pressure.			
21. I have at least three different sex partners each month, or have had multiple partners in the past.			
22. For women only: I have had problems getting pregnant in the past, or have never been pregnant. For men only: Past partners have had problems getting pregnant; I have never impregnated anyone.			
23. I live in a warm climate.			
24. There are bitter odors in the air I breathe at home or at work.			

To Score Your Lifestyle Fertility Quiz, simply total your A's, S's and N's, assigning them points as shown below:

  A responses: 10 points each
  S responses: 5 points each
  N responses: 2 points each

Add your total score and use the Fertility Scorecard below to determine the current status of your reproductive health.

Fertility Scorecard

50–100 points: Your fertility is likely in good shape, or at least your lifestyle habits are not making significant contributions to future problems. It is also likely you are a well-balanced person who does everything in moderation. If you maintain your current lifestyle, it's likely you will preserve your fertility and your sex life for many years to come.

101–150 points: You're not quite as careful as you would like to think! While your reproductive health is probably not in any imminent danger, if you keep on doing what you're doing, or add a few more excesses, you may find your fertility in trouble within the next few years. Turn to the Fertility Protection Update following this quiz to find out where you can make some important lifestyle changes.

151–200 points: You are in the danger zone! If you're not already having problems conceiving, it's likely because you haven't tried! This high score should tell you that changes need to be made if you want to preserve both your fertility and your sex life for the coming years. Do read the Fertility Protection Update that follows and make changes right away.

201–250 points: You are in serious danger. Not only is your fertility in jeopardy, your general health is in danger as well. If you are able to conceive, your chance of miscarriage and birth defects is probably higher than average. If you are also above age thirty and have been living this way for some time, you are at especially high risk for infertility or a problem pregnancy. Read the next section and begin to make changes in the way you live, work, and play.

The Fertility Protection Update 2000:
What You Need to Know Now

Because your reproductive health is a cumulative biological function, to what extent you are affected by your environment has much to do with how long negative aspects have been a part of your life and to what degree they are present right now. It's also important to remember there are often exceptions to even the most hard and fast rules. Some men and women continue to be fertile and produce healthy children despite being in poor health themselves or indulging in practices and habits that are detrimental to fertility. At the same time, some couples who scrupulously avoid anything that could harm their fertility find they cannot conceive. Science, it seems, can show us the smartest course of action, but nothing can give us guarantees.

With this mind, I have prepared the *Fertility Protection Update 2000*— a guide to what the very latest research shows will and won't affect your reproductive health. By checking the guide for factors present in your lives, you and your partner can determine where changes should be made.

The factors listed are in alphabetical order, and placement does not indicate ranking, in terms of ability to harm you or the degree of damage they may cause. How much or how little each factor affects you can vary greatly, depending on the number of negative factors present in your life.

Factor: Air Travel

Effects on fertility:

Female: For many years we have known that radiation, in almost any form—including that which comes from flying in an airplane—can be detrimental to fertility. Now, however, planes fly at much higher altitudes than ever before, so exposure to atmospheric radiation is even greater today than in the past. In women who fly a great deal, particularly flight attendants, this constant exposure has been shown to cause irregular ovulation, difficulty in conceiving, and a higher risk of miscarriage.

Male: Since sperm is exceptionally vulnerable to the effects of all types of radiation, excessive air travel may cause a variety of fertility problems, including a decrease in sperm count, an increase in the number of abnormal sperm, and sperm that are too immature to bring about a natural fertilization.

For maximum fertility protection: Both you and your partner should avoid all unnecessary air travel three to five months before attempting conception. Once you become pregnant, limit air travel as much as possible, not only to avoid exposure on the plane itself but also to escape the dangerous effects of X-ray equipment now used at all major airports. This is particularly important if you are at high risk for infertility or if you currently have irregular menstrual cycles or a history of miscarriage.

Factor: Alcohol

Effects on fertility:

Female: The more alcohol a woman drinks, the less likely she is to get pregnant. That's the 1998 finding published in the *British Medical Journal*. Here, a study on four hundred couples revealed that even moderate drinking—one glass of beer or wine a day, for example—could cut a woman's chance for conception by as much as 50 percent. A similar study from the University of Washington revealed that even if you do conceive, taking just one drink a day before getting pregnant could cause your baby to have an exceptionally low birth weight, which, in turn, could cause a variety of lifetime health problems. Although researchers aren't sure what the link between alcohol and female fertility is, they theorize that it may interfere with ovulation or the transport of the egg down the fallopian tube. Alcohol may also prevent a healthy implantation. Additionally, when combined with marijuana (see the section on drug use later in the chapter), alcohol may affect your fertility to an even greater degree.

Male: Although the effects of alcohol in a man's body are slightly less dramatic, the newest studies have shown that as little as four drinks a day can lower sperm count significantly—particularly important if your partner has a marginal or low-normal sperm count. New evidence also links alcohol to sperm defects, resulting in an increased risk of serious developmental problems in your baby.

Additionally, researchers now believe that consuming alcohol before conception can cause subtle genetic changes in sperm that increase the risk not only of a low-birth-weight baby but also of a variety of developmental delays. This is consistent with studies on the offspring of alcoholic fathers, which show many of these children suffer selective intellectual and functional impairment.

For maximum fertility protection: It's a good idea to somewhat limit alcohol consumption for several months before attempting conception, particularly in the four weeks before you plan to conceive. If either you or your partner have even a marginal fertility problem, you should avoid alcohol completely for at least two weeks before conception.

If your lifestyle is such that avoiding alcohol altogether is not possible, at least do so for forty-eight hours before you plan to conceive. In addition, increase your nutrient intake several weeks before attempting conception, paying special attention to the fertility vitamin and mineral guide featured later in this book. This may help balance some of the effects of alcohol, which can deplete key nutrients necessary for a healthy conception and optimum fertility.

Factor: Bodybuilding Drugs (Steroids, Creatine)

Effects on fertility: Over the past several years a number of substances, both prescription and over-the-counter, have been popularized by bodybuilders and others looking to increase muscle stamina. Aside from other warnings about health effects, I believe that at least two of these product categories have the potential to harm fertility: steroids and the natural supplement creatine.

Female: Used on even a temporary basis, bodybuilding steroids can cause:

- Menstrual irregularities
- Lack of ovulation
- Cessation of menses
- Permanent infertility

Male: In addition to increasing the risk of heart problems, deep depression, and excessive rage and psychosis, bodybuilding steroids taken on a regular basis may cause:

- Testicle atrophy (testicles shrink in size and deteriorate)
- Drastic reduction in sperm count
- Complete inability to make sperm
- Sterility

Men should also be wary of using the much-touted natural supplement known as creatine. Sold under various product names, and sometimes as part of a bodybuilding formula, creatine can have myriad health effects. In terms of fertility the most dangerous problem appears to be an imbalance of electrolytes. These are body minerals such as sodium and potassium that help regulate fluid retention, which in turn helps control the volume of blood plasma. When blood plasma is reduced, it can affect your partner's ability to perform, as well as dissipate body heat—and that, in turn, may affect sperm production.

For maximum fertility protection: Although the male fertility problems resulting from steroid use can sometimes be reversed when the drugs are discontinued, these substances can cause dangerous psychological and biochemical changes. They are rapidly addictive and can be deadly, so they should be avoided at all costs. If a man is already using steroids or creatine, he should stop at least three months before trying to conceive a child and allow his body to cleanse itself of all residues.

Even more important: In almost every instance, damage to female fertility caused by bodybuilding steroids is irreversible, so *women should never use these substances under any circumstances.* Research concerning links between creatine and female fertility is too limited to form any solid conclusions. However, I would advise any woman of childbearing age to avoid use of creatine supplements without a doctor's OK.

Factor: Cell Phones, Portable Phones, Beepers

Effects on fertility — male and female: All three of these devices rely on some type of radio frequency or remote transmission device in order to work—and therein lie the major concerns. Not only are radio frequencies suspected of causing certain fertility problems, but some researchers believe they also have links to cancer and other catastrophic ills.

To be fair, it's important to realize that some fairly exhaustive studies continue to verify that these concerns may be unfounded. To date, there is no clear-cut evidence that talking on a cell or portable phone, or using a beeper, can affect your health. That said, it's also important to note that many studies did produce disturbing results worthy of further research. What does that mean to you? In essence, all of the facts are not in. And while it may turn out that these devices offer convenience without health threats, we simply can't guarantee that yet. This is particularly the case when the effects of the radio frequencies are measured in relation to other health threats in your life, including other sources of radiation. There are, in fact, some scientists who are certain a "synergistic" effect does exist, meaning that certain negative factors bolster each other's harmful effects. Taken singly, each may be safe, but together, they could bring out the worst in each other, and the worst in our physiology.

For maximum fertility protection: The answer is really a matter of common sense: If you are at all concerned, limit cell phone use or replace cordless phones with corded models. Don't carry your beeper or phone in the area of your genitals, and when possible, don't keep it on your body at all. Again, there is no research to show that this will protect you, but it couldn't hurt. Additionally, if you are having problems getting pregnant you should investigate whether you work or live near a broadcasting transmitter of any type (including those used to transmit TV or radio broadcasts, as well as beeper signals), or particularly a mobile telephone base station. Although exposure to radio frequencies remains fairly low, even in the direct vicinity of the transmitters, there are widespread health concerns for those who are in direct and constant contact with these facilities. If you find you are in close proximity, consult an environmental engineer about what steps you can take to protect your home or office from assault.

Factor: Color Televisions

Effects on fertility — male and female: Like microwave ovens (see below) and computer terminals (see previous chapter), color televisions emit low levels of nonionizing radiation, which some experts believe is linked to various physiological disturbances that can result in infertility. Although color television is not considered a prime risk for fertility, when exposure is combined with other radiation sources, it is my opinion that watching too much TV may have residual effects on your ability to conceive.

For maximum fertility protection: Because color TVs manufactured today emit much lower levels of radiation than those made before 1975, if you have a newer set, you have far less to worry about. However, if you do watch a lot of TV, and also spend a lot of time around other radiation sources, such as a computer terminal, take an extra precaution by sitting at least ten feet from your television. This will significantly minimize any risks and give you an extra measure of fertility protection.

Factor: Heating Pads and Electric Blankets

Effects on fertility — male and female: Both of these common household items have two major threats in common: They produce heat, and they emit low-voltage electromagnetic fields. Both factors have been linked to detrimental effects on fertility. More specifically, studies show that use of an electric blanket before conception increases the risk of certain birth defects, particularly a congenital abnormality of the urinary tract. This effect seemed most prominent in women who had difficulty in conceiving. And the more the electric blanket was used, the greater the risk of problems if conception did occur.

Perhaps even more disturbing, however, are studies indicating that the rise in body temperature caused by both electric blankets and heating pads has the potential to cause egg damage, upset ovulation, and decrease conception odds. In men, the excess heat may decrease sperm count and even affect motility.

For maximum fertility protection: Don't use heating pads, particularly in your genital area when you are trying to conceive. If you normally use this appliance for relief of menstrual cramps, try a hot water bottle instead, or one of the new microwave heat packs. Keep temperatures moderate—opt for warm, never hot—and use for as short a time as possible. The same is true for your partner, who should bypass a heating pad in favor of a warm wet cloth or hot water bottle to relieve sore muscles.

In addition, do not use an electric blanket while you are trying to conceive—particularly do not have intercourse under the blanket if it is plugged in, especially if it is turned on.

Factor: Home Decorating and Repair Products

Effects on fertility:

Female: If you are planning home renovations there is something you should know: At least some of the chemicals found in common home decorating and repair products may interfere with both male and female fertility. Although the effects are generally cumulative—you are far more likely to be affected only after months of exposure—still, in those who are sensitive to chemical pollutants, problems could occur within a short time. According to studies conducted at the University of California at Berkeley as early as 1991, the most detrimental products are paint thinners, paint strippers, and glycol ethers, which are chemicals found in many paints. All can significantly increase the risk of miscarriage, so much so that you may be losing your pregnancies before you are even aware that you are pregnant. If you are over age thirty-five when trying to conceive, studies published in the *Harvard Health Letter* in 1992 indicate that household exposure to glues (like the kind used to put up paneling or lay carpets) or oil paints can dramatically decrease fertility. Meanwhile, an impressive Australian study of more than six hundred couples found exposure to household glue can dramatically increase the risk of miscarriage.

Male: In men—who often do a lot of home repair work—studies at the University of North Carolina at Chapel Hill found that chemicals and solvents contained in many paint products have been shown to cause defects in sperm that lead to abnormalities in the central nervous system of the children they produce. Other studies show that when Dad is exposed to these chemicals before conception, children may be born with a higher risk of brain tumors as well as childhood leukemia. When exposed to household glues for an extended period of time a man may increase his partner's risk of miscarriage.

For maximum fertility protection: As much as you want to build that nursery, or repaint your hubby's old crib and your childhood rocking chair, I caution you not to do so—at least not at the same time you are trying to get pregnant. This is particularly true if you are already having problems conceiving. If you must do some home repairs, make certain there is adequate ventilation while the repair work is being done, and for up to five days afterward. A good rule of thumb: If the products you are using have an offensive chemical odor, you probably should not be inhaling them. Furthermore, the stronger the odor, the longer your living space must remain ventilated. This, by the way, is true for odors coming from new carpets or furniture, particularly if it contains particle board and is emitting formaldehyde gases. If possible, get your redecorating and

home repairs out of the way at least three months before attempting conception—and, if possible, avoid home repairs while you are
pregnant.

Factor: Household Cleaners

Effects on fertility — male and female: Evidence continues to mount
that some of the most common products used in the home every
day can have cumulative detrimental effects on reproductive health,
particularly if other fertility factors are present, such as endometriosis or a hormone imbalance. In fact, one of the most significant new studies—a look at some twelve hundred men and
women by genetic scientists at Queen Elizabeth Hospital in Australia in 1994—found that chemicals lurking in a wide variety of
household products caused a 33 percent increase in the inability to
conceive. For those who do get pregnant, chemical exposure could
increase the risk of pregnancy loss by some 75 percent.

Indeed, while most folks are concerned with pollution out of
doors, the truth is the Environmental Protection Agency found that
in many homes the levels of a dozen or more pollutants are three to
five times higher than they are outside—and many of these pollutants can and do harm our fertility.

The most likely culprits are found in:

- Rug or upholstery shampoo
- Furniture polish
- All-purpose cleaners
- Bug sprays
- Bathroom cleaners
- Room deodorizers

Since manufacturers of most household products are required by
law to list only those ingredients that have been proven hazardous
(most of which are ambiguously identified as simply "poisons" or "ir-

ritants"), it's difficult to say with certainty which of these products can have specific reproductive effects. However, many contain substances that have been shown to decrease fertility in men and women alike, including organic solvents such as benzene, petroleum distillates, and formaldehyde.

To maximize your fertility potential: Whenever possible, replace chemical household products with nontoxic and organic substances. Bon Ami, for example, is an excellent all-purpose cleanser that is also fairly nontoxic. Oxi-Clean is another excellent organic household cleaner that has no odor and is considered nontoxic. In addition, mail-order catalogs such as Walnut Acres, Harmony, and Healthy Home offer a number of home cleaning solutions that are considered nontoxic and therefore safer for your fertility. Remember too, that exposure and effect are cumulative. So, if you must use traditional chemicals in your home, do so as little as possible.

Factor: Medications

Effects on fertility:

Female: Generally speaking, when properly used, most medications will not interfere with your ability to get pregnant. However, because everyone's body responds to drugs in a slightly different manner, it's sometimes difficult to predict the exact reaction your reproductive system will have to any given medication. For this reason, always advise your ob-gyn, and particularly your fertility specialist, of any drugs you are taking regularly. This includes both prescription and over-the-counter medications such as:

- Allergy pills
- Cold remedies
- Cough medicines
- Gastrointestinal aids
- Pain relievers
- Antibiotics

In addition, you must mention if you regularly take medication for any chronic health concern, such as diabetes, high blood pressure, kidney or thyroid disorders, arthritis, heart problems, depression, anxiety, or allergies.

Since many drugs on the market today have been linked to a variety of birth defects if they are in your system at the time of conception, check with your doctor about eliminating all unnecessary treatments for at least one month before attempting conception, and when possible, discuss drug substitutions. In many instances your doctor may be able to replace a questionable medication with a safer one, in terms of the risk of birth defects or even fertility-related consequences.

Male: The same general advice concerning medications that applies to women also applies to men. In fact, many drugs can have an even greater impact on male fertility, since the residue of every medication a man takes passes through a portion of his reproductive tract before leaving the body. In addition to the general precautions—including avoiding all unnecessary medications in the weeks before conception—the following drugs have been known to cause specific fertility problems in men:

- Clonadine and other blood pressure drugs can cause a decrease in sex drive and temporary impotence.
- Chemotherapeutic agents can cause injury to the testes, resulting in sterility.
- Methotrexate, used in the treatment of psoriasis and cancer, can damage the testes and stop cell growth.

In addition, the following drugs have been reported to lower sperm count, as well as causing a variety of other reproductive problems in men. Needless to say, the effects can be particularly devastating if your partner is already experiencing sperm-related problems.

- Cimetidine (Tagamet) used in treatment of duodenal ulcers as well as heartburn or acid stomach
- Salicylazosufapyridine (SASP), used in the treatment of irritable bowel syndrome

- Phenytoin, used in the treatment of seizures
- Sulfasalazine, used in the treatment of ulcerative colitis
- Colchicine, used in the treatment of gout

In addition, while the subject is rarely discussed, according to reports published in the *Journal of Urology* as far back as 1974, overuse of both penicillin and tetracycline can depress sperm production.

For maximum fertility protection: Because many medications work by accumulating in the body, some can remain in your system for as long as a month after the last dose is taken. While the drugs themselves may not directly affect your ability to get pregnant, their presence in your body could affect the quality of your conception. Sperm tainted with drug residue can be generally unhealthy and could impede or even block fertilization.

For this reason both you and your partner should consult your physician about ways to clear your system of any unnecessary medication for at least one to two months before attempting conception.

Important Warning for Women

Among the most often prescribed drugs for men is Proscar (finasteride), a medication used to shrink an enlarged prostate gland. If your partner, father, or any male in your home or office is using this drug, and you are actively trying to conceive or are already pregnant, never touch this medication, particularly if the pill is crushed. Known to cause severe birth defects in pregnant or nursing women, this drug has effects that can be so potent that merely touching it can cause devastating results. In addition, if you are having sex with a man who is taking Proscar, be certain that he always uses a condom, every time, and avoid performing oral sex on him. Since traces of Proscar have been found in semen, you can ingest harmful amounts of this drug during sexual activity. If your partner is using Proscar, do not try to conceive. Instead, insist he speak with his doctor about a substitute medication.

Can Aspirin Help or Harm Your Conception?

Pain relievers commonly used to treat everything from an occasional headache to muscle strains and sprains can have powerful effects on ovulation. But whether those effects are positive or negative depends largely on whose research you are reading!

Indeed, several small studies conducted in 1995 and 1996 have shown that, when used regularly, medications known as nonsteroidal anti-inflammatory drugs — common treatments such as aspirin, Advil, and Aleve — can keep your follicles from bursting and releasing from your ovary. The problem — medically known as "luteinizing unruptured follicle syndrome" (LUF or LUFS) — can make natural conception impossible.

Conversely, information published in the journal *Fertility and Sterility* in mid-1999 suggests the exact opposite may be true — at least when you are undergoing fertility treatments such as IVF (in vitro fertilization).

Indeed, the new study, which looked at 149 women enrolled in an IVF program, found that small daily doses of aspirin (about 100 mg or one baby aspirin a day) actually improved ovarian responsiveness as well as increased blood flow to the ovaries and uterus. Not only were the women able to make more and stronger eggs, pregnancy rates were nearly doubled. Previous studies have also shown that taking one baby aspirin a day may also reduce the risk of miscarriage, as well as prevent fetal growth retardation.

What is behind the research conflicts? One possibility is that problems are linked to dosage rather than the drug itself. In the first series of studies, the aspirin and other drugs were taken in far greater amounts; in the new study, only a minimal amount was used. Another theory suggests that what may work for IVF does not necessarily translate to natural conception.

Finally, it's also possible that in certain women, those who already have an undiagnosed ovarian-related fertility problem, the treatment could have the detrimental rather than beneficial effects.

What should you do? Certainly, limit the use of large amounts of aspirin and other drugs in this category. If there is any detrimental effect, it stands to reason the larger the dose, the more dramatic the consequences.

At the same time, I also believe you can safely take one baby aspirin a day, both before and after you get pregnant. Do, however, confirm this with your doctor, and let him or her know what you are doing. More important, listen to his or her advice, particularly if he or she doesn't believe this therapy is right for you.

Factor: Microwave Ovens

Effects on fertility — male and female: In the past twenty-five years the safety of microwave ovens has improved dramatically. Most important has been the virtual elimination of dangerous radiation leaks—which have been associated with incidence of cancer, nervous system disorders, and sterility in both men and women. Today, oven doors are sealed shut, and dangerous leakages are rare. However, since the overall effects of microwave radiation are still under investigation, anyone having difficulty conceiving should avoid direct or constant exposure.

For maximum fertility protection: Limit the use of microwave ovens if you have any of the following:

- Menstrual irregularities
- Ovulation problems
- Trouble conceiving
- A history of miscarriage

If you must use a microwave oven stand at least six feet away from the unit while it is turned on. Since sperm production and quality are extremely sensitive to the effects of all types of radiation, men, even more than women, must obey microwave precautions.

If you suspect your microwave may not be properly sealed (if the edges of the rubber or cloth sealer are frayed, for example), you might purchase one of the various types of home testing kits available and determine if there is a radiation leak. Periodic checks are one way to ensure your fertility is not being compromised.

Factor: Oral Contraceptives

Effects on fertility — female: While there remains much speculation about whether fertility is compromised following the use of birth control pills, the consensus of medical opinion says it is not. That said, it's still important for you to know that should you get pregnant while pill residues are still in your body, there is a slight increase in the risk of birth defects. Since it can take up to one month, or sometimes even longer, to clear all traces of oral contraceptives from your body, I believe it's a good idea to stop pill use two to three months before you want to conceive, and to use another form of birth control—such as a condom—during that time.

You should also know that studies show that stopping the pill can have a wide variety of effects on your reproductive hormones, sometimes making it more difficult to get pregnant for up to several months. Of course, in some women the exact opposite happens—they stop the pill and get pregnant immediately. In either case, it's still a good idea to use a condom for several months before you plan to conceive.

For maximum fertility protection: Birth control pills that vary the dosage of hormones throughout the month (collectively called triphasic pills) have been implicated as having a link to the formation of ovarian cysts in some women. If you have a tendency to this problem, especially if you have poly cystic ovarian disease (PCOD), you should avoid using this form of birth control in the months or years before conception.

Personal Care Products and Your Fertility

During the process of manufacturing a number of paper products—including personal care items such as tampons and sanitary napkins—a chemical by-product called dioxin is formed. Unfortunately, residues of dioxin may remain in these products even after processing. Why is this important? Worldwide studies have shown it has an important link not only to cancer but also to endometriosis (see Chapter 3) as well as male and female infertility. Even more potentially damaging is that dioxin is not only found in paper products (which also include toilet tissue, coffee filters, tea bags, and paper towels), but is also present in varying degrees in soil, water, and air.

Since the effects of dioxin are suspected to be cumulative, the more you are exposed the greater the impact may be when you do use the paper products in question.

However, there is still another concern and another fact that you should know: Personal care products containing dioxin, such as tampons and toilet paper, come in direct contact with the genitalia, and in the case of women, the vaginal mucosa, one of the most porous areas of the body. Indeed, a tampon placed inside a woman's body may release any residues that are present directly into her system.

While manufacturers of tampons and some napkin products vehemently deny any dangers associated with these products, in reality, the only testing we have to verify safety are studies ordered by the manufacturers themselves. Meanwhile, many independent studies are starting to raise questions, with some researchers solidly convinced that these products, as they are now made, do represent a clear threat to a woman's reproductive health. Further, new studies have shown that when environmental dioxin makes its way into a man's body, not only can sperm production plummet, but the risk of testicular cancer increases significantly.

Currently, several legislators have introduced bills into the U.S. Congress calling for more unbiased studies on the effects of dioxin, particularly as it relates to female personal care products. In the near future we may begin to piece together the dioxin picture with far more accuracy.

In the meantime, however, I caution you, as I do all my patients, against the overuse of these products, particularly if you are already having problems conceiving or if you suffer from endometriosis. When possible, look for sanitary personal care products made from organic cotton and manufactured without dioxin. (Check the Resource section at the end of this book for sources.)

If this is not possible, then do restrict tampon use to only the first day or two of your menstrual period, then switch to pads, which will lessen the contact with vaginal mucosa. In addition, try to use tampons only during the day and use a pad at night instead.

In addition to the risks posed by these sanitary products, you should also avoid regular douching if you are trying to conceive. The reason? Research shows it can reduce your fertility by a significant margin. In one study, data on more than eight hundred women collected by the National Institute of Environmental Health Sciences in 1996 revealed douching can reduce the overall chance of getting pregnant by some 30 percent.

For younger women, aged eighteen to twenty-four, the risks were even greater, reducing the chance of conception by some 50 percent. Interestingly, the study, published in the *American Journal of Public Health*, found conception was equally affected by both commercial douches and homemade vinegar and water compounds. Indeed, even douching with plain water appeared to have a negative affect on fertility.

Factor: Pesticides, Fungicides, Insecticides

Effects on fertility — male and female: Since its creation in 1970, the EPA has banned dozens of pesticides, fungicides, and insecticides. Yet by 1982, 880 million pounds of toxic chemicals were still being routinely sprayed on the most commonly eaten fruits and vegetables, including tomatoes, apples, onions, potatoes, grapes, melons, lettuce, celery, carrots, broccoli, oranges, and peaches. Today, more than seventy pesticides, insecticides, and fungicides are actively in use in all parts of the world, despite the fact that animal studies have shown they are carcinogenic. Almost daily, evidence mounts that they may have the same effect on the human body.

Now, however, another dangerous health risk is coming to light: These same chemicals can wreak havoc on our reproductive health. This occurs, experts say, when chemical exposures disrupt the action of hormones that regulate reproduction. The result is a variety of potentially harmful or even deadly effects.

- In men, sperm counts can plummet, while the risk of testicular cancer soars.
- In women, uterine abnormalities lead to implantation problems and ultimately a frightening increase in the risk of miscarriage.

While hard evidence is still difficult to come by (one reason is that in the past, the definition of what constitutes reproductive toxicity was very narrow), that, however, will soon change. Indeed, during the late 1990s, both the American College of Occupational and Environmental Medicine in the United States and a similar organization within the European community have greatly expanded the definition of what constitutes damage to our reproductive health.

I believe we can expect to see many more chemical manufacturers who now sell their products without warnings confront the truth about what their products can and will do to human reproductive potential. This includes not only the effects on a developing fetus, but also the fertility-related problems that can effect Mom and Dad, including:

- Menstrual irregularities
- Impotence
- Decreased sex drive
- Reduced sperm count
- High potential of abnormal sperm

Also, when present in your body, through either inhalation or toxic residues left on your foods, your breast milk can be contaminated, leading to kidney damage, depressed immune system function, and cancer in a baby you breast-feed during this time.

For maximum fertility protection: Whenever possible, avoid eating fruits and vegetables that could be contaminated with sprays. Purchasing organically grown produce can help. If this is not possible opt for frozen or canned vegetables. The reason? Although they may be subjected to an initial dousing of pesticides while being grown, they will avoid subsequent exposures that occur during shipment to the distributor, at the distribution warehouse, and again when they arrive at the store.

You should also try to avoid all use of pesticides and insecticides in the home, particularly when you are actively trying to conceive. If it becomes necessary to use these products, try to vacate your home for at least twenty-four to forty-eight hours when the products are initially in use. Whenever possible, substitute organic or nontoxic solutions, such as Borax powder to deter roaches and herbal candles and sprays to help control other insects, including fleas on your cat or dog.

Haunted Houses and Your Fertility

If your home was built before 1980, the very air you breathe could be the culprit behind a delay in getting pregnant. The reason? Rampant use of a common termite pesticide called chlordane. Not only is direct and immediate exposure suspected of harming fertility, but once used in the home, it can continue to give off vapors for decades. Indeed, a recent study found that approximately 75 percent of all U.S. homes contain at least some level of chlordane in the breathable air. Over 5 percent of homes built before 1988 and up to 20 percent of those built before 1980 contain levels above the safety limit, which is five micrograms per cubic meter of air. Although, to date, we have only animal studies to indicate a clear-cut risk to fertility, still, results are convincing enough to at least warrant a warning. If you are having problems conceiving, particularly if no medical reason for your fertility problems can be found, you might consider the possibility that air pollution inside your home may be adding to your conception problems. Fortunately, you can help remedy this problem, not only by having your home tested for chlordane levels (look for an environmental engineer in your area) but also by making sure that your home is well ventilated and that fresh air is allowed to circulate throughout all of your rooms daily.

Factor: Small Appliances, Clock Radios, Personal Stereos

Effects on fertility — male and female: Similar in their effects to cell phones and beepers (see previous listing), the concerns about small personal appliances is that they not only produce potentially harmful electromagnetic fields, but that they are often in use either on the body or in close proximity.

Some researchers believe that these two factors, combined with additional sources of electromagnetic stimulation (coming from cell phones, beepers, and electronic office equipment), may have a cumulative effect on reproductive health. Greatest concern remains for those who are already having a problem conceiving.

Truthfully, however, research remains slim in this area. So while

I do not want to mislead you into thinking that these items are immediately harmful to your ability to get pregnant, I do believe that it is wise to give the limited research some credence by suggesting that you reduce your exposure to at least a few sources of electromagnetic stimulation if you are having problems getting pregnant.

For maximum fertility protection: Take a few small steps to protect yourself: Whenever possible, remain at least six feet away from any appliance while it is in use; unplug all appliances when they are not in use; if you use a clock radio in the bedroom, make certain it's at least an arm's distance from your bedside. If you live in a confined space and must have your home office in your bedroom or living room, you should not only turn off but unplug all equipment, particularly your computer, when not in use.

Factor: Tobacco

Effects on fertility: While the ill effects of cigarettes on both our heart and lungs have long been known, in the past several years we have learned about still more important health risks linked to smoking—and they involve our reproductive health. Certainly, mothers who smoke put their developing baby at great risk, and fathers who subject their pregnant wives to secondhand smoke share the blame.

Now, however, new research has revealed the powerful effects that smoking appears to have on male and female fertility.

Female: Although it is nicotine that has garnered much of the negative attention in the last century, cigarette smoke actually contains several hundred potentially dangerous substances, including many carcinogens and mutagens. The degree to which you have problems getting pregnant is in direct proportion to the amount you smoke, with the most significant damage beginning with about sixteen cigarettes a day. The younger you are when you start smoking, the greater your chance of suffering at least some type of tobacco-related fertility disorder.

According to the most recent studies:

- Smokers are four times more likely to take longer than a year to conceive.
- The fertility of light smokers (fewer than twenty cigarettes daily) was 75 percent that of nonsmokers.
- The fertility of heavy smokers (more than twenty cigarettes daily) was 57 percent that of nonsmokers.
- The overall rate of pregnancy per cycle was only 22 percent in smokers, compared to 32 percent in nonsmokers.

The newest studies have also shown that smoking may be a significant factor in the failure of some laboratory-assisted pregnancies including IVF (in vitro fertilization) and GIFT (see Part Three of this book).

Smoking harms a woman's fertility by affecting the inside of the fallopian tubes. This in turn leads to difficulties in egg transport, implantation, delivery to the uterus, and transport timing. Any one of these can not only affect the ability to get pregnant, but also increase the risk of tubal inflammation and infection. This, in turn, increases the risk of ectopic pregnancy, the leading cause of maternal death worldwide. Indeed, a study of more than one thousand women by the World Health Organization showed that smokers had higher rates of ectopic pregnancy overall.

Male: Tobacco is an equal-opportunity fertility thief. In studies conducted in both Greece and the United States, researchers found:

- The sperm of heavy smokers was of much poorer quality than that of nonsmokers.
- Smoking also appeared to cause changes in the shape of the sperm, making it more difficult to achieve conception.

But the reproductive effects of smoking are not limited to the sperm—it can also affect the seminal plasma, the fluid in which sperm resides. In studies reported in the journal *Fertility and Sterility*, simply incubating the sperm of nonsmokers in the seminal

plasma of smokers was enough to cause significant damage.
Smoking can also cause:

- A decrease in sperm count
- Increased risk of miscarriage in partner
- Increased risk of birth defects
- Decrease in sperm motility
- Decrease in the ability to fertilize an egg

Young Men Affected Most by Cigarettes

If you think that a man has to smoke for a long period of time in order for
his fertility to be affected, guess again. New reports in the journal *Fertility and Sterility* revealed the fertility of men as young as eighteen can be
adversely affected when they smoke. Indeed, studies on more than two
dozen eighteen-year-old male smokers revealed an increased proportion
of abnormally shaped sperm and sperm with genetic defects, when compared with young men who did not smoke. Since smoking is often accompanied by alcohol consumption, the researchers theorize that
together, the two factors may be especially detrimental to male fertility.

CIGARETTES, CANCER, AND YOUR BABY

Even more disturbing than the effects of cigarettes on fertility is the potential harm that smoking can cause to any baby you conceive. Among
the newest research is a 1998 Chinese study on the health of children
of men who smoked. What the researchers discovered: Babies whose fathers smoked at any time in their lives were 30 percent more likely to develop a childhood cancer. Ironically, the length of time the father smoked
appeared to have greater impact on the children's cancer rates than the
number of cigarettes smoked.

In case you're wondering whether the secondhand smoke inhaled
by these men's pregnant partners also played a role in their children's
cancer risk, you're not alone: Researchers wondered the same thing.

However, subsequent studies revealed this isn't likely. More specifically, research on women who smoked during their entire pregnancy did not reveal any increase in the rate of childhood cancers. Studies conducted in England backed up these findings with research suggesting that a father's smoking habit—but not a mother's—increased the risk of cancer death among British children.

Although this is the newest research in this area, studies dating as far back as the 1960s found the death rate among newborns was nearly 50 percent higher when their fathers smoked. Other studies found that birth defects were more likely in children of fathers who smoked.

If you are trying to get pregnant, most researchers agree that the longer a man is smoke-free the more likely he is to conceive a healthy baby.

For maximum fertility protection: The good news here is that if you stop smoking you can halt most of the damaging effects on your fertility, and in many instances reverse those which may have already occurred, usually within four months after your final cigarette.

If your partner quits smoking and remains cigarette-free for just six months before attempting conception, your chances for conceiving a healthy baby significantly increase. In fact, I often tell my patients that giving up cigarettes is the most inexpensive and effective form of "fertility therapy" they can try!

If your partner is still resistant to giving up smoking, this should get his attention:

New studies show that 56 percent of men who smoke are likely to develop permanent impotence.

In addition, both you and your partner must avoid smoke-filled rooms while you are actively trying to conceive. First, new evidence shows that secondhand smoke can be nearly as detrimental as smoking a cigarette. Even more important, it is likely that you may be pregnant weeks before you know it. Avoiding secondhand smoke during the critical early stages of pregnancy can help you avoid many serious complications, including abnormal placenta implantation and early miscarriage.

Factor: X-Rays

Effects on fertility — male and female: Heavy exposure to the ionizing radiation of X-rays can have major mutagenic effects on the reproductive organs of men and women alike, causing both biological and genetic damage. A man's testes and a woman's ovaries can both undergo severe damage with even minimal exposure, including:

- A change in the genetic material present in sperm and egg, increasing the risk of miscarriage and birth defects
- Genetic effects that can inhibit the ability of the sperm and the egg to be fertilized

These can have a profound effect on fertility, in many cases rendering you or your partner sterile. The testes, in fact, are so sensitive to the effects of radiation that even small amounts can bring about serious damage.

In addition, adults who were exposed to a great deal of X-ray radiation as a child can give birth to babies with a higher incidence of chromosomal abnormalities and Down's syndrome, a form of mental retardation.

For maximum fertility protection: Because the effects of radiation are cumulative, the more exposure you have, the greater your risk of reproductive damage, especially if your genitals are directly in the line of the X-ray beams. For this reason, a lead apron should always be used to protect your reproductive organs whenever any type of X-ray is taken.

In addition, any woman of childbearing age who must undergo a diagnostic pelvic or abdominal X-ray should, if possible, have it during the first ten days following the start of a menstrual cycle. This will help prevent any newly fertilized egg from receiving X-ray exposure.

Finally, for ultimate protection, choose an ultrasound exam or an MRI (magnetic resonance imaging) scan in place of an X-ray.

Drug Abuse and Your Fertility

Currently it is estimated that 5 to 10 percent of all women of childbearing age use illicit drugs or abuse prescription medications, such as tranquilizers or barbiturates. The statistics for men are equally alarming. Although the reproductive risks of any drug largely depend on the substance itself and the individual way in which your system metabolizes it, several other factors also play a role, including:

- Extent of drug use
- Amount of the drug used
- Frequency of use
- Amount of active ingredient
- Length of time the drug is used

Regardless of the substance, however, the potential for damage does increase with frequency of use. A single dose of any drug will not be likely to cause your reproductive system any damage, whereas regular or habitual use can be extremely harmful. In addition, the younger you are when you begin abusing drugs the more potential reproductive damage you can experience.

How Drugs Can Affect a Woman's Fertility

One of the most common illegal drugs is, not surprisingly, also one of the most harmful to fertility. It is marijuana, and according to a number of new studies, it can have a major effect on ovulation. Both animal and human studies show that regular use of marijuana causes a disruption of ovary function, making it far more difficult to get pregnant. When combined with alcohol—as it often is—marijuana can significantly reduce your chance for conception.

But that should not be your only concern. If you should conceive while both marijuana and alcohol are in your body, there is a strong chance that your pregnancy may end in crisis. Indeed, according to the

Research Institute on Alcoholism in Buffalo, New York, animal studies showed that the combination of these two drugs increased the rate of miscarriage as high as 100 percent.

Of even greater consequence, however, are the effects of the drug cocaine on a woman's reproductive system. Indeed, evidence has begun to mount that, with regular use, this drug may cause damage to the inside of the fallopian tubes, so much so that the chance for natural conception may be lost.

Stoned Sperm: How Drugs Affect Male Fertility

Even in moderate amounts marijuana and cocaine can have debilitating effects on your partner's fertility, as well as cause a number of serious birth defects in your baby.

More specifically, laboratory tests conducted at the University of Buffalo in New York revealed that compounds in marijuana inhibited the release of enzymes that help sperm penetrate the egg's outer shell. Moreover, it can also cause sperm to act "stoned"—swimming in circles rather

---

The Most Common Prescription Drugs to Cause Birth Defects

In addition to causing conception problems, some of the most commonly prescribed tranquilizers and sedatives can, when used by the mother during pregnancy, cause the baby harm. These include:

- Valium: Causes cleft palate
- Quaalude: Causes musculoskeletal defects, cardiac and circulatory problems, cleft lip and palate, dislocated hips
- Xanax: Causes assorted congenital anomalies
- Librium: Causes neonatal depression, "floppy baby" syndrome
- Elavil, Tofranil, Asendin, and other tricyclic antidepressants: Cause face, head, limb, and central nervous system defects as well as newborn withdrawal symptoms.

than heading straight for the egg. If, in fact, they do manage to get their directions straight, compounds in marijuana can prevent sperm from binding to the egg, a step that's necessary for conception to occur.

As with women, of even greater concern, for men, are the effects of cocaine on conception. In addition to the cardiovascular and other health risks this recreational drug can cause, according to studies published in the *Journal of the American Medical Association,* it may also affect embryo development. Specifically, while cocaine won't affect sperm directly, it can attach itself to the tail and literally "ride" into the egg, triggering a variety of developmental problems. Indeed, animal studies have shown that male mice exposed to either cocaine or methadone (a drug used to help cocaine addicts quit) appear to have a higher rate of birth defects and neurological problems than mice born of drug-free conceptions.

While these studies are still considered preliminary, the warning is considered serious enough to heed. Fortunately, avoiding cocaine, particularly for two weeks before conception, should clear the drug from the body and help avoid at least some of the reproductive consequences.

How Climate Affects Fertility

Can the weather affect your ability to get pregnant? Some believe that it can. Studies conducted by the Chemical Industry Institute of Toxicology and Glaxo, Inc., in Research Park, North Carolina, in conjunction with the Fertility Institute of New Orleans and the Fertility Institute of Louisiana, found that sperm undergoes an annual reduction every summer, due to a rise in temperature. In addition, summer weather induces:

- Depression in semen quality
- Low sperm concentration
- Fewer sperm per ejaculate
- Lower percentage of motile sperm
- Higher percentage of abnormal sperm

Other fertility studies have shown that women who live in warmer climates generally have an early menopause, with a premature end to their childbearing years. They also have a higher rate of pregnancy complications and problems with delivery timing when the first trimester of pregnancy takes place in summer months (a spring conception).

In one of the most recent studies, conducted at the National Institute of Environmental Health Sciences, researchers found a seasonal pattern to miscarriage. In studies on more than two hundred North Carolina women over a three-year period, it was learned that early pregnancy loss (within the first six weeks) was greatest when conceptions occurred anywhere from July through October, when weather in this area is considered seasonably warm. This seasonal pattern, the researchers say, appears to indicate that environmental factors, including weather, do play a role in pregnancy health.

The Time to Protect Your Fertility Is Now!

One important misconception about infertility is that it only happens to "older" people. Actually, lifestyle and other problems linked to infertility can begin to affect you almost any time after puberty.

While many of the reproductive villains you are reading about in this book—such as alcohol, drugs, and nutritional deficiencies—do have cumulative effects that build over time, remember, the younger you are when you start abusing your body, the faster the consequences will become evident.

Keep in mind that it is never too early in life to begin protecting your fertility!

Part II

The Fastest, Easiest Ways to a Safe, Natural Conception

Chapter Eight

The Pre-Conception Exam 2000: Getting Ready to Get Pregnant

While it was once believed that obstetrical treatment should begin only after a conception is confirmed, today most forward-thinking physicians recognize that many problems can be prevented when the same care begins before you get pregnant. The concept is known as pre-conception counseling, a form of nurturing care in which you, your partner, and your doctor work together on a program personally tailored to:

- Encourage a quick and easy conception
- Ensure your health and safety during pregnancy
- Decrease your risk of miscarriage
- Help your baby avoid birth defects

Although preparation for these goals ideally starts about six months before you want to conceive, scheduling a pre-conception exam at any time before getting pregnant can offer a multitude of benefits to you and your baby.

How Pre-Conception Counseling Works

The basis of pre-conception counseling is multifaceted. It takes into consideration not just factors affecting *your* reproductive health, but the joint fertility status of you *and* your partner, as well as a host of shared physical, psychological, and social factors capable of affecting your fertility including:

- Age
- Fitness
- Occupation
- Weight
- Lifestyle
- Family history
- Nutritional profile
- General health
- Reproductive history

Evaluating information from many areas of your life, your pre-conception specialist formulates a risk assessment profile of your pregnancy and determines where potential problems might lie. To help accomplish this, your first visit should include a detailed health and lifestyle history of both you and your partner. If your gynecologist is also your pre-conception specialist, much of this information about you is probably already on file. However, it's still a good idea to discuss your medical history with your doctor at the time of your pre-conception exam, and to make certain to inform him or her of any pertinent factors about your partner as well.

The Personal Facts Your Doctor Needs to Know

To help prepare for your initial visit, write down key information, then give these notes to your doctor. I have found this to be extremely helpful, especially in getting to know a new patient, and I often refer to these personal notes throughout the course of treatment. Here's what your doctor needs to know.

Your reproductive history: Because your reproductive history can influence the future of your fertility, it's important that your doctor have an accurate, detailed account of any conception-related events that might have occurred, including:

- Miscarriages: How often, how many, and when
- Abortions: How often and how many
- Reproductive surgeries, including laparoscopies, D&C, and treatment for ovarian cysts
- Whether your mother took DES
- Number of previous pregnancies and their outcome
- History of fetal death, neonatal death, infants with birth defects
- History of vaginal bleeding
- Ectopic pregnancies

In addition, your doctor should know something about your partner's reproductive history, including:

- If he has fathered any children
- If any previous partners had miscarriages
- If he has fathered children with birth defects
- If his mother took DES

Family history: We now know that the family history of both parents can influence the outcome of a pregnancy. Conditions to look out for in your background and your partner's include:

- High blood pressure
- Diabetes
- Birth defects
- Inherited diseases associated with birth defects (for example, sickle cell anemia, Tay Sachs disease)
- Mental retardation
- Cystic fibrosis (CF)

Personal medical history: Because so much of what is happening in your body today is the result of biological conditions and events that occurred in the past, it is important for your doctor to have a personal history of both you and your partner regarding diseases, conditions, or infections that could have a residual effect on fertility, including:

- STDs (gonorrhea, chlamydia, syphilis, genital herpes)
- Infections of the reproductive tract, especially PID
- High blood pressure
- Diabetes (type, for how long, any treatment received)
- Exposure to X-rays (when, what areas of the body)
- Heart disease
- Exposure to AIDS
- Epilepsy
- German measles (important to you)
- Mumps (important for your partner)
- Any medications you or your partner regularly take, including allergy pills or shots, insulin, and antacids
- Any chronic health threats that exist now, or have existed in the past, including colitis, arthritis, high blood pressure, high cholesterol, heart problems, weight problems

Other Vital Information Your Doctor Must Have

Since your fertility, your pregnancy, and the health of your baby can also be affected by factors *outside* the realm of personal biology, your doctor should have information about aspects of your life that could influence your reproductive health. This includes where you and your partner live and work, how each of you earns a living, and how you spend your leisure time, both together and apart. More specifically, your physician needs to know:

- How much alcohol you and your partner regularly consume
- Your eating habits and your partner's, the number of calories consumed daily, vitamin supplements (if any)
- If either of you smoke, and if so, how much
- If either of you has used recreational drugs, and if so, what and when
- If you or your mate work with radiation or are exposed to any toxic chemicals or substances (see Chapters 6 and 7)
- If you own a cat (see toxoplasmosis, p. 198)
- If either of you has or has had sexual relations outside your marriage

The T.H.E. 2000 Physical Exam: What It Must Include

One of the most important aspects of your pre-conception exam is the physical. Unlike gyn exams of the past, however, the new pre-conception exam is more practical and applicable to your life and your lifestyle. Not only does it pay attention to your fertility, it can also offer you a greater degree of overall preventative care.

In fact, I often refer to the new pre-conception exam as T.H.E. 2000—short for **Total Health Evaluation.** Besides your personal and family health history, it involves several important diagnostic steps, vital to the protection of your reproductive health. It all begins with a comprehensive, head-to-toe physical evaluation to assess your current state of health and identify future problems for which you may be at risk.

- Neck: Your doctor should check for thyroid malfunctions and swollen glands by examining your neck. Both can be linked to conditions responsible for infertility.

- Skin and Hair: Tone and condition can be indications of anything from a thyroid disorder to hormonal disturbances, even serious infections.

- Weight: Because of the links between weight and fertility (see Chapter 9), keeping accurate records is one way your gynecologist can remain actively aware of your fertility status.

- Blood pressure: Although this has no direct link to fertility, levels that stray too far from the norm, either high or low, can be one of the first signs of other conditions that can ultimately affect your chances to conceive.

- Abdomen: Not to be confused with an internal or pelvic check, an abdominal examination takes place outside the body; the physician checks for any suspicious abnormalities, including lumps, tumors, or protrusions.

Don't Overlook Any Symptoms

Your exam should also include an investigation of any symptoms or complaints you have, no matter how unrelated to gynecology they might seem. Sometimes symptoms can be deceiving, with the real problems obvious only to the trained eye.

- Do you suffer from stomach cramps, gas, or constipation? It could be an ulcer, a nervous stomach, or the first signs of endometriosis or ovarian cysts.
- Is your throat sore, and are you running a low-grade fever? It could be tonsillitis or signs of an STD.
- Pains in your lower back, upper thighs, or shins? May be the result of too many hours on the Stairmaster at the gym, or the beginning of one of several serious pelvic problems capable of destroying your reproductive health.

The point to remember is this: While your gynecologist may not treat every ailment that strikes you, he or she is capable of at least evaluating your total health picture to determine if, indeed, you need additional or speciality care.

The New Breast Check: Why Self-Exams Are No Longer Enough

Every year nearly 150,000 new breast malignancies are diagnosed in the United States alone. Right now, one in nine women will develop breast cancer some time in her life—and one-third of those will die.

While there is no doubt that self-examination is one of the best preventative steps you can take against this catastrophic disease, I firmly believe that the burden of diagnosis must not be yours alone. Your doctor *must* participate in this vital diagnostic procedure, and it must be a part of every initial T.H.E. 2000 exam.

If your doctor does not include a breast exam as part of your checkup, find a new doctor. It's that simple and that vital.

Breast Cancer and Motherhood

Recent research has uncovered important new links between breast cancer and motherhood:

- The longer you wait to conceive, the greater your risk of breast cancer. Women who never have children have the highest risk.
- Breast-feeding reduces the risk of breast cancer; and the earlier you get pregnant and the more children you bear, the less your risk.

Breast Cancer and Your Fertility

Formerly, doctors believed that any woman even suspected of having breast cancer should not conceive. Because the high estrogen levels of pregnancy are capable of stimulating dormant breast cancer tissue, as well as increasing the risks associated with an existing breast cancer, conception was considered a life threat for these women. While it still may not be advisable in many cases, according to Dr. Phillip Kivitz of the Breast Evaluation Center in San Francisco, studies show that in certain instances pregnancy *is* okay, providing the cancerous tissue no longer exists. Indeed, when the first edition of this book was published in 1990, I had the great pleasure to appear on the Geraldo Rivera show with the wonderful television actress Ann Jillian, who, at the time, had survived breast cancer and then went on to become a mother. Today, Ann is healthier and more beautiful than ever—vivaciously living out her parenting dreams!

All this is to say that breast exams are a very important part of not only your regular gyn care, but also your pre-conception exam.

The Pelvic Exam: An Important Fertility Evaluation

Clearly, the pelvic exam remains a cornerstone of the new T.H.E. 2000 exam. To ensure that your fertility and your reproductive capabilities are well protected, the exam should include a check of the following:

- The vulva: The outside portion of your vagina, where the first tell-tale lesions and sores caused by some STDs begin to appear
- The inside of your vagina: Where your doctor will look for additional sores or lesions and for the presence of abnormal discharges or odors
- The uterus: Which must be checked for growths, tumors, cysts, and signs of endometriosis, as well as abnormalities in size and shape. During this portion of the exam your ovaries and tubes should be manually examined as well, to help ensure no damage has occurred there.

If any abnormalities *are* found, your doctor should evaluate them further, using either ultrasound or MRI imaging—nonradiation ways of looking inside your body. In some instances you may also require a laparoscopy, a minimally invasive exploratory surgery during which your doctor may also render treatment, such as the removal of endometrial lesions (see Chapters 3 and 17).

The Newest Diagnostic Tests: What You Need, When You Need It

Regardless of whether any abnormalities *are* found in your pelvic exam, but most especially if they are, the next step in T.H.E. 2000 is a series of vaginal screenings designed to eliminate the most obvious threats to your reproductive health: STDs and cancer. These tests should include:

- **The Pap smear/Thin Prep:** The traditional Pap smear used to detect cervical cancer just got better, via two new technologies designed to improve the rate at which early disease is diagnosed. First, new brushes designed to sweep the inside of the cervix with far more accuracy than the traditional swabs ensure a better, more accurate collection of cells. Studies show that more efficient cell sampling with the brushes nearly doubles your chance of catching cancer at its earliest, most easily treated stage. Equally important is a brand-new way of preparing Pap smear slides, one that helps doctors to find even the slightest abnormality in the size or shape of the cervical cells. The method, called Thin Prep, is very successful at identifying even the very earliest precancerous cell changes. With proper treatment, you can then actually prevent cancer from occurring. Although many doctors advise a Pap smear every two years, to maintain your best line of defense before conception consider being tested every six months, particularly if there is a family history of cervical cancer. If any abnormalities are found, the test should be repeated immediately. If results are still questionable, a colposcopy (a test explained later in this book) should be performed.

• **The ViraPap:** For venereal warts. If you are sexually active, this test needs to be taken every six months. If results show you are at high risk for venereal warts, the test should be repeated every four months.

• **The Chlamydia test:** Because this sexually transmitted disease can lie silently in your system for many years, it is imperative that you be tested before you want to conceive and continue to be tested every six months until you are pregnant. The reason: Undiagnosed chlamydia can be a leading cause of very early miscarriage (see Chapter 5).

T.H.E. 2000 Blood Evaluation

In addition to the vaginal tests you receive during your exam, the new T.H.E. 2000 should also include the following blood tests:

• **The SMA 12:** A comprehensive blood chemistry profile to evaluate your overall health status. This includes a test for anemia, a fairly common condition that develops when your oxygen-carrying red blood cells decrease due to any number of causes, including poor nutrition, iron deficiency, or heavy menstrual bleeding. Getting anemia under control via iron supplements before conception can prevent a number of serious birth defects.

• **CA 125:** In the event your doctor discovers a certain type of ovarian cyst during your exam, this test can help rule out the risk of ovarian cancer.

- **T3, T4:** Used to measure basic thyroid function, these tests can help uncover "hidden" fertility problems.

- **Estrogen, progesterone, FSH, LH:** These hormonal assays are important if you suffer from PMS or other menstrual disorders, particularly cycle irregularities.

You should also be given blood and urine testing for any specific complaints you bring to your doctor's attention during the history portion of your exam, even if your reproductive system does not seem to be involved.

The Extra Tests You Need Before Getting Pregnant

A comprehensive T.H.E. 2000 exam should also include a blood pressure and weight check, and your doctor should investigate any potential heart problems or symptoms of an undiagnosed cardiac or vascular condition. If you have a family history of diabetes or if you are exhibiting symptoms of this disease (including weight loss and excessive thirst or urination), you should receive a glucose tolerance test.

Most important, however, are tests for what are called the "TORCH Diseases"—which stands for toxoplasmosis, rubella, cytomegalovirus, and herpes.

When contracted during pregnancy, any of these diseases can affect the health of your unborn baby and increase the chance of a number of serious birth defects. Testing beforehand gives you the chance to be treated before conception and provides your doctor with important information that can be helpful should you become exposed to these infections during your pregnancy.

Toxoplasmosis

An infection linked to a parasite found in the intestines of cats, sheep, cattle, and pigs, toxoplasmosis makes its way into your body when you eat undercooked or rare meat or when you come into contact with the feces of an infected animal. This can occur when emptying your cat's litterbox, for example, or when working in the garden, where contaminated stools may have been deposited. Toxoplasmosis is most dangerous in the first trimester of pregnancy, when the virus can attack the fetus and cause a number of serious birth defects.

In adults and children symptoms can often be so mild that the virus can go completely unnoticed. Once infected, however, you will develop antibodies, and that is precisely what your pre-conception blood test is designed to measure.

If that test shows you do not possess toxoplasmosis antibodies, once you are pregnant watch diligently for these symptoms and report them to your doctor immediately:

- Fever
- Slight rash
- General flulike feeling

While there is no treatment, if you contract the virus during pregnancy your baby must receive immediate medical attention directly after birth. The most common therapy is folic acid and sulfur, and occasionally corticosteroids. While the effects of the virus cannot be reversed, additional problems can sometimes be prevented with immediate medical care.

There is no vaccine for toxoplasmosis, but you can avoid the disease both before and after conception:

- Make certain all red meat and pork is throughly cooked.
- Avoid cat litterboxes.
- Wear heavy protective gloves while gardening.

RUBELLA (GERMAN MEASLES)

In addition to causing a number of serious birth defects, when contracted during pregnancy, rubella is also one of the most common causes of miscarriage and infant death. Fortunately, if you have had this virus in the past, it is almost impossible for you to be reinfected, so your baby is probably safe. If you have not had rubella, there is a highly effective vaccine capable of protecting you and your unborn child.

If your prepregnancy test shows that you have no rubella antibodies (indicating you have not had this virus), you should be vaccinated before conceiving. However, because the rubella vaccine is "live," you must wait a minimum of three months after receiving it before attempting conception. Whether or not you have been vaccinated, should any of the symptoms of rubella appear during your pregnancy (including a red skin rash and a slight fever), see your doctor immediately.

CYTOMEGALOVIRUS

Caused by a parasite thought to live silently in the bodies of up to 80 percent of the population, this virus is passed via intimate contact with an infected person. It is usually found in body secretions, such as breast milk, saliva, semen, cervical mucus, urine, and transfused blood, and it is most often transmitted from children to adults who care for them, in daycare centers, schools, or especially hospitals.

For the most part, the virus remains dormant until stress, a lowered immune system, or some unknown factor triggers it into activity. If it becomes activated during your pregnancy, birth defects or miscarriage can result.

Because it often resides in the body silently, with no symptoms, testing before pregnancy is imperative. When symptoms do appear, they usually resemble flu, including fever and general aches and pains. There is currently no treatment, but since the disease usually attacks only those women who are in poor health or under prolonged stress, you can protect yourself by getting adequate rest, eating nutritious foods, and taking vitamin supplements to support your immune system. In addition, if you work with children, wash your hands frequently and give special attention to hygiene on the job.

HERPES

Although an outbreak of this virus during pregnancy won't affect your baby, should it occur just before your delivery date, your child could be infected during the birthing process. Up to 25 percent of all babies born with herpes can die, and many more are blinded for life when the virus attacks their eyes.

Since your initial outbreak is always the most severe and lasts longer than any subsequent infections, your doctor needs to know before your pregnancy if herpes is present in your system. Should you have an outbreak when you are ready to deliver, a Cesarean section will minimize the threat of contamination to your baby. The treatment regimen for herpes can be found in Chapter 5 of this book.

The Hepatitis Virus

When contracted during pregnancy, this virus generally does not cause birth defects, but it can do devastating, sometimes permanent damage to *your* liver. In addition, it can make your gestational time uncomfortable and uneasy. Moreover, your baby's immune system does not fully develop until after birth, so if this virus is contracted during any stage of your pregnancy, it can easily be passed to your developing fetus, causing weakness and, in rare cases, death.

Should symptoms develop during your pregnancy (including fatigue, lethargy, nausea, vomiting, and jaundice) a pre-conception blood test for hepatitis antibodies will help your doctor determine the true source of your problem. Other conditions sometimes mistaken for hepatitis include mononucleosis, a drug allergy, or a mild jaundice that sometimes develops when the weight of your baby presses on your gallbladder.

A protective vaccine may be advisable if you are in a high-risk profession, such as doctor, nurse, dentist, or other medical worker.

The Pre-Conception Blood Test That Protects Your Baby

In addition to testing for diseases, it's also important that your doctor have on file—and that you know as well—not only your blood type (A, B, or O) but whether you have the Rhesus (Rh) factor, a substance that is found on the surface of red blood cells in the majority of the population.

- If you have the Rh factor, your blood type carries the suffix "positive," as in A, B, or O positive blood.

- If the Rh factor is missing, as it is in 15 to 20 percent of the population, your blood type carries the suffix "negative," as in A, B, or O negative blood.

Whether negative or positive, the Rh factor has no influence on your health. However, if your blood is Rh negative, pregnancy-related problems can occur.

How Your Blood Type Can Affect Your Baby

Although for most Rh negative mothers pregnancy is healthy and normal, problems can develop if your partner's blood is Rh positive. In such a case, your baby's blood can be Rh positive. Why is this a problem?

If, during the course of pregnancy, your baby's Rh positive blood makes its way into your Rh negative system (as can happen, for example, during amniocentesis, a test used to determine the risk of birth defects), your body will react as if it were being invaded by a virus or bacteria— it will begin creating antibodies. Should those antibodies make their way into your baby's bloodstream, they will begin destroying the blood supply. The result is a severe type of anemia known as Rhesus disease. If left undiagnosed, severe birth defects and even fetal death can occur. Deprived of precious oxygen-carrying red blood cells, your baby's brain and body may literally starve to death.

How to Protect Your Baby — Right Now

Because the effects of Rh antibodies are cumulative (building in your system each time your body is infused with positive blood), there is very little risk that your first Rh positive conception will be affected. In fact, most of the time serious problems don't set in until after the second or third Rh positive pregnancy. Today, however, precautions can be taken to protect these pregnancies as well. Among the most important is the Rhogam injection, a treatment that absorbs any Rh positive blood cells that enter an Rh negative system, offsetting the body's need to manufacture antibodies. To be effective, however, Rhogam must be administered within three days following any event that could allow the passage of Rh positive blood cells into your body, including:

- The delivery of an Rh positive baby
- Amniocentesis of an Rh positive baby
- Miscarriage or abortion in which the blood type of your baby was unknown
- A stillbirth of an Rh positive baby
- An ectopic pregnancy

If you are Rh negative and fall into any of the above categories and have not been given Rhogam injections, make your doctor aware of this during your pre-conception interview. Once you are pregnant, be checked frequently for rising levels of antibodies and receive a Rhogam injection in your seventh month. Every Rh negative mother-to-be should get this injection even if the baby's Rh factor is unknown.

Testing for Genetic Diseases

Although everyone carries four to six genes that have the potential to cause birth defects, most often they remain harmless. However, if you and your partner both carry the same defective gene, your child is at increased risk. Currently we can identify more than 250 genetic defects, but except under extraordinary circumstances (such as a history of genetic diseases in both partners' families), pre-conception testing should remain limited.

Because, however, certain genetic diseases do occur more regularly in certain groups, if you and your partner fall into any of the following categories your pre-conception exam should include blood tests for their related conditions:

- Asian and Mediterranean: Test for Thalassemia major (also known as Cooley's anemia)
- African-American: Test for sickle cell anemia, Cooley's anemia
- Jewish: Test for Tay-Sachs disease

(Although there are many other important genetic diseases that can be inherited, these are the most common.)

Because many families are not aware of the presence of certain diseases in their family history, I also suggest genetic testing if my patient or her partner have any of the following factors in their family history:

- Mental retardation
- Intellectual impairment
- Physical deformities present from birth
- Physical disabilities present from birth

Get Tested — But Don't Panic

In order for a genetic birth defect to occur, both parents must carry the recessive gene. Even then, the odds of problems occurring can range from as high as one in two to as low as one in ten thousand or more. For this reason, even a positive genetic test does not mean that your baby will be born defective.

If, however, your pre-conception tests or your family histories indicate the possibility of a problem, I suggest you seek sophisticated analysis at a genetic counseling center. These are specially equipped laboratories staffed with medical personnel who specialize in gene-related disorders. They can perform special blood tests and provide other background screening tests before conception, as well as fetal tissue and fluid sampling as early as nine weeks after conception to detect the possibility of a genetic disorder. If a problem is found, specially trained counselors can review all possible threats to your baby, and if necessary assist you in exploring alternative ways to achieve parenthood.

The Final Evaluation

Perhaps the most important part of your pre-conception exam is the time your doctor takes to explain his or her findings to you. Indeed, every ob/gyn exam you receive should conclude with a doctor-patient conference, at which time your physician should inform you of the following:

- Specific problems or signs of impending disease, as well as any suspicions about any aspect of your health, particularly those involving your ability to conceive
- Why certain tests have been taken and what your doctor is looking for
- When you can expect test results
- If, based on the exam, there are signs or symptoms you should watch out for

If medication has been prescribed, ask specifically what it is for, what the side effects are, and whether it is safe to take while trying to conceive. Also important is whether this prescription has any restrictions in regard to any other medications you are taking. If you drink alcohol (and I must remind you that you should limit consumption while you are trying to conceive), ask if this will affect your medication.

If you don't understand the diagnosis, and especially if you don't understand your problem or why you have it, please ask your doctor to explain things to you further, in a way you can understand.

Most important, don't let your doctor duck out of these end-of-exam talks; instead, ending your visit with empty assurances and a gratuitous pat on the head. This will not do. When it is *your* health and *your* fertility, not to mention *your* future on the line, you deserve to know and understand all you can about whatever your doctor believes is true for you.

It's also important that you speak up about any aspect of your treatment or care that you feel is lacking, or about any procedure you feel is unduly painful. Why is this important? If you are in pain, you can tense your body to such a degree that subtle but significant internal symptoms can be missed or mistakenly identified.

Also remember: Today's gynecologist must show you that he or she is as interested in preventing problems as in treating them. You must not settle for any physician who offers you less than an equal partnership of quality care.

Some Final Advice: Take Charge of Your Pregnancy!

Although sometimes it may seem as if there are more chances of things going wrong with a pregnancy than going right, I can promise you this is not the case. And the concept of pre-conception counseling is not suggested to frighten you into believing that every pregnancy requires specialized care. In fact, if you are young and both you and your partner are basically healthy, you probably won't have any problems conceiving or delivering a healthy baby all on your own. However, we cannot deny that there are factors in today's world, and maybe even in your personal life, that *can* sometimes act as an obstacle to getting pregnant, making conception and even delivery more difficult than it has to be.

By giving you the opportunity to overcome these obstacles before they have the chance to present problems, pre-conception counseling offers you an *extra* measure of protection and safety, and a new kind of *complete* control over your childbearing options.

Chapter Nine

Body Fat, Dieting, and Fertility: How Your Weight Affects Conception

One of the most important steps you can take to ensure you are biologically ready for a fast and easy conception is to pay careful attention to your weight, particularly in the months and weeks before you plan to get pregnant. In fact, much research has shown that by reaching the proper weight six months before you want to conceive (and we'll tell you how to find your correct fertility weight later in this chapter), you can exert a powerful force over your ability to get pregnant.

What's the connection? Studies continue to reveal important links between body fat and the reproductive hormones. More specifically, women who are either underweight or overweight can suffer a hormone imbalance that disrupts or even blocks ovulation. Indeed, according to new studies published by the University of Washington, Fred Hutchinson Cancer Research Center in Seattle, as much as 12 percent of all primary infertility caused by ovulation dysfunction is the result of incorrect weight—a fact a patient of mine recently discovered when she set out to have a baby.

Too Thin to Get Pregnant?

Certain that the success of her modeling career depended on remaining ultraslim, Jan dieted constantly and worked out frantically. Repeatedly ignoring my warnings that her usual 110 pounds were far too slight for her large frame, when work became exceptionally demanding she sometimes allowed her weight to drop as low as 102 pounds.

While her menstrual cycle was always in question (she continually reported scanty bleeding and irregular periods), it wasn't until recently that Jan herself began to see the error of her high-fashion ways.

Although she looked, felt, and indeed was healthy, Jan discovered she was unable to get pregnant. By the time she confided her problem to me she was in a state of depression. "I can't believe that after a year and a half of trying nothing is happening," she said.

Since she had been my patient for some years, I was able to reassure her that there were no structural problems behind her inability to conceive. She was free of all tumors and cysts and her organs were in good shape.

However, a series of blood tests revealed what I had warned her about for several years. Jan's low weight had led to a hormone imbalance that nearly shut down her entire reproductive system. Jan was just too thin to conceive a child.

How Your Body Fat Affects Your Fertility

Although research into the connection between weight and fertility is still considered new, overwhelming evidence continues to show us that how much a woman weighs when she attempts conception can have an enormous influence on the production of key reproductive hormones, particularly estrogen.

How does this work? Each fat cell in your body is a kind of miniature hormone factory. Using a unique biochemical process it converts certain body chemicals (primarily the adrenal hormone androgen) into estrogen, which you already know is one of the key factors necessary for egg production and release. In fact, while some estrogen is made in your ovaries, up to one-third of your body's total supply (and sometimes up to 80 percent at certain key times of the month) is formed in your fat cells.

- The more fat cells you retain, the greater estrogen-making power your body has.

- The fewer fat cells you retain, the less estrogen you can make.

But just having estrogen in your body is not enough to ensure conception success. If you are to achieve your maximum fertility potential, your estrogen must be present at a specific level. Whenever that level rises too high or falls too low—as it can when you have too many or two few fat cells—you can have a problem getting pregnant.

What Turns Fertility On and Off

- Complete hormonal shutdown can occur if your body fat falls just 10 to 15 percent below the norm of 29 percent.
- Even a slight drop in body fat (below 22 percent) can disrupt hormone levels and cause infertility.

Weak Estrogen – Strong Estrogen

According to another theory, not all estrogen is alike. Subdivided by your body into two types, weak and strong, each type of estrogen must be maintained in a certain amount. Dr. Jack Fishman, professor of endocrinology at Rockefeller University in New York City, maintains that when levels of body fat change, the ratio of weak to strong estrogen is disrupted, resulting in a hormone imbalance that can also lead to infertility.

Brain Messages and Infertility

In still other studies, researchers found that weight loss, as well as low weight, can decrease important hormonal messages sent from the brain to the ovaries. When this process is disrupted, you may still ovulate, but you may not produce enough estrogen to build a uterine lining strong enough to allow a fertilized egg to implant and grow. In more severe cases, when weight is exceptionally low, ovulation may not occur at all.

Eat Your Heart Out—and Get Pregnant!

Although there are a variety of fertility medications that can counter some reproductive problems caused by being underweight (and you'll learn more about what they are in Part Three of this book), for the most part, you are far better off taking the natural route—and that is gaining enough weight to restore your reproductive health to normal status. Indeed, a fascinating report filed in the 1980s by Dr. G. William Bates, a prominent professor of obstetrics and gynecology at the Medical University of South Carolina at Charleston, revealed this is not only possible, but perhaps easier to achieve than you realize.

Specifically, Dr. Bates worked with twenty-nine ultraslim women, each no more than 91 percent of her ideal weight. All had been infertile at least four years, and some had undergone fertility treatments with drugs or surgery, all to no avail. Each also had a partner whose sperm tested normal.

Dr. Bates's theory was that the percentage of body fat on these women had dropped so low that their estrogen was in dangerously short supply and affecting all their other hormones in the process. He decided to try what was then a rather revolutionary fertility treatment—weight gain.

Can Ice Cream and Milk Shakes Make You More Fertile?

Dr. Bates asked the women in the study to try a high-calorie weight-gain diet, which he believed might raise estrogen levels, put hormones back in balance, and increase conception odds. Although three of the women refused the dietary changes, twenty-six agreed to give weight gain a try. Each worked to gain one-half to one pound per week until she reached 95 to 100 percent of her ideal fertility weight.

When they did, ovulation kicked in! Within one to three years later, twenty-four of the twenty-six women became pregnant. The average gain that made the difference? A mere 8.2 pounds. And more than 90 percent of the women in the study were able to conceive naturally, requiring neither drugs nor surgery.

The Foods That Make You Fertile

Dr. Bates's high-calorie fertility diet for underweight women consisted of generous meals containing meat, pasta, whole milk, fish, and cheese. In addition, the women were encouraged to snack frequently on ice cream, pastry, milk shakes, and beer.

Overweight and Infertile? The New Links

Just as too few fat cells can disrupt estrogen levels, so can too many. By flooding your system with an estrogen overload, your excess fat cells cause your body to react as if it's on birth control, preventing ovulation from occurring.

According to the American Society for Reproductive Medicine, being overweight can also cause insulin levels to rise, which in women may cause the ovaries to overproduce male hormones, such as testosterone, which in turn can cause ovarian problems that block egg release.

Even more important than the amount of excess fat cells is where in your body they lie. Indeed, studies published in both the *British Medical Journal* and the journal *Reproductive Fertility Developments* found that women with a high waist-to-hip ratio (an "apple" shape) had far more difficulty conceiving than those with a low waist-to-hip ration (a "pear" shape).

Losing Weight and Gaining Fertility

To help verify the links between not only excess weight and infertility but also weight loss and reproductive health, once again Dr. Bates called on a special food plan.

This study involved thirteen *overweight* women, all infertile and averaging 169 pounds. He placed them on a diet designed to encourage weight loss of about one pound per week. The results:

- An average loss of just twenty pounds per patient restored ovulation in eleven women.

- Ten of the women were able to conceive naturally after losing the weight.

Getting Your Body Ready for Pregnancy

After I explained the body-fat–fertility connection to my patient Jan, she decided to give weight gain a try. I'm happy to report that just seven and a half pounds and nine weeks later, tests showed her ovulation patterns and her menstrual cycle were normal, perhaps for the first time in years. Three months after that, she was able to conceive.

Finding Your Ideal Fertility Weight

In the past, most physicians used something called the Metropolitan Height and Weight Standards chart to decide whether a patient was overweight or underweight. With the push toward living on the lean side, however, some health professionals, particularly cardiologists, began to think these numbers were too high. I, however, along with many other fertility specialists, believe that, at least for the purpose of conceiving, the Metropolitan Standards are correct. Based on these numbers, the following chart can help you find your ideal fertility weight.

Men, Weight, and Infertility

Although most of the research concerning weight and fertility has been centered on women, there is some evidence that being underweight or overweight can harm a man's reproductive potential as well. According to reports by the American Society for Reproductive Medicine:

- In men, low weight or weight loss may lead to decreased sperm function or low sperm count.
- Being overweight may affect a man's testes, causing sperm production to be affected as well.

Your Fertility Height and Weight Guide

IF YOUR HEIGHT IS :	YOUR PRE-CONCEPTION WEIGHT SHOULD BE:
4'10"	109 to 121
4'11"	111 to 123
5'0"	113 to 126
5'1"	115 to 129
5'2"	118 to 132
5'3"	121 to 135
5'4"	124 to 138
5'5"	127 to 141
5'6"	130 to 144
5'7"	133 to 147
5'8"	136 to 150
5'9"	139 to 153
5'10"	142 to 156
5'11"	145 to 159
6'0"	148 to 162

Note: Height includes one-inch heels; weight includes three pounds of clothes.

Important: Figuring your body type: To accurately figure which numbers indicate your correct weight, you must determine whether you have large bones or small bones. Use this formula:

- Small bones: A wrist measurement of 5.5 inches or less; ankles 8 inches or less
- Large bones: A wrist measurement of 6 inches or more; ankles 9 inches or more

For small bones, use the lower weight as your guide, for large bones, use the higher weight.

How to Calculate Body-Fat Levels

Although keeping your weight under control will generally keep your body fat at the right level, sometimes relying strictly on the numbers on your scale can be deceiving. Why? Muscle mass weighs more than fat, so it's possible that you might be at the optimum fertility weight but still be short on body fat. Likewise, you may be thin, but all your weight may be fat and not muscle, so you might very well have enough estrogen to keep ovulation going.

While there are a number of sophisticated laboratory tests that can determine body-fat levels, and several home scales available to take these measurements as well, there is also a simple no-cost way for you to do the same and monitor levels whenever you want to conceive. The method is called the body mass index or BMI.

Measuring Your Body Fat: What to Do

Using metric system measurements, BMI calculations begin with an accurate reading of your weight and height. Once you have established these, you must convert them to the metric system. The following formula can help:

1. To convert your weight from pounds to kilograms, divide the number of pounds you weigh by 2.2. For example, 125 pounds divided by 2.2 equals 56.8 kilograms.
2. To convert your height measurement from inches to meters, divide the number of inches by 39.4. For example: Height 60 inches divided by 39.4 equals 1.5 meters.
3. You must then square your height measurement by multiplying it by itself. In this case, 1.5 times 1.5, equaling 2.25.

To calculate your percentage of body fat: Divide your body weight in kilograms by your squared height in meters. The result will be your BMI or Body Mass Index. Continuing to use our 125-pound woman as a guide, the calculations looks like this: 56.8 kg (weight) divided by 2.25 (squared height) equals 25.2 BMI.

Calculate your risk:

- If your BMI falls between 19 and 25, congratulations! Your body is ready to conceive right now.
- If your BMI is over 27.5 you need to lose body fat to optimize your fertility potential. If your BMI is over 31.5 your weight loss needs to be medically supervised.
- If your BMI falls below 19, you need to increase body fat to maximize your fertility potential.

Achieving Your Fertility Weight Goals

Whether you need to lose or gain body fat, the latest research suggests that *how* you obtain your pre-conception weight goals can also affect your fertility. What should you avoid? Any diet or exercise program that promotes exceptionally rapid gain or loss. Why?

Each significant shift in weight, whether up or down, causes a corresponding shift in hormone production. Because many reproductive functions take their cue from the amount of certain hormones in your bloodstream, levels that change too abruptly can confuse the signals being sent from your brain to your body. The result—your reproductive system falls into biochemical chaos, and you're infertile. Even more important, continual fluctuations in weight keep hormone levels constantly on the move.

Studies show that victims of the yo-yo diet syndrome, hopelessly caught in the lose-gain-lose groove, are at higher risk for reproductive problems when compared with those who lose weight more slowly and keep it off. I have observed that many patients who have problems stabilizing their weight also have problems getting pregnant. Even short-term dieting can affect your fertility. Studies at the Institute of Psychiatry in Munich, Germany, recently revealed that if your weight falls within the normal range, trying to lose even a few pounds can cause your menstrual cycle to become so irregular that ovulation is impaired, causing at least temporary infertility.

Enhancing Your Fertility: What to Do

The good news is that by following a few simple guidelines, you can *safely* achieve your pre-conception weight goals and enhance your fertility at the same time. What should you do?

   • If you need to lose body fat, eat balanced, nutritious meals of no fewer than twelve hundred calories a day. Avoid liquid diets, high-fiber quick-loss products, or any diet that uses just one food group, such as all-protein, all-fruit, or all-vegetable meals.

   • If you need to add body fat, add complex carbohydrates to your diet—foods such as whole grain pasta, fruit, and vegetables. Even when you are trying to gain weight you should limit your intake of high-fat foods and continue to avoid all foods containing tropical oils.

   • Avoid the use of all diet pills and commercial weight control products. Because every woman's physiology is different, it's difficult to tell if what you are taking could have residual effects on your reproductive system.

   • Whether you need to lose or gain weight, be certain to get adequate amounts of protein every day, at least 46 grams (or about 180 calories' worth). The latest studies show this can help reduce your risk of ovulatory problems.

   Finally, remember to give your body adequate time to adjust to your new weight before trying to conceive. If possible, allow at least one month of dieting time for every six to eight pounds you need to lose or gain. Once you reach your goal, plan on six to eight weeks of maintenance time before attempting conception.

   By making sure weight changes are gradual and then giving your reproductive chemistry time to readjust, you will not only remain healthy while you are dieting but ensure that your body will be in great shape when you reach your fertility weight goals—ready when you are, to conceive and deliver that healthy baby.

Chapter Ten

Fitness, Stress, and Getting Pregnant

Every day I find more evidence that being physically fit before you get pregnant can help you have a healthier pregnancy. If your muscles are strong and toned and your cardiovascular system is in peak order before conception, you have a good chance of sailing through your pregnancy with few problems, and your delivery is likely to be natural and problem-free.

However, as beneficial as working out can be, studies show, and my patients have proved as well, that some strenuous activities work against female fertility. Likewise, so can overdoing even the most otherwise beneficial fitness routines. In either case, sometimes exercise can cause a variety of negative reproductive effects, from menstrual irregularities to outright infertility. What are these activities? Endurance workouts, including:

- Marathon running
- Excessive jogging
- Frequent high-energy aerobics
- Triathlon training

In fact, studies show that any workout regimen that promotes extreme physical or emotional stress can be detrimental to your reproductive health. When performed on a regular basis, especially in the months before attempting conception, such workouts can affect your ability to produce eggs, encourage irregular ovulation, or even stop egg release completely.

If you should conceive, serious implantation problems could result. In some cases, studies show endurance workouts can compromise your fertility to the point of infertility.

Although no one is certain why this occurs, the latest studies point to the hypothalamus as one possible source of the problem. This is the gland that secretes gonadotropin-releasing hormone (GnRH), which helps initiate the entire egg-production-release process. Some research has shown that workouts that require you to push your body too hard for too long a period of time may inhibit the functioning of your hypothalamus gland, and in the process upset the function and timing of all reproductive hormones necessary for conception.

Endurance training is also thought to alter the way your body metabolizes thyroxin, the hormone produced by your thyroid gland and linked to the reproductive process. Eventually this important gland can malfunction to such an extent your entire body chemistry is adversely affected and your fertility comes to a complete halt.

The Body-Fat Connection

Even more important are the effects of endurance workouts on body fat, often forcing you to burn massive amounts in a relatively short amount of time. Like strenuous dieting (see Chapter 9), manic fitness activities can burn so much body fat that your estrogen levels drop dangerously low. When this happens, your reproductive system can actually return to a prepubescent stage. I have seen a number of patients who, after losing excess body fat, developed such an irregular menstrual cycle that ovulation eventually stopped. Sometimes it was difficult or even impossible to recharge their reproductive systems and rejuvenate their fertility, even with medication.

A recent study found that marathon runners with continuously low levels of body fat had almost no estrogen in their bodies and consequently no menstrual cycle. Even after they were given estrogen replacement therapy, damage to their reproductive system had progressed to such a degree that the other hormones necessary for conception remained too low for pregnancy to occur.

Working Out: The Silent Dangers

What can complicate things even more is that unlike dieting, in which weight change can signal that hormone levels may be dropping too low, the effects of endurance workouts can be dangerously silent. Why? As you lose pounds, you build new muscle mass, which can allow your weight to actually remain the same. Since it is body fat and not just pounds you need in order to be fertile (again, see Chapter 9), you can be fooled into believing your weight is adequate for optimum fertility when, in fact, it is not.

Often female athletes with the most severe reproductive problems are near or at their correct body weight. But since that weight is mostly muscle mass and not fat, they remain infertile.

Only a small dip in fat stores (just a few percentage points below normal) is enough to trigger menstrual irregularities, so it doesn't take very long for endurance workouts to affect your ability to get pregnant.

Super Hazards for Young Athletes

Research shows that the earlier in life you become involved in endurance training, the more likely you will be to suffer conception-related difficulties, sometimes even permanent reproductive damage. In fact, before puberty, each year of endurance athletic training a woman engages in delays the onset of the menstrual cycle by an average of three months. It is also not unlikely for some female athletes who begin training at a very young age to never get a menstrual cycle at all.

In fact, even dancing, when done to excess, has the potential to harm a young girl. Studies show that some ballerinas who begin rigorous training or professional dancing before puberty may never get a menstrual cycle. Many older ballet (and other) dancers lose their menstrual period for months or even years on end while performing on a regular and rigorous schedule.

For this reason I always advise my patients who have young daughters to see that they practice caution and moderation when participating in sports and other demanding physical activities. More important, these girls should cut back whenever any sign of impending reproductive damage becomes apparent—such as a significant delay in the onset of the menstrual cycle (past age fourteen or fifteen would be a sign of trouble). If they are already menstruating, a cycle interruption of more than three consecutive months would also indicate problems. Remember, damage to the reproductive system can occur at almost any age, and it's never too early for a girl to begin caring for her fertility.

How Exercise Can Protect Your Fertility: The Good News

Even with its dangers, there is no doubt that some degree of physical activity is not only safe but essential to a healthy body. In addition to protecting your heart and your overall good health, research shows that if you are athletically active in your twenties and thirties you will have a lower lifetime incidence of:

- Breast cancer
- Uterine and ovarian cancer
- Cervical and vaginal cancer
- Benign tumors of the reproductive system
- Benign breast disease

The Center for Population Studies at the Harvard School of Public Health published findings that show reproductive cancers occurred 2.5 times less often in athletic women than in those who led sedentary lives.

Many types of exercise can also help you alleviate tension and stress, and thus keep your hormones in balance and your menstrual cycle regulated. And that's one of the best ways to ensure your reproductive health.

The Workouts That Can Encourage Your Fertility

The key to your workout success depends on the activities you choose, especially if you are planning to conceive in the near future. Doctors and fitness experts agree that you can derive the greatest overall benefits from noncompetitive, mildly aerobic activities that condition your whole body, without placing strain on any particular muscle group. It's also important that you choose activities that can be sustained for long periods of time without exhaustion.

These include:

- Swimming
- Dancing
- Bicycling
- Moderate aerobics
- Walking
- Stretching
- Tennis (in moderation)
- Weight lifting

When done in moderation, all these activities can help keep you in great shape without disturbing the delicate body chemistry needed for a fast and healthy conception.

How Yoga Can Help You Get Pregnant

You should also note the positive power that *passive* muscle-toning workouts can have on your ability to get pregnant. Many of my patients have reported great success with yoga, a form of exercise that uses a series of body positions (rather than moves) maintained for increasing lengths of time to condition and tone the muscles. According to some experts, yoga can help encourage your fertility by decreasing stress levels, which in turn can help promote healthier functioning of your hypothalamus (the area of your brain involved in stimulating hormone production), and by having a positive effect directly on your reproductive organs. Many of the yoga movements increase the amount of blood flow and circulation to your ovaries and uterus, and that, in turn, can help maintain better reproductive health.

Indeed, studies have shown that practicing yoga regularly may help promote more regular menstrual cycles, keep reproductive hormones in balance, and alleviate the symptoms of premenstrual syndrome.

If you have never participated in yoga fitness before, you need professional guidance. Books, videotapes, and especially a personal instructor can get you started in the right direction and help you master the yoga postures that can encourage your fertility.

Make All Your Workouts Work for You

Regardless of your choice of activity, you can be sure that your fitness regimen continues to work *for* and not *against* your reproductive health if you follow a few simple guidelines:

- Practice moderation. Limit workouts to three times weekly with at least one day of rest in between.
- Keep each workout session short—no more than forty-five to sixty minutes per session.
- Avoid becoming *compulsive* about your workouts by avoiding heavy competition, even with your own records.
- Don't be afraid to cut back whenever you feel excessive body or brain strain.

Most important, take steps to ensure that your workout is not burning too much body fat. Use the BMI (see Chapter 9) to monitor body-fat levels every ten days, cutting back on activities whenever weight or body fat falls below the accepted norm.

Stress, Anxiety, and Infertility: What You Need to Know

In much the same way that the chronic stress of a bad relationship can affect your fertility, the ways in which your body processes and deals with all kinds of stress can also have a significant effect on your ability to get pregnant. How?

It begins with the functions of your hypothalamus, the area of the brain responsible for the flow and timing of all reproductive hormones. As it turns out, this gland is extremely sensitive to both emotional and physical tensions, so much so that almost any type of stress has an immediate effect on its functions. When this occurs, a variety of menstrual-related problems can develop—from a temporary change in your ovulation pattern, to complete ovarian shutdown. If you have ever experienced a temporary menstrual upset during times of stress—a period that is delayed or comes on too quickly, for example—then you already have some idea of how stress can affect your reproductive health.

Although the effects of short-term stress usually cause only a temporary bout of infertility, distress that goes on for long periods of time can have more serious, long-lasting effects. Not only can long-term stress lead to a higher incidence of fertility-robbing diseases, such as endometriosis, vaginitis, and some STDs, it can also throw your reproductive hormones into prolonged biochemical chaos. Often these imbalances cause even more stress, which in turn affects your hypothalamus even further, thus creating a kind of vicious cycle of fertility-related consequences. Ultimately they can bring your childbearing options to a halt, and sometimes it can be difficult or even impossible to reverse that damage.

Stress and Infertility: The Latest News

Although I and many fertility specialists have long believed in the stress-infertility link, it wasn't until the late 1990s that we really began to see the proof behind our theory. The researcher who made a real difference was Harvard's Alice Domar, Ph.D., now head of the Mind-Body Center for Women's Health at Beth Israel's Deaconess Medical Center in Boston. As far back as 1987, Dr. Domar began assembling groups of white-collar women in their thirties and forties who had been unsuccessful at getting pregnant for a number of years. Her goal at that time was to establish stress-reduction workshops to help these women deal with their feelings about being infertile.

Then, something quite amazing began to occur. As stress levels began to fall, the women in the study began getting pregnant. At first, Dr. Domar reportedly viewed it as simply a pleasant "side effect" of the coping therapy. Still, month after month, year after year, the phenomenon continued. Finally, she began formally tracking the women and ultimately presented her findings to the American Society for Reproductive Medicine.

Those results: of 174 severely infertile women who participated in the stress management program, up to 60 percent were able to conceive.

Finally, we had the beginning of the solid scientific proof we needed to seriously embrace the idea that stress and infertility had an undeniable link.

Ultimately, Harvard University granted Dr. Domar "seed money" to begin the Mind-Body Center for Women's Health, a place where she continues her research on stress and infertility and on the vital role that depression and anxiety may play in the development of many diseases that affect women's overall health, including lupus, chronic fatigue, eating disorders, heart disease, even breast cancer.

Stress, Depression, and Infertility

Among the most outstanding, if not surprising, of Dr. Domar's study conclusions established a new link between depression and infertility.

Among the tests that Dr. Domar administered to the infertile women before starting the stress-reduction program was an evaluation called the Beck Depression Inventory. Here, the women answered questions designed to calculate their level of distress. At the conclusion of the program, the women were tested again, with some surprising results.

Not only did the de-stressing program improve their fertility status, but those who tested as being the most depressed at the start of the program turned out to have the highest conception rate at the end of the program—nearly 60 percent!

What's more, their new Beck Inventory tests showed their level of depression was on a par with that of healthy women who had no problems conceiving, showing, for the first time, not only that stress and depression can be linked to infertility, but that relieving those problems can lead to pregnancy success.

Stress and Fertility Treatments: What You Need to Know

Ironically, research has begun to show that the very fertility treatments developed to help you conceive may, in some couples, be so stressful that they actually work against conception, increasing anxiety to the point where reproductive health is even more compromised than it was before treatment began.

Indeed, once diagnosed with infertility, many couples feel a sudden and overwhelming loss of control over their bodies, or even their lives, which in turn increases their stress by a considerable proportion. This, combined with the fact that infertility treatments can be physically, emotionally, and financially draining and can disrupt some sense of the intimacy partners previously shared, can mean that fertility treatments themselves become the source of much stress.

In still other instances, patients undergoing fertility treatments have developed post-traumatic stress disorder (PTSD). Although this diagnosis usually pertains to those who experience war or natural disasters, there have been a number of infertility patients who developed PTSD following either a very dramatic high-risk pregnancy or particularly grueling infertility treatments. The classic symptoms can include the re-experiencing of the stressful events in the form of nightmares, flashbacks, and intrusive thoughts, all of which can be triggered by fertility-related events such as seeing a pregnant woman walking down the street or visiting a doctor's office. Avoidance symptoms include a reluctance to discuss fertility issues, including the failure of treatment to bring about a pregnancy. When fertility treatments have resulted in the birth of a child, PTSD symptoms can include a delay in bonding with the baby, or even great anxiety or aversion at the thought of holding the baby.

If, at any time, you, or those close to you, begin to feel that either fertility treatments or the inability to conceive is causing you undue stress, please talk to your doctor immediately. Although it is my hope that if this does happen to you, your doctor will be vigilant enough to recognize the signs, this isn't always the case. In many areas of the country, fertility centers are vast, impersonal clinics, and the patient is seen briefly by many different members of the medical team, so that no real bond is formed with any one doctor. As such, it can be easy for those women who are troubled to slip through the cracks, and consequently end up even more infertile than when they started, simply because of the stress they have placed on themselves (or others have placed on them) to get pregnant.

Eliminating Stress in Your Life

The good news is that by keeping stress levels in check and remaining as relaxed as possible in the months and weeks before you want to conceive, you can significantly increase your chances for a healthy conception. The most obvious place to start? By identifying the causes. Once you know what your stressors are, you can begin to reduce them or eliminate them from your life. Certainly, such factors as an irritating boss, disarming in-laws, financial problems, or worries and fears about the health of loved ones aren't going to go away overnight. However, if you look into your life, you may see that many of the major stresses are made worse by *smaller* stresses, things that very often you *can* control.

One way to do just that is by taking extra time for yourself whenever possible. The restorative effects of a relaxing herbal bath, for exam-

---

Stress: The Most Common Causes

While almost anything you personally find stressful can bring about negative changes in your menstrual cycle, and ultimately your fertility, the most common major stresses are:

Job tensions
Relationships with lovers, kids, parents
Sexual problems
Loneliness
Guilt or grief
Fear of failure
Excessive competition

ple, or a facial or a massage, or even a half-hour "me" break where you do something you really enjoy (reading a book, window shopping, gardening, baking, scrapbooking, or knitting) can have powerful stress-busting effects that can go a long way in helping you both biologically and psychologically to deal with the major problems in your life.

The Scent of Relaxation

Many of my patients have recently begun using aromatherapy to reduce their stress levels, particularly when undergoing fertility treatments. Based on the ancient practice of using fragrances to influence mood, today it is often used to affect everything from our stress levels to our appetite, even our sex drive. The "science" behind the smell theory is based on the idea that the nose is a direct pathway to the brain and that smelling certain fragrances can have an immediate effect on brain chemicals, which, in turn, influence not only our behavior but our stress levels.

When it comes to inducing relaxation, the two scents that my patients say are the most effective—and that some scientific studies have proven to work as well—are vanilla and lavender, either alone or together. In one hospital study it was found that lightly scenting a diagnostic room with a natural vanilla spray lowered patients' stress levels enough to allow them to endure a lengthy and somewhat traumatic medical test with far greater ease.

For you, taking just a few minutes several times a day to "stop and smell the vanilla" may, in fact, work wonders in reducing your overall stress levels, particularly if you can't afford a lavish holiday weekend to break your tension.

If you try aromatherapy, my advice is to select products that are natural—for example natural vanilla- or lavender-scented items as opposed to synthetic. My patients have reported particular success with a line of organically grown, naturally scented items by a company called Perlier—particularly their vanilla-based line of products, as well as many lavender and vanilla products for the home and the body found at The Body Shop (see Resources section at the end of this book).

Watch Out for Hidden Stress!

One of the most frustrating aspects of stress is that it can be so deceptive. In our busy lives, we can get so used to feeling tense, rushed, and fatigued, and even somewhat depressed, that we begin to view tension as a normal state of being. Many of my patients don't even realize how much tension is a part of their lives until a diagnosis of stress-related infertility is made!

For this reason it's important that you listen to your body for signs of *hidden* stress that could be affecting your reproductive health. The best way to do that is to use your menstrual cycle as a guide. Regardless of how you feel, if you begin to experience irregular cycles (or other possible stress-related menstrual problems such as cramps, backaches, or sore breasts) arrange for a consultation with your doctor. If no precise physical problem can be isolated as the cause of your menstrual concerns, you should begin to suspect stress as the culprit. If hidden stress is a problem, your doctor can help you uncover the source and map out a plan to reduce tensions.

How Stressed Are You?

Ask yourself these important questions:

- Am I tired all the time, regardless of the number of hours I sleep?
- Do I have trouble falling asleep, or do I wake easily, unable to get back to sleep?
- Do I have frequent headaches?
- Do I catch a lot of colds, the flu, or sore throats?
- Am I prone to vaginal infections or herpes outbreaks?
- Is my menstrual cycle on time?
- Do I find myself losing patience with my coworkers or family?

If you answered yes to any of these questions, stress may be a problem in your life. If you said yes to three or more questions, your reproductive health may already be in jeopardy.

The Good News: Stress Doesn't Have to Harm You

The important thing to remember is that, even if you are experiencing great stress, help is available. In many instances, programs like those offered by Dr. Domar can go a long way in helping you deal with the stress in your life and can encourage your fertility at the same time. (You can find contact information about her center in the Resources section at the end of this book.)

In other instances, a regimen of diet and nutrients (much like those found in the Fertility Food Plan later in this book), along with adequate rest, fresh air, and mild exercise, may help your body overcome many of the physical manifestations of stress, which in turn may help you to better cope with your anxiety about getting pregnant. And that, in turn may increase your fertility.

Finally, if your stress levels really climb, and particularly if you are also suffering severe depression or PTSD, your doctor can prescribe a short regimen of antidepressant medication. Although I generally recommend that you avoid tranquilizers, sedatives, and even antidepressants while trying to conceive, when this medication becomes necessary, it should be considered. After several months it can be discontinued and you can resume your fertility treatments, often with great success.

The main thing to remember: Advancements in fertility treatment being what they are today, you are far more likely to get pregnant than to not conceive, providing you don't compound your problems by worrying about the fact that it may never happen.

Smile More—and Get Pregnant Faster!

Finally, don't forget to smile—even when you don't feel like it. The reason?

Studies show that when the muscles of the face form a smile a biochemical message is relayed to the brain to produce endorphins, powerful mood-altering natural substances that not only work to immediately make you feel better, but also work long-term to help you combat stress and even promote fertility.

Chapter Eleven

Fertility Diet 2000:

The Foods That Enhance Your Fertility and Protect Your Pregnancy

Since almost the dawn of time, food and fertility have been intimately entwined. From meals that increase potency to desserts that drum up desire, throughout history we can find hundreds of references to aphrodisiac foods that are credited with boosting fertility, sexual performance, or both.

The truth is, however, if any of these foods had the power to enhance fertility at all, it is my guess that they did so by providing some basic elements of good nutrition—factors that we now know *can* influence fertility potential. How can food help you get pregnant?

Recent studies conducted or reported by numerous health organizations have shown that eating nutritiously can help you counter some of the fertility-robbing effects of many toxic influences, such as cigarette smoke, alcohol, drugs, birth control pills, and air pollution. Further, independent studies continue to reveal that diets that are nutritionally balanced and meet the minimum daily requirements of vitamins and minerals can also help decrease your risk of pregnancy-related problems, such as prolonged labor, hypertension, gestational diabetes, preeclampsia, infection, and excessive bleeding.

Not coincidentally, these same nutrients are the foods that can also play a role in helping to ensure your baby's health, both before and after conception. Certainly, my own patients have proved time and time again that good nutrition has not only improved the outcome of their pregnancy but also helped enhance their fertility. Indeed, some of my patients completely overcame their infertility problems simply by changing their eating habits.

The Fertility Power Boost: What to Eat to Get Pregnant

Later in this chapter you will find a meal plan I devised to help my own patients meet the nutritional and caloric needs of conception and pregnancy.

However, more generally speaking, I have found that many of my patients were able to have a faster and easier conception when they increased their protein intake by about 10 to 12 percent, particularly in the form of lean red meat or poultry. How can this help?

Studies show that all meals high in protein, but especially those containing lean, red meat, promote ovulation. Conversely, diets that are deficient in protein can disrupt the menstrual cycle and cause at least a temporary and sometimes a longer-lasting bout with infertility. According to the American College of Obstetricians and Gynecologists

---

Are You Eating Enough to Get Pregnant?

As important as what you eat when you are trying to get pregnant is how much you eat—in the form of daily caloric intake. According to the U.S. Department of Agriculture (USDA) Nationwide Food Consumption Survey, women are currently consuming two hundred calories a day fewer than they did in the past. The study also shows that more than three-quarters of the participants did not meet the basic nutritional requirements for proper body functioning.

If you are not underweight or overweight, the U.S. Department of Health maintains that a woman's body needs about 2,100 calories a day to function properly. Just before conception that need can rise as high as 2,300 calories a day, while just after conception you should be consuming 2,500 to 2,700 calories a day.

(ACOG), an adequate amount of protein in your diet (at least two hundred calories daily) can increase your developing baby's birth weight and may protect you from premature delivery.

You may also want to add more complex carbohydrates (such as whole-grain breads, fruits, vegetables, and pasta) to your diet, while at the same time reducing your intake of simple carbohydrates (such as white bread, cake, and sugary snacks). New studies show this may promote more efficient functioning of neurotransmitters, the biochemical messengers that carry hormonal signals and other important reproductive data from your brain to your body.

Most important, remember that nutrition is an interdependent concept. Each food you eat needs components of other foods in order to be of maximum value. When your diet is balanced all the calories you consume are super-effective. Without this nutritional teamwork, depletions capable of harming your fertility can eventually develop.

Indeed, you can make almost any eating plan more beneficial for your fertility if you follow these simple dietary guidelines for the meals you prepare each day:

- Carbohydrates: 45 to 55 percent (Recommended Daily Allowance)—about 1,200 to 1,400 calories daily
- Protein: 12 to 14 percent (Recommended Daily Allowance)— about 45 to 50 grams or 200 calories daily
- Fat: 30 percent or less (American Heart Association)—about 50 to 60 grams or 500 calories daily
- Sodium: 1,000 to 3,000 mg daily (USDA)
- Cholesterol: 300 mg daily

The Antifertility Foods: Can Peas Make You Infertile?

As powerful as some foods can be in increasing your fertility potential, there are also some that, when consumed in large amounts, may delay or in some cases even prevent you from conceiving. One of these foods is peas, and its history as an antifertility food goes back at least as far as 1949.

It was then that scientists noted that the people of Tibet maintained one of the most stable populations in the world. Since one of the foods most prominent in their daily diet was peas, researchers theorized that perhaps this vegetable was working as a kind of "national contraceptive," limiting the growth of their population. Soon, researchers began to back up these ideas with scientific fact.

What they discovered was that a natural chemical found in peas—called m-xylohydroquinone—did appear to have contraceptive effects. In studies conducted in India, capsules containing m-xylohydroquinone were found to cut the pregnancy rate by up to 60 percent. In men who took the pea capsule, sperm counts dropped by some 50 percent.

Back here in the United States, studies conducted in the 1990s at the University of Illinois helped establish the antifertility effects of pea-oil—so much so that it is now being studied as a possible natural contraceptive. So it's easy to see how a diet high in peas could keep you from conceiving.

Soy Foods and Pregnancy: What You Should Know

Like peas, soybeans may also disrupt your ability to get pregnant. The reason, experts say, has to do with their high content of phytoestrogens—essentially, a plant form of estrogen that mimics the way your own supply of this hormone reacts in your body. In fact, one of the reasons that soy-based foods are thought to be so beneficial for women experiencing menopausal symptoms is because of their estrogenlike effects. For those trying to conceive, however, this excess estrogen activity is enough to induce a hormone imbalance that may affect egg production and ovulation.

Early evidence of links between soy and infertility came when researchers were studying why a particular breed of exotic cats housed at the Cincinnati Zoo seemed unable to reproduce. It wasn't long before the researchers discovered the cat chow zoo officials were feeding the animals was half soybeans. When these legumes were replaced with chicken, cat fertility began to rise.

Generally, soybeans and foods containing soy are good for a woman's health, with some studies indicating they may possess some powerful anticancer properties. However, when it comes to your fertility, it may be a good idea to reduce your intake of soy-based foods beginning about six months before you want to conceive. Do remember, too, that soy comes in many forms and is often "hidden" in some products, such as oils, lecithin, flour, powder, and milk, as well as tempeh (made from fermented soybeans). TVP, texturized vegetable protein, is also made from soy and often found in frozen fast foods or even soups. You will also find soy in the form of tofu, which is often included in imitation meat products, particularly vegetable patties and sausages.

More Foods You May Want to Avoid

In addition to the foods already mentioned, there are a number of others suspected of harming your fertility—either because of specific ingredients, or because they can rob key fertility nutrients from your body. When eaten on a regular basis, they may even cause your baby real harm.

What should you avoid when you are trying to conceive? Although in many cases reports are still largely inconclusive, I advise my patients against the following:

- **Artificial sweeteners:** Particularly avoid saccharin, which, according to studies presented to the American College of Nutrition, may not be safe to consume either before conception or after you are pregnant. Studies on aspartame (sold under brand names Nu-traSweet or Equal) are still being conducted, but it is my personal suggestion that you avoid these products as well until reports are more conclusive.
- **Soda, high-sugar fruit drinks, and candy:** Excessive sugar can exacerbate hypoglycemia (low blood sugar), which in turn can upset levels of reproductive hormones.
- **Peanut butter and spinach:** These should be avoided because of their ability to deplete calcium. According to Cedric Garland, Ph.D., director of the epidemiology program of the Cancer Center at the University of California at San Diego, the latest research shows that these foods, along with those high in sugar, can cause a

---

Health Foods Make a Healthier Baby?

Although studies on this subject are scarce, it is my *personal* belief that the fewer chemicals, toxins, and pollutants you put into your system around the time of conception, and certainly after you are pregnant, the healthier your baby will be.

---

potentially dangerous depletion of calcium, a mineral that is essential for your baby to develop and grow.

- **Rare red meat:** Avoid it because of its link to toxoplasmosis, a virus that often resides in undercooked meat and can harm your baby.
- **Frankfurters, bologna, salami, lunch meats:** These foods contain nitrates and nitrites, which some researchers maintain can exacerbate the growth of some reproductive cancers. Although in recent years newer studies have shown that if these ingredients do have cancer-causing effects they are far less potent than what we once thought; still, if you are at high risk, you should probably limit your consumption of foods containing these ingredients.

Finally, while it's important to include some fats in our diet, meals that are high in saturated fats (especially dishes that are fried or contain large amounts of tropical oils such as palm or coconut) should be avoided.

In addition to basic health concerns (like heart disease and cancer) fatty foods have also been linked to an estrogen overload, which in turn may exacerbate such conditions as endometriosis and some forms of breast disease, including breast cancer.

Food Additives and Fertility

A common food additive found in everything from Asian cuisine to potato chips and other snack foods is monosodium glutamate, better known as MSG. Although it has long been known to cause a variety of sensitivity reactions in both men and women, new studies show it may also have the potential to affect fertility. In animal studies conducted by Northeastern University's Department of Psychology, it was noted that ingesting MSG before attempting conception reduced male mating success by up to 50 percent. Further, when pregnancy did occur, offspring were shorter in length, while male babies had smaller testicles. In addition, as the animals developed, they tended to be overweight, while eating less than normal. This, say researchers, indicates a possible defect in the area of the brain responsible for controlling body weight.

In addition, the common preservative BHA, found in a variety of products including many baked goods and snack foods, was found to cause fertility problems by mimicking the effects of estrogen, thus confusing the body's natural hormone receptors. And, in fact, studies published in the journal *Environmental Health Perspectives* suggest that any form of environmental estrogen (that which mimics the effects of natural estrogen in the body) can result in fertility problems for both men and women.

Because this entire area of research is brand-new, studies linking either MSG or BHA to infertility in humans are clearly limited. In the case of MSG, there are no clear-cut indications that human reproductive health is affected at all. However, in my personal experience, factors that do affect animal reproduction are often later found to affect human fertility as well. For this reason I suggest you avoid eating any foods with either MSG or BHA in the weeks before conception. This is particularly important if you already experience even a slight sensitivity to foods containing these ingredients.

Caffeine and Infertility: An Important New Link

One of the most widely debated food-fertility links involves just how much, if any, caffeine can affect your reproductive health. While some studies clearly show a problem, others do not. Among the most impressive research in this area, however, was a 1990 study of nearly two thousand women conducted by Yale University. Here it was revealed that the risk of not conceiving over a twelve-month period is 55 percent higher if you drink as little as one cup of coffee per day. Increase coffee consumption to between one and a half and three cups per day and that risk goes up by 100 percent. Finally, drink more than three cups of coffee per day and the risk of not conceiving within a year jumps by 176 percent.

Perhaps even more disturbing, however, were 1993 studies from McGill University in Quebec, Canada, which clearly revealed that drinking two to three cups of coffee per day before conception could double the risk of miscarriage.

If you are absolutely "hooked" on caffeine (which is found, by the way, in not only coffee, but tea, chocolate, cola, and some medications), try to minimize the amount you consume for about six weeks before you want to conceive. If you must have coffee during the day, try to avoid other sources of caffeine, such as chocolate or cola. In any event, you should avoid all caffeine for at least forty-eight hours before attempting conception, and for at least seventy-two hours afterward.

Switch from Coffee to Tea — And Get Pregnant Faster

Can merely switching from coffee to tea help encourage your fertility? According to research published in the *American Journal of Public Health,* women who drink more than one half-cup of *caffeinated* tea every day (such as orange pekoe or black tea) may actually increase their odds of conceiving. In fact, of the two hundred women studied, those who sipped tea daily were twice as likely to get pregnant as those who did not.

Researchers believe the link may be aromatic polyphenol compounds found in this brew. They work, say experts, by inhibiting the development of chromosomal abnormalities, which in turn decreases the number of what doctors call "nonviable embryos"—conceptions that are simply too weak to survive.

In addition, a second chemical found in tea—a compound known as hypoxanthine—also appears to be a component of follicular fluid, the liquid that surrounds the egg and helps foster maturation and even fertilization.

But before you "belly up to the tea bar," remember, links between

How Much Caffeine Do You Get Every Day?

Although coffee contains among the highest levels of caffeine (one 5-ounce cup can have 115 mg or more), what you might not realize is how many other foods and beverages contain large amounts as well. When trying to control your overall caffeine intake, keep these numbers in mind:

Tea: One 5-ounce cup contains 40 to 60 mg of caffeine.
Cola: One 12-ounce glass contains up to 40 mg of caffeine.
Chocolate: Each ounce contains 5 to 10 mg of caffeine.
Cocoa: Each 5-ounce cup has about 4 mg of caffeine.

Many pain relievers also contain significant amounts of caffeine, ranging from 30 mg per tablet and up. If you are trying to conceive, you should avoid taking:

Excedrin, Extra Strength
Maximum-strength Midol
Vanquish
Anacin
Amaphen

Finally, note that many over-the-counter diet pills, such as Dexatrim, and stimulants, such as No-Doz and Efed II, can contain up to 200 mg of caffeine per dose, as do many diuretics. Also, check the ingredients of cough medicines, over-the-counter cold pills, and especially allergy pills, all of which may contain significant amounts of caffeine per dose.

To protect your fertility: Remember that single-dose or even short-term use of any caffeine-rich products are not likely to harm your fertility. However, large amounts, particularly taken over a long period of time, may affect your ability to conceive. Cut out caffeine when you can, and when you can't, minimize consumption by taking into account your total daily intake from all sources.

infertility and caffeine are still an issue, so you certainly don't want to overdo the amount of caffeinated tea you consume in the days and weeks before conception. Instead, drink tea in moderation, when possible, substituting it for coffee until you conceive.

Vegetarian Diets and Your Fertility

If you are currently on a vegetarian diet, careful meal planning is necessary if you are to conceive and deliver a healthy child. Often, vegetarian diets are low in calories and sometimes deficient in complete proteins, both of which can lower conception odds. In addition, *strict* vegetarian diets can sometimes lack four important fertility nutrients normally found in meat, fish, and poultry: zinc, Vitamin B_{12}, iron and folic acid.

To make your vegetarian diet work for and not against your fertility, do take nutritional supplements. In addition, make a special effort to raise the protein levels of the food you eat by mixing and matching, in as many meals as possible, complementary food sources to form a complete balance, such as:

- Legumes and grains
- Legumes and nuts
- Grains and dairy foods

Finally, you should simply eat more food, more often. By increasing your intake of complex carbohydrates and grains you can add substantial calories to your daily diet. Eating six or seven smaller meals a day can help you take in more calories than if you try to eat three large meals.

A Food Strategy for Getting Pregnant

Based on the guidelines for prenatal care set down by the American College of Obstetricians and Gynecologists, as well as many years of personal experience involving thousands of my own patients, I have devised

What's Your Food IQ?

Living in the weight-conscious, diet-crazed world that we do, it's some-times easier than we realize to become undernourished. To discover if you are undernourished right now, answer **yes** or **no** to the following ques-tions:

1. Do you eat at least 45 grams (180 calories) of protein daily?
2. Do you eat two servings of vegetables per day?
3. Are you a nonsmoker, and do you drink alcohol rarely?
4. Do you take a prenatal supplement or super-high-potency vitamin every day?
5. Do you eat two pieces of fresh fruit daily?
6. Do you eat at least four foods a day high in calcium?
7. Have you avoided birth control pills for at least three months?
8. Do you avoid processed foods and frozen prepared foods?

If you answered **no** to even one of the above questions, you could be lacking an important nutrient. If you answered **no** to three or more, your nutritional deficiencies may be significant.

a Fertility Food Plan, a diet that has helped many of my patients enhance their fertility and give birth to healthier babies. Some of my patients who previously suffered from unexplained infertility were able to conceive within just six months of following this food plan and taking vitamin sup-plements.

Unlike other diets that use specific recipes and rigid structured meals, the Fertility Food Plan 2000 takes a more progressive approach by offering you great freedom of personal choice. Assuming that you have already achieved your proper pre-conception weight (see Chapter 9), this diet has only two requirements:

1. You must choose the recommended number of servings from each food group every day.
2. Your food intake goal must be between 2,100 and 2,300 calories per day.

As long as you meet these requirements, you can personalize this diet in any way that suits your appetite and your lifestyle.

- You can eat any of the foods in any of the groups at any time of the day, and you can vary your meals according to your appetite and your lifestyle. One day you can have a large breakfast, a small lunch, and a medium dinner; another time you can eat lightly in the morning and have a heavier meal at midday or at dinnertime.

- You can also split your meals any way you like, eating as often as you like as long as you remain within the calorie count. As mentioned, I advocate six or seven small meals rather than three large ones, to help keep blood sugar at a stable level. Studies show this may have beneficial effects on reproductive hormones as well as alleviating some of the symptoms of PMS.

- You can also use any healthful recipes you like in preparing your meals. For variety, try combining ingredients from more than one food group in one dish, such as pasta and vegetables or macaroni and low-fat cheeses. Or combine different items in one food group—for example, in fruit salad or in a health salad. Use your imagination and do feel free to experiment.

Fertility Food Plan 2000

Caloric Goal: 2,100 to 2,300 Calories per Day
Number of Meals: 6

GROUP 1: MEAT, POULTRY, AND BEANS

These foods ensure adequate protein intake, as well as providing iron and other essential nutrients.

Recommended amount: Three 3- to 4-ounce servings per day

Average number of calories per day: 600

Suggested sources:

- White meat chicken, no skin
- White meat turkey, no skin
- Turkey leg, no skin
- Veal, any style
- Lean beef, any style
- Tuna, packed in water only
- Dry beans, lentils (avoid peas and soybeans)

You can also have any type of broiled or baked fish, including flounder, cod, sole, shrimp, scallops, or lobster. You should also include a portion of any type of liver in your diet at least once a week, broiled or baked. Two eggs, cooked well to avoid bacterial infections, can be eaten up to three times weekly. (Hard boiled eggs are the safest.)

GROUP 2: COMPLEX CARBOHYDRATES AND GRAINS

These foods provide energy, and studies show they may help encourage the flow of reproductive hormones by promoting better functioning of body-to-brain signals. They also provide important vitamins and minerals.

Recommended amounts: Five or more 1-cup servings per day

Average number of calories per day: 600 to 800

Suggested sources:

- Whole-grain pasta
- Potato (one medium, baked)
- Rice
- Oatmeal
- Cereal (dry), 1 ounce
- Oat, wheat, or bran muffins (one average muffin equals one serving)
- Whole-wheat bread (one slice equals one serving)

GROUP 3: CALCIUM

These foods provide not only calcium, but phosphorus, protein, and important vitamins necessary for the healthy functioning of your reproductive system.

Recommended amount: Four or more servings

Average calories per day: 400 to 500

Average serving size: 1 cup (or equivalent)

Suggested sources:

- Low-fat milk (one 8-ounce glass)
- Low-fat yogurt (12 ounces)
- Low-fat cottage cheese (1 1/3 cups)
- Low-fat cheese (1 1/2 ounces or 1 1/2 slices)
- Broccoli (1 cup)
- Sardines (3 ounces)
- Kale (1 cup)
- Low-fat ice cream (1 1/2 cups)

GROUP 4: FRUITS AND VEGETABLES

These foods help you fight off infections that can disrupt fertility, in addition to providing vitamins and minerals. Select at least one serving rich in vitamin A (a dark yellow or leafy green vegetable) and one rich in vitamin C (for example, a citrus fruit). Fresh, organic produce is best, but be sure to wash it thoroughly and then eat it raw or lightly steamed.

Recommended amount: Four or more servings per day

Average number of calories per day: 300 to 400

Serving size: Vegetables, 1 cup raw, 1/2 cup cooked; fruits, 1 medium-sized fruit, 1/2 cup fruit juice, 1/2 cup cooked fruit

Suggested sources:

Vegetables: Cabbage, brussels sprouts, carrots, green beans, broccoli, winter squash, cauliflower
Fruits: Oranges, grapefruits (one-half per serving), apples, bananas, cantaloupe (one-half per serving), honeydew melon (one-half per serving), strawberries (1/2 cup per serving)

GROUP 5: LIQUIDS

Recommended amount: 8 to 10 cups daily, including milk and fruit juices

Choose from the following:

- Spring water
- Tap water
- Low-sodium bouillon
- Herbal tea
- Seltzer (plain or flavored)
- Low-sodium clear soup

GROUP 6: FATS

Recommended amount: About 2 teaspoons daily

Average number of calories per day: 100 maximum

Choose from the following:

- Butter
- Margarine
- Polyunsaturated oil
- Low-sodium salad dressing

Sample Meal Plan for One Day

MEAL 1

Orange juice (1 cup) (group 4)
Toast (two slices) (group 2)
Milk (8 ounces) (group 3)
Eggs (two) (group 1)

MEAL 2

Cantaloupe (one-half) (group 4)
Veal patty with cheese on whole-wheat toast (groups 1, 2, 3)
Lettuce-and-tomato salad (group 4) with cold-pressed sesame seed oil
    and vinegar dressing (group 6)
Spring water (8 ounces) (group 5)

MEAL 3

Broccoli (1 cup) (group 4)
Pasta (1 cup) (group 2)
Milk (8 ounces) (group 3)
White-meat turkey (3 to 4 ounces) (group 1)
Apple (one) (group 4)

MEAL 4

Bran muffin (one) (group 2)
Milk (8 ounces) (group 3)

MEAL 5

Yogurt (8 ounces) (group 3)
Vegetable juice (1 cup) (group 4)
Whole-wheat crackers (four) (group 2)

MEAL 6

Ice cream (1 1/2 cups) (group 3)
Spring water (8 ounces) (group 5)

In addition, add one to two glasses of spring water, herbal tea, or bouillon between meals.

Chapter Twelve

Mother Nature's Bounty:

All-Natural Ways to Increase Your Fertility
(Including the Vitamins, Minerals,
and Herbs That Can Help)

There is no question that some of the most futuristic fertility procedures and treatments have become realities today.

Still, we must never forget that at the core of all these technological advances remains one of the most *natural* biological functions, and that is conception.

For this reason, I have always believed that one of the best ways in which to encourage fertility is to rely on Mother Nature herself. And one of the most important ways to do just that is with vitamins and minerals, nutrients that are becoming increasingly valuable as a way to fine-tune your fertility potential as well as protect your baby from the moment of conception.

While eating good, nutritious meals—like the kind featured in the previous chapter—will go a long way, it can only do so much. Food processing, along with environmental and lifestyle factors you read about earlier in this book, can rob you of the nutrients you do eat, allowing even the most nutritious diet to come up dangerously short. This is where vitamin and mineral *supplements* can help.

What should you be taking in the weeks and months before you want to conceive?

Most fertility specialists now agree that one to two prenatal vitamins daily (the kind normally taken by women who are already pregnant) starting six months before you want to conceive is a must. Sold under brand names such as Stuart Natale Plus One, Natabec RX, and Natalins RX, these vitamins are available by prescription only. So, if your doctor does not automatically recommend prenatal vitamins, do bring them to his or her attention.

In addition, many over-the-counter companies are now offering prenatal vitamins that come close to, or even exceed, the formulas offered in the prescription versions. Since the cost is generally lower, do talk to your doctor about whether these are okay for you.

The Vitamin You Need Most: Folic Acid

No doubt you have already heard about the power of this wonder vitamin to safeguard your baby from some major birth defects.

In just one study of some twenty-three thousand women conducted at the Boston University Center for Human Genetics we learned that by simply meeting a dietary requirement of just 1 mg of folic acid daily in the first six weeks of pregnancy, you can decrease your baby's risk of neural tube defect, a serious congenital malformation that often results in infant death.

Additionally, the National Institute of Child Health and Human Development reports that adding folic acid to your diet during your reproductive years can reduce your baby's risk of both brain and spinal cord defects by almost half. In fact, even increasing your intake of folic acid by a small amount—just 100 mcg (micrograms) a day—can reduce certain birth defects by up to 22 percent. Up your intake to just 400 mcg a day and cut your baby's risks up to 71 percent.

Since you may be pregnant six, eight, or even ten weeks before knowing it, building adequate pregnancy nutritional reserves ahead of time can help ensure that your body will always be ready to protect your baby, regardless of when conception occurs.

But that's not all this powerful nutrient can do for you. A number of clinical trials have shown that taking adequate folic acid before conception may also boost fertility—as much as 4 percent in many women!

(See the Vitamin-Mineral Support Guide later in this chapter to determine how much folic acid you should be taking.)

Folic Acid and Miscarriages: What You Need to Know

Although overwhelming evidence of the positive benefits of folic acid has dominated the news, it's possible you may have also heard one or two isolated reports concerning links to an increased risk of miscarriage. Since this is such a vital nutrient for pregnancy as well as fertility, it's important that you fully understand how and why these reports came about.

It's true that at least one study—a research program conducted in Hungary on some twenty-eight hundred women—found that those who took folic acid had a 16 percent increased risk of miscarriage when compared with women who took no supplements. However, many researchers believe strongly that the pregnancies that were lost were destined to produce children with severe birth defects. Some studies now suggest that the way in which folic acid protects against birth defects is by helping the body to recognize and subsequently naturally abort a fetus with severe defects. This, in fact, may be the basis of the pregnancy losses noted in the Hungarian study.

More Fertility Nutrients: What You Need to Know

Yes, folic acid and other prenatal vitamins can get you off to a good start. But if you are planning to get pregnant and any of the following factors are present in your life, you may need to increase your nutrient intake over and above what your prenatal vitamin supplies.

Think about taking additional vitamin supplements if:

- Your regular diet has consisted primarily of carbohydrates, processed sugars, and artificially sweetened foods.
- You eat a lot of chocolate and drink coffee, tea, or colas.

- You smoke more than ten cigarettes a day.
- You consume more than two alcoholic drinks a day (or fourteen drinks per week).
- You currently take birth control pills, or took them for a long period of time.
- You live or work in a highly polluted or industrialized area.
- You have fibroid tumors, excessive menstrual bleeding, or anemia.

To find out exactly which extra supplements you may need, see the following Fertility Vitamin-Mineral Support Guide.

The Fertility Vitamin-Mineral Support Guide

Vitamins

NUTRIENT: VITAMIN A

ACOG recommendation: Up to 100 micrograms retinol equivalents daily

Effects on fertility: Although studies linking vitamin A to fertility are scarce, there is evidence that in some women deficiencies can contribute to symptoms of PMS by affecting levels of estrogen and progesterone. Since these same imbalances can also contribute to biochemical infertility, researchers theorize that vitamin A deficiencies may, in some women, also be linked to infertility.

Because vitamin A is essential to sperm production, deficiencies in men have been directly linked to infertility. Although treatment with vitamin A will not improve the fertility status of men who have no deficiency, if a lack of this vitamin does exist, supplements can restore sperm count and improve potency.

Role in pregnancy: Forms baby's tooth enamel and hair, helps growth of the thyroid gland

Signs of deficiency: Night blindness, rough, dry skin, decreased sense of smell, fatigue, skin blemishes

My recommended supplements:
Men: Up to 10,000 IU daily
Women: Take only the amount found in a prenatal vitamins. An excess of vitamin A can lead to increased risk of birth defects
My suggested food sources: Fish, egg yolks (no more than three a week), fortified low-fat milk (check the label), dark green and yellow vegetables and fruits (particularly cantaloupe and apricots).

NUTRIENT: VITAMIN B$_1$ (Thiamin)

ACOG recommendations: 1.1 mg daily
Effects on fertility: No information available
Role in pregnancy: Aids in baby's growth and development, contributes to successful breast feeding
Signs of deficiency: Easy fatigue, loss of appetite, irritability, emotional instability
My suggested supplements: Men and women: 100 mg of B-Complex supplement daily
My suggested food sources: The most potent source of this nutrient is fresh, lean pork, followed by whole grains, dried beans, nuts, and seeds.

NUTRIENT: VITAMIN B$_2$ (Riboflavin)

ACOG recommendations: 1.2 to 1.5 mg daily
Effects on fertility: No specific information available
Role in pregnancy: Aids in general growth and development of fetus; deficiencies in mother during pregnancy linked to birth defects in baby, including cleft palate, heart malformations, lack of growth of arm and leg bones, eye problems
Signs of deficiency: Sore mouth, including cracks in lips, red and sore tongue, visual disturbances, eye fatigue, scaly skin, dizziness
My suggested supplements: Men and women: 100 mg of B-Complex daily
My suggested food sources: Low-fat dairy products (including milk,

cheese, and yogurt), plus liver, beef, fish, and fortified breads and cereals (check the labels)

NUTRIENT: VITAMIN B₃ (Niacin)

ACOG recommendations: 13 to 16 mg daily

Effects on fertility: Because niacin is necessary for the synthesis of the sex hormones needed for conception, researchers theorize that fertility will suffer if this nutrient is in short supply.

Role in pregnancy: Builds brain cells and transfers energy to your baby

Signs of deficiency: Muscular weakness, general fatigue, loss of appetite, indigestion, bad breath, insomnia, depression

My suggested supplements: Men and Women: 100 mg B-Complex daily

My suggested food sources: High-protein foods such as chicken, beef, fish, and nuts, and niacin-enriched breads, cereals, and pasta

NUTRIENT: VITAMIN B₆

ACOG recommendations: 2 to 2.5 mg daily

Effects on fertility: Reports indicate that vitamin B_6 improves fertility by increasing levels of serotonin and dopamine, two brain chemicals that influence the production of reproductive hormones FSH and LH, both necessary for ovulation. When levels of B_6 are low, studies indicate these reproductive hormones may also be in short supply.

When, however, deficiencies of other B vitamins are present, particularly B_2, B_6 may actually yield a negative effect, leading to hormonal disruption rather than harmony. For this reason, be certain to always take B_6 in conjunction with a full B-Complex supplement, as well as adequate supplies of magnesium, a mineral necessary for the body to use B_6.

Interestingly, reports issued as early as 1979 showed that unexplained infertility could be overcome when women consumed between 100 and 800 mg of B_6 daily. Because the study was relatively small, these results are in no way considered conclusive. However, it is further indication that B$_6$ has at least some influence over a woman's reproductive system.

Role in pregnancy: Aids in development of healthy fetus; helps ease morning sickness during first trimester of pregnancy; deficiency during pregnancy can lead to edema (swelling) and high blood pressure as well as increased risk of cleft palate in your baby

Signs of deficiency: Depression, dermatitis

My suggested supplements: Men and women: Up to 500 mg daily, in balance with 100 mg of B-Complex daily. Stop supplements and rely only on the amount of B$_6$ found in prenatal vitamins once your pregnancy has been confirmed.

My suggested food sources: Fish, poultry, beef, chickpeas, potatoes, and bananas

NUTRIENT: VITAMIN B$_{12}$

ACOG recommendations: 3 to 4 mg daily

Effects on fertility: Although studies linking vitamin B$_{12}$ and fertility are scarce, those that do exist continue to show that a deficiency can exacerbate menstrual disturbances, including irregular cycles. The connecting factor: the ability of B$_{12}$ to influence regular ovulation.

Role in pregnancy: Aids in development of baby's red blood cells; helps avoid oxygen deprivation, which in turn can lead to birth defects, especially brain damage

Signs of deficiency: Nervousness, body odor, menstrual disturbances, difficulty in walking

My suggested supplements: Men and women: 100 mg of B-Complex daily (including at least 3 to 4 mg of B$_{12}$)

My suggested food sources: Brewer's yeast, oysters, sardines, eggs (no more than three times weekly), beef, and low-fat cheese.

NUTRIENT: VITAMIN C

ACOG recommendation: 60 mg daily before pregnancy; 80 mg daily after conception

Effects on fertility: As we age, our sex glands develop a greater need for vitamin C. If supplies are limited, our body will draw what it needs from whatever tissues harbor the most. Once those sources are depleted, however, your sex glands can become so severely impaired it can affect your ability to reproduce.

Conversely, when vitamin C intake is too high, it can also increase your risk of reproductive problems, causing, among other problems, infertility, premature birth, and miscarriage.

In men, studies show vitamin C can affect sperm motility, viability, and ability to mature. One reason: Seminal fluid, as well as sperm cells, contains high levels of all antioxidant vitamins, particularly vitamin C. (See Chapter 4 for more information on how vitamin C affects sperm.) The good news: When a deficiency exists, just 500 mg every twelve hours was shown to restore male fertility in just four days!

Additionally, when antioxidant vitamins, particularly vitamin C, are added directly to sperm during preparation for laboratory conception (read more about this in Part Three), it may increase the likelihood of conception. If you plan on a laboratory-aided conception, talk to your fertility specialist about the possibility of adding antioxidant vitamins directly to your partner's sperm before it is mixed with your eggs.

Finally, studies at the University of Texas Medical Branch in Galveston found that vitamin C may help the body rid itself of lead, nicotine, and other toxic substances capable of affecting fertility.

Role in pregnancy: Aids in the development of baby's skin, tendons, and bones through the formation of collagen; maternal deficiencies can cause abnormalities in baby's bones and teeth

Signs of deficiency: Shortness of breath, impaired digestion, bleeding gums, tendency to bruise, slow healing of wounds

My Suggested supplements:

Men: Up to 1,500 mg daily

Women: Up to 1,000 mg daily over what a prenatal vitamin offers until pregnancy is confirmed, after which time, two prenatal vitamins daily supply all your basic needs. **Important:** Depleting factors include regular use of aspirin, birth control pills, stress, tobacco, alcohol, and recreational drugs.

My suggested food sources: Citrus fruits and juices, broccoli, red peppers, strawberries, tomatoes

NUTRIENT: FOLIC ACID

ACOG recommendations: 400 mcg (micrograms) daily before conception; up to 800 mcg daily after conception

Effects on fertility: See "The Vitamin You Need Most," above

Role in pregnancy: See above

Signs of deficiency: Prematurely gray hair, inflamed tongue, gastrointestinal disturbances, anemia

My suggested supplements:

Men: None—a multivitamin containing folic acid meets requirements.

Women: Up to 1 mg (1,000 mcg) daily total

My suggested food supplements: Beans, green vegetables, whole grains, and orange juice

NUTRIENT: VITAMIN D

ACOG recommendations: 10 to 15 mcg daily

Effects on fertility: Because some vitamin D receptors are found in the hypothalamus gland and in the ovaries, deficiencies might impair the reproductive functions of both, in women as well as men. (See "How the Sun Can Help You Get Pregnant," in Chapter 13.)

Role in pregnancy: Works with calcium to help your baby build strong bones and teeth

Signs of deficiency: Tetany (a form of muscular weakness), numbness, tingling, and muscle spasms

My suggested supplements:

Men: Up to 400 IUs daily

Women: Only that which is present in one to two prenatal vitamins daily. Excess vitamin D during the first twelve weeks of pregnancy has been linked to birth defects

My suggested food sources: Fatty fish such as herring, salmon, and tuna are rich in this vitamin. However, the best source still remains fortified milk—and you should choose the low-fat or no-fat variety.

For your information: A fat-soluble vitamin that is not readily excreted, vitamin D is now added to many foods, so single supplements are rarely necessary. It is also made naturally in your body when you are exposed to sun, although production does stop when you get a suntan. Because pregnancy can make some women highly sensitive to vitamin D, toxic levels (espccially those linked to birth defects) can occur if you take as little as two to three times the recommended daily allowance.

Nutrient: Vitamin E

ACOG recommendations: Up to 10 mg daily

Effects on fertility: A number of studies have shown that a severe vitamin E deficiency is linked to increased risk of premature labor and miscarriage. Additionally, getting enough vitamin E may help regulate menstrual flow and rhythm, leading some researchers to believe it may increase fertility by helping to promote more regular ovulation.

Studies involving male fertility have shown that a deficiency in vitamin E may increase the risk of the degeneration of testicle tissue, affecting sperm production and maturation. Should this type of damage occur, restoring nutrient levels won't help, so it's essential that your partner never allow even a slight dip in E levels, particularly when you are trying to conceive. Also important: Vitamin E is stored in the liver, fatty tissue, heart, muscles, testes, uterus, blood, and adrenal and pituitary glands. However, it only remains in the body for a short period of time, with up to 70 percent excreted in the feces. And that means a deficiency may occur faster and more easily than you realize.

Role in pregnancy: Promotes lung maturation. When premature births are the result of vitamin E deficiency, infants can be born susceptible to anemia. When the child's E quotient is low, hemorrhaging can occur. The blood cells of E-deficient babies are also prone to weakness.

Signs of deficiency: Gastrointestinal distress, anemia, rupture of red blood cells

My suggested supplements:

Men: Up to 800 IUs daily total

Women: Up to 400 IUs daily, in addition to prenatal supplement (a total of about 800 IUs daily) until pregnancy is confirmed. Once you are pregnant, stop all extra supplements and rely only on prenatal vitamin.

My suggested food sources: Wheat germ is an excellent source, with just 2 tablespoons offering some 50 IUs of E. Also most vegetable oils, nuts, seeds, green leafy vegetables, and whole grains contain significant amounts of this vitamin.

The Essential Minerals

In addition to vitamins, the following four minerals have special importance in relation to fertility and pregnancy:

Calcium

ACOG recommendations: 800 to 1,600 mg daily

Effects on fertility: When calcium is in short supply, the output of estrogen decreases, affecting egg production and ovulation. Since your reproductive health depends not only on the presence of estrogen but on precise amounts of this hormone, calcium is a key to good reproductive health.

Role in pregnancy: Beginning in the second trimester, calcium is used to form your baby's skeletal system and teeth. It is also essential for lactation (breast feeding). A deficiency can cause your baby to develop bones that are less dense and weaker than normal.

Signs of deficiency: Numbness and tingling in arms and legs, cramps in muscles, joint pains, heart palpitations, slow pulse rate, tooth decay, insomnia, excessive irritability of nerves and muscles, menstrual pain, PMS.

My suggested supplements:

Men: Up to 800 mg daily

Women: Up to 500 mg daily, in addition to what your prenatal vitamin supplies, depending on depletion factors

My suggested food sources: Low-fat or nonfat dairy products, which, ounce for ounce, actually contain more calcium than the higher-fat varieties. Fortified orange juice is also a good choice, as well as broccoli, collard greens, and almonds.

IRON

ACOG recommendations: 18 mg daily before pregnancy; up to 75 mg daily after pregnancy

Effects on fertility: By causing anemia (a reduction in your supply of red blood cells), an iron deficiency can disrupt the menstrual cycle, in some cases bringing it to a complete halt. (Some believe this disruption might be your body's natural defense system for conserving depleted red blood cells.) If your menstrual cycle is affected by iron deficiency anemia, the timing and function of ovulation and all reproductive hormones can be thrown out of kilter, affecting fertility.

Role in pregnancy: Needed by your baby to form his or her own blood cells and to build a stored supply. Most fetal iron is obtained through the placental blood flow, but some can be taken directly from your body as well. The fetus, the placenta, and your own expanding blood volume during pregnancy require considerable iron, so supplements are always recommended.

It is extremely vital that you correct all iron deficiencies before conceiving, since a depletion that continues could be a sign of anemia. The latest studies show if you are anemic when you conceive, the risk of premature birth and other pregnancy complications is higher.

*Signs of depletion:*Anemia, pale skin, abnormal fatigue, constipation, lusterless and brittle nails, difficulty in breathing. Calcium and iron are the most commonly deficient nutrients in women. Before pregnancy, your body absorbs about 10 percent of the iron you take in, but by the time you are into your second trimester, your iron intake increases threefold. (Absorption is also increased by vitamin C, folic acid, and vitamin B_{12}.)

My suggested supplements:

Men: Unless anemia exists, a multivitamin should cover all needs. If signs of depletion exist, see your doctor before taking supplements.

Women: One to two iron pills a day, depending on depletion factors

My suggested food sources: Lean red meat, liver, clams, oysters, mussels, broccoli, peas, beans, dried apricots and raisins, pumpkins, squash, and sunflower seeds

Magnesium

ACOG recommendation: 300 to 450 mg daily, or one-half the amount of calcium supplement

Effects on fertility: Works with B$_6$ to regulate hormone production and control PMS

Role in pregnancy: Allows your baby to absorb adequate calcium for development of bone and teeth

Signs of deficiency: Apprehension, muscle twitch, tremors, confusion, disorientation

My suggested supplements:

Men and women: One-half the amount of your calcium supplement

My suggested food sources: Whole grains, nuts, legumes, dark green leafy vegetables, and shellfish

Zinc

ACOG recommendations: 15 to 20 mg daily

Effects on fertility: As early as puberty, a deficiency of zinc can affect the development of the sex organs, inhibiting both growth and maturation. Later in life, a zinc deficiency has been associated with various types of reproductive problems in both men and women.

In fact, if your partner experiences even a minimal zinc deficiency he can also suffer from both low testosterone and a low sperm count—enough to cause infertility. It also can lead to unhealthy changes in the size and structure of the prostate gland, which contains more zinc than any other part of the body. In prostate illness, especially cancer, zinc levels drop, leading to infertility. Ironically, too much zinc can have a toxic effect on sperm and also result in infertility. (For more information on zinc and male fertility see Chapter 4.)

Role in pregnancy: Deficiencies during pregnancy can result in a variety of birth defects, including skeletal and brain malformations, cardiovascular problems, and defects in the central nervous system of your baby. A zinc deficiency can also cause you prolonged labor, excess bleeding, eclampsia, higher risk of infection, and hypertension during your pregnancy.

Signs of deficiency: Abnormal fatigue, loss of normal taste sensitivity, poor appetite, and suboptimal growth

My suggested supplements:

Men: Up to 100 mg daily

Women: Up to 20 mg daily, in addition to what is supplied in your prenatal vitamin, depending on depletion factors

My suggested food sources: Lean beef, pork, dark meat poultry, eggs, seafood (especially oysters), cheese, beans, nuts, and wheat germ

Megadosing: Too Much of a Good Thing?

A number of years ago some researchers began advocating supplement megadosing, the practice of using excessively large amounts of vitamins and minerals (more than ten times the recommended daily allowance per dose) to treat everything from stress to immune system deficiencies to disease—even infertility! Can massive doses of vitamins help? And more important can they harm you or your baby?

The facts are thus: It is easier to develop toxic effects from the fat-soluble vitamins—A, D, and E—because they are stored in the body. So, megadosing of these nutrients may harm your fertility as well as your overall health and the health of your baby. The water-soluble vitamins—C and B-Complex—leave your body within twenty-four hours, so they are considered relatively safe in all but the most grossly excessive amounts.

While hard evidence linking nutrient megadoses and fertility or pregnancy problems is scarce, the following has been reported:

- Vitamin A: Taken in excess of 25,000 IUs daily during pregnancy, it increases your baby's risk of bladder malformation, cleft palate, eye damage, and webbed fingers and toes.
- Vitamin D: More than ten times the RDA may decrease sexual desire.
- Vitamin B_6: 2,000 to 6,000 mg daily may cause nerve damage.
- Vitamin C: 12,000 mg or more daily during pregnancy may cause your baby to be born with an abnormal dependance on this nutri-

ent, leading to a condition called "rebound scurvy." This causes irritability and pain in the arms, legs, bones, and muscles. In addition, excessive vitamin C can decrease the absorption of copper, a trace mineral essential to ovulation. It can also cause a false positive in certain urine and stool tests.

- Zinc: An excess of more than 2,000 mg daily can cause gastrointestinal distress and may upset the balance of other important minerals, bringing about deficiencies that can affect fertility and the health of your baby.

By sticking to the formulas found in prenatal vitamin prescriptions (and following your physician's advice about supplements), you can be sure you are giving your body the most positive nutritional power available.

The Fertility Plants: The Herbs and Flowers That May Help You Get Pregnant

Although many Western doctors are just beginning to turn to the Eastern practice of using herbs and other plants for medicinal purposes, I have long believed in the power of Mother Nature's bounty to aid a number of medical conditions, among them infertility. While no one plant or herb can have the power of, for example, a commercial fertility drug, they can, in many instances, have a cumulative healing effect that ultimately may increase your ability to conceive. This is particularly true if your infertility problems are caused by certain hormone imbalances, or if your doctor has diagnosed you with "unexplained" infertility.

You should, however, also know that, unlike Western medications, which are largely synthetic or chemical preparations, natural substances derived from plants and flowers can cause very individual reactions in each person who tries them. This is particularly true in regard to dosages and the speed and success with which they work. For this reason, you may need to take some time to learn about your own body and its reaction to certain natural ingredients before you can determine the precise herbal combinations that may work for you.

With that information in hand, you may very well be able to take advantage of some of the best Mother Nature has to offer!

Vitex: The Fertility Herb

Although its name sounds more like that of a modern pharmaceutical, Vitex is, in fact, one of nature's most powerful herbs. Short for *Vitex agnus-castus L*, and also known as "chasteberry," this flowering plant of Mediterranean origins has been used for hundreds of years in the treatment of a variety of gynecological complaints. In Germany, chasteberry is one of the foremost remedies "prescribed" by medical doctors for the treatment of PMS—and therein lies its link to fertility.

It is thought to work by affecting the function of both the pituitary and hypothalamus glands—each of which is responsible for the production and release of various hormones that stimulate egg production and ovulation, including GnRH, FSH, and LH. In the process, Vitex also exerts a stabilizing effect on both estrogen and progesterone. In studies conducted at the University of Göttingen in Sweden, researchers learned that although Vitex does not contain either hormone, it can help regulate their production.

Studies have also shown Vitex may be particularly helpful if you are diagnosed with a corpus luteum deficiency, or an excess of prolactin, another hormone that can affect fertility. (Read more about these conditions in Part Three of this book.)

In the very latest Vitex research—a double-blind, controlled study of nearly two hundred women—German researchers found it was so effective in reducing the symptoms of PMS, it worked far better than vitamin B_6, long used to help control symptoms. Although women who wanted to get pregnant were excluded from this study, a nice "side effect" of the research was five pregnancies.

For supplementation: The typical dosage for Vitex in several studies is between 3.5 and 4.2 mg daily. Some naturopathic physicians, however, recommend the chasteberry extract form, in strengths from 175 mg to 225 mg per day. As with all natural products, there is always the chance for side effects, which, in the case of Vitex, can include headaches, gastrointestinal upsets, and lower abdominal complaints.

The British Fertility Herb

Among the most popular British fertility remedies is the little-known herb *Chamaelirium luteum*. As a tonic, it is often prescribed to tone the uterus and ovaries, and has been used to help rebalance a variety of reproductive hormones in both men and women. In men, tea made from this flowering plant has been known to have curative powers over impotency. When taken during pregnancy, it may also help reduce the risk of miscarriage, mostly by helping to prevent uterine hemorrhage.

The American Indian Fertility Remedy

I'll never forget one of my very first fertility patients, a young woman of American Indian origin. She had come to see me when, after a little more than a year of trying, she was unable to conceive. She was concerned, she said, that some structural abnormality, such as a fibroid tumor or ovarian cyst, might be behind her infertility.

After examining her, I reassured her this was not so. "Now," she said, "I can do what my great-grandmother suggested, without hesitation." And what, I couldn't help but ask, had her grandmother told her to try? "An old Indian herbal remedy known as black cohosh," she said. Although it wasn't the first time I had heard of this herb—I had long known it to be useful for menopausal complaints—it was the first time I had heard it suggested as a treatment for infertility.

Sure enough, however, a little more than six months later, this young woman was back in my office, with a decidedly telling "glow" on her face. She was indeed pregnant, a feat that she is convinced was due to her daily regimen of black cohosh. While I'm not so certain it was the herb alone that helped her—perhaps just knowing that she had no serious problems helped her relax enough to get pregnant—still, I cannot discount the fact that this particular herb can have some powerful hormonal effects.

How black cohosh works: As I already mentioned, the black cohosh plant has been used for many generations as a natural treatment for menopausal complaints, particularly the hormonal fluctuations responsible for hot flashes, night sweats, and mood swings. It has also worked as an antispasmodic, to relieve menstrual cramps. In terms of enhancing fertility, I believe it may work in one of two ways. First, by normalizing hormonal activity, it may help foster more regular ovulation. In addition, its antispasmodic effects on the reproductive tract may prevent a newly fertilized egg from being pushed down the fallopian tube too quickly, before the uterus is ready for a healthy implantation.

For supplementation: Although the newest edition of the *PDR— The Physician's Desk Reference for Herbal Medicines*—says that there is no scientific evidence to show this herb does work on a woman's reproductive system, still, I continue to see patients who tell me that it does, indeed, make a difference. If you are going to try black cohosh, look for supplements that are "standardized" to contain 1 mg of triterpenes (sometimes noted on the package as 1 mg 27-deoxyacteine), the active ingredient in this herb. The usual dosage is between one and two tablets (up to 2 mg of 27-deoxyacteine) daily.

The Herbal "Cocktail" to Boost Fertility

Using its own unique methods of diagnosis and prescription, traditional Chinese medicine often focuses on ways to unblock energy pathways in the body. When energy flows freely from our brain, down our spine, and throughout our body, Chinese medicine practitioners believe we can obtain optimum health. Likewise, when something blocks an energy pathway, disease can result.

One of the most important ways in which Chinese medicine works to restore both energy and harmony to the body is through the use of various herbs. In terms of reproductive problems, those herbs include a specific quartet of plants that are believed to work synergistically to enhance reproductive energy and health.

These four herbs are:

- Dong Quai (*Angelica sinensis*)
- Ligusticum
- Rehmanii
- White peony

The Herbal Tea That Can Harm Fertility

If you are like many of my patients, you probably enjoy the relaxation and health benefits of a steaming cup of herbal tea. While I often recommend just such a remedy—particularly for women undergoing the stress of trying to conceive, there are several ingredients commonly found in many commercial herbal teas that can actually reduce your ability to conceive.

These include the Mexican herb known as zoapatle, as well as the more common hibiscus flower, the latter of which is often found in many herbal tea "blends."

In the case of zoapatle, a period may be induced, thus causing you to immediately lose any embryo that you have conceived. In the case of hibiscus flower, you may experience an actual reduction in the production of certain key fertility hormones, particularly those produced by the pituitary gland. In men, hibiscus may negatively affect the testes, reducing sperm production.

If there is any chance that you might be pregnant, you should also avoid the following herbs, which may increase the risk of miscarriage:

- Southernwood
- Wormwood
- Mugwort
- Barberry
- Celandine
- Golden seal
- Feverfew
- Tansy
- Mandrake root
- Blood root
- Broom
- Juniper
- Pennyroyal
- Nutmeg (in large amounts)
- Arbor vitae
- Senna

Collectively, they are often known as Dong Quai Four and are frequently sold that way in Chinese or health food stores. (Other, similar formulas are sold as "Women's Precious" or "Eight Precious Pills".) Since dosages can vary widely depending on the strength of the product you buy, always follow the directions on the label.

How does Dong Quai Four work? Together, these four herbs are said to promote pelvic circulation, and in doing so, restore blocked energy passages that otherwise block fertility. Because of their stimulating effect, these herbs should not be used during an active menstrual cycle (stop taking the pills as soon as your period begins and resume after the last day of bleeding), and they should not be taken during pregnancy. In fact, if you try this remedy to help you get pregnant, stop as soon as you believe you may have conceived.

Other herbs that often work with Dong Quai Four include Vitex, false unicorn root, partridge berry, and camp bark.

The Helpful Herbs That May Harm Fertility

Perhaps you or your partner have already joined the millions of consumers worldwide who regularly use a variety of herbs to treat such common ailments as colds, flu, mild depression, or memory loss. But did you know that some of these popular preparations can also have a devastating effect on fertility? It's true. Laboratory studies published in 1999 in the journal *Fertility and Sterility* revealed that in high concentrations, the most commonly used herbs—**Saint-John's-wort**, **Echinacea**, and **Ginkgo Biloba**—were found to affect an egg's capacity to be permeated by sperm and should be avoided by couples trying to conceive.

- **Saint-John's-wort**, which is often used to treat mild depression, was also found to have mutagenic effects on sperm—causing a damaging change in the DNA structure. At this point, no one is certain why this occurs. Additionally, this herb may also affect a gene known as BRCA1, a tumor suppressor that, when mutated, could increase a woman's risk of both breast and ovarian cancer.

- **Echinacea,** an herb frequently used to help prevent colds, appeared to have no direct effect on eggs, but it did alter the head of sperm, changing the chemical composition of the enzymes needed to penetrate an egg's outer shell. It also appeared to affect the basic DNA of sperm.

- **Ginkgo Biloba,** often used in the treatment of memory loss, appears to cause eggs to degenerate and affects the ability of sperm to penetrate the shell. Although this herb is considered a powerful antioxidant—which in most instances is a plus for sperm—in this instance it had a clearly detrimental effect.

In addition to these three herbs, the study also looked at the effects of **saw palmetto**, often used in the treatment of benign prostate disease. The good news: It was not found to have any negative effects on fertility, and it did not appear to affect the DNA of sperm.

If you are trying to get pregnant, I suggest that both you and your partner avoid using Saint-John's-wort, Echinacea, and Ginkgo Biloba for a minimum of three months, and if possible, longer, before attempting conception. Once you are pregnant, you should also avoid these three herbs, and continue to avoid them if you are at high risk for either breast or ovarian cancer. While these studies were conducted in a laboratory, and not on human beings, which means that they may very well be proven wrong sometime in the future, the results are alarming enough to warrant cautious and judicious use until more research can confirm or deny these findings.

All-Natural Male Fertility Boosters

In much the same way that some herbs can boast female fertility, so too can several herbs boost your partner's ability to father a child.

As with your own reproductive health, I do not believe he should forgo medical treatment, and particularly diagnosis, in favor of using only the "natural" approach. However, I do believe he should thoroughly investigate all his options, including whatever Mother Nature has to offer.

What the French Know About Male Fertility

France is not only famous for giving us some of the world's greatest lovers, now it may also be responsible for giving us healthier, more fertile sperm! The reason is a little-known nutrient called pycnogenol, which just happens to come from the bark of pine trees indigenous to certain regions of France.

In a small but significant study conducted by an independent fertility clinic in New Jersey, it was learned that men who took just 200 mg of pycnogenol daily from French pine tree bark, for just ninety days, were able to increase the health of their sperm by a whopping 99 percent! The highly controlled study, which excluded men who had used any hormone-enhancing medications, as well as those who smoked or drank alcohol, also insisted the participants take no other vitamins, minerals, or herbs during the ninety-day period. After measuring sperm samples for count, motility, and overall health, both before and after the ninety days of pycnogenol therapy, astounding results were seen. The researchers were so impressed with their results they concluded that in some men daily use of pycnogenol may help couples avoid costly laboratory conception procedures in favor of far less expensive and easier methods of conception.

Although there are no long-term studies on the effects of pycnogenol specifically on fertility, long-term usage has shown it to be safe and effective overall, when taken in amounts up to 200 mg daily.

Boost His Fertility with Amino Acids

Amino acids are the biochemicals that help our body use protein. Research shows, however, they can also play a role in fertility. Among the most important to men is L-carnitine, which is found in both seminal plasma and sperm. Acting as a ready source of energy, it is L-carnitine that permits sperm to swim through a woman's reproductive tract to her egg. When levels are low, studies show, sperm motility can suffer. This can easily occur if your partner limits his consumption of red meat, and particularly if he is a vegetarian.

Fortunately, problems can be reversed simply by taking L-carnitine supplements. In studies conducted at the Clinic of Urology in Belgrade, Serbia, doctors reported that when men with clinically low sperm counts took daily doses of L-carnitine supplementation, sperm count as well as motility dramatically increased.

How Much L-Carnitine Should Your Partner Take?

Although no studies exist on the regular or long-term use of this amino acid, research shows most men can safely take up to 2,000 mg daily, in two doses, in a regimen of three weeks on one week off.

However, the *Physician's Desk Reference* suggests doses be limited to no more than 1,200 mg, three times daily, an amount I also feel more comfortable recommending. Be certain, however, that your partner checks with his doctor before using L-carnitine; he should also avoid this supplement if he suffers from liver or kidney disease or diabetes.

A second amino acid your partner should consider taking is arginine, which is necessary for the body to manufacture cells and is essential for the formation of sperm. If, in fact, your partner's sperm count falls below 20 million/ml of ejaculate, it's very likely that arginine supplements may offer a fertility boost. My recommendation is four grams per day for a period of at least three months before attempting conception.

The Chinese Male Fertility Herb

Chinese medicine specialists have long believed that ginseng holds the key to male potency. Current research shows that at least two types of ginseng—Panax and Siberian—have the best overall effects on treating male infertility. Although most of the clinical data is based on animal and not human studies, still, the evidence is impressive enough for most proponents of natural medicine to recommend this herb when male fertility is at stake. What do the animal studies show? An increase in reproductive capacity and sperm count, an increase in sperm development and growth, an increase in testosterone levels, and finally, an increase in what scientists call "mating desire," or as we know it in human terms, sex drive!

Since ginseng supplements can vary widely in potency, simply have your partner follow the directions on the label of his supplement.

Acupuncture and Fertility

If your partner has been diagnosed with low sperm count, or even sperm motility problems (see Part Three of this book), the Chinese medicinal practice known as acupuncture may help. Here experts use a series of needles to stimulate specific points on the body, which in turn are believed to open energy pathways and restore health.

In studies recently presented at the world conference of the American Society for Reproductive Medicine, researchers from Yugoslavia revealed that acupuncture can increase both the number of sperm available for fertilization and sperm motility. A total of ten treatments was needed by the men to yield the full impact. Indeed, the results were so positive that the researchers are now suggesting that all men undergo at least a few acupuncture sessions before participating in any laboratory-assisted reproduction.

Although there are few studies showing acupuncture has a similar positive effect on female fertility, many believe that it does—particularly England's royal family. Currently, Prince Edward's lady love, Sophie Rhys-Jones, has sought treatment with a midwife who specializes in acupuncture (before pregnancy, as well as during pregnancy and childbirth) at the Hale Clinic in London, which features both traditional and alternative medical practitioners. Other royals who have sought treatment at Hale Clinic include the late Princess Diana and Sarah Ferguson, Duchess of York, as well as many top celebrities.

Taking the Natural Approach: A Final Word

There is no question—at least in my mind—that natural products can impact your overall health, as well as affect your fertility. And, for many of you, the natural route will turn out to be the fastest and easiest way to encourage a pregnancy.

That said, I also feel obligated to warn you against what I call the "charlatans" of natural medicine. Whether they be product manufacturers, or so-called alternative medicine experts, they can play on your strong desire to get pregnant and thus promise or guarantee you conception success. I am here to tell you that nothing, not a single product, natural or pharmaceutical, and no one person, not an alternative medicine doctor or even a renowned fertility expert, can give you that guarantee. While your chances for getting pregnant today are far greater than they were even five years ago, in the end, it is still Mother Nature who deals the final hand.

Remember: If you don't get pregnant within six months of using any natural treatment or alternative therapy, see a fertility specialist.

Chapter Thirteen

Making Love and Making Babies: How to Get Pregnant Fast!

Do you make love with the lights on . . . or in the dark?

What position do you most often use when making love?

What do you do right before you have sex . . . and what do you do right afterward?

When do you make love—and how often do you have an orgasm?

While Mother Nature may play the most important role in getting pregnant, there are also many practical aspects of making love that can influence how quickly and easily you conceive. And later in this chapter I will share some of the newest findings about this, as well as pass along some helpful suggestions from my own patients.

However, the first and most important way to ensure that you will get pregnant right away is to make love as close to the time of ovulation as possible. Why is this important? From the moment your egg is released it begins to age. Once ovulated, it remains at peak fertility for only a very short time—for most women, no more than twenty-four hours.

In fact, one of the first large-scale studies on conception—a 1999 report featured in the *New England Journal of Medicine*—found that even one day after ovulation, the chance of getting pregnant drops so dramatically it is almost impossible to conceive. At the same time researchers from the National Institute of Environmental Health Sciences in Research Park, North Carolina, also discovered that to ensure conception, the best time to begin making love is five days prior to ovulation, as well as the day of egg release. Why does this new six-day "window of opportunity" work so well?

Although your egg is fertile for less than twenty-four hours after it is released, sperm can live in your reproductive tract for up to five days. So, making love before you believe you will ovulate is one way to ensure that sperm is on hand and ready for conception whenever your egg arrives.

Predicting Ovulation: How to Tell when You Can Get Pregnant

Needless to say, these new findings have somewhat altered the way we think about charting the course of conception. If, in fact, a pregnancy is most likely to occur if you make love beginning five days before you ovulate, then you will need to be more precise than ever in approximating when your ovulation will occur.

Unfortunately, some of the standard methods for predicting egg release, such as ovulation predictor kits, may not be quite as useful as we once thought. Still, they, along with several other methods, can play a role in helping you to chart an ovulation *pattern* that, ultimately, can help you estimate your most fertile time.

Method One: Using Your Body Temperature to Predict Fertility

As you have already learned, ovulation is governed by a pattern of hormones that are released at various times throughout the menstrual cycle. There are also distinct temperature changes that go along with these hormonal fluctuations, changes that, not coincidentally, can tell you something about your ovulation timetable.

This method of ovulation prediction is called the basal body temperature guide or BBT. Using the BBT involves taking your temperature every day for at least two months. The best way to ensure the success of this method is to start on the first day of a new menstrual cycle.

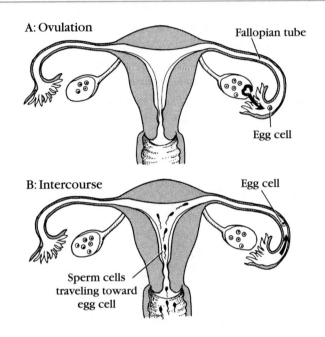

A: Ovulation

Fallopian tube

Egg cell

B: Intercourse

Egg cell

Sperm cells
traveling toward
egg cell

How Conception Occurs

In order for you to get pregnant, you must release an egg from your ovary (Step A: Ovulation). As it pops from its shell, the egg is "caught" by the fimbria, the fingerlike ends of the fallopian tube, and then gently swept inside. There it waits for sperm to arrive. Once you have intercourse (Step B), sperm rush through your cervix into your uterus and swim down

Be sure to take your temperature as soon as you wake up each morning, before getting out of bed, and before eating, drinking, or smoking. Also keep a written record of your temperature changes to help make ovulation patterns clear. (See the sample grids in this chapter.)

To discover your fertility curve—the time of the month when you are most likely to conceive—look for specific drops in body temperature (occurring just before ovulation), followed by a distinct rise (occurring after your egg is released).

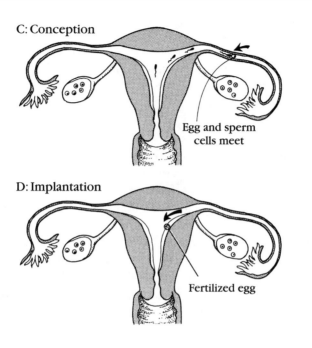

C: Conception

Egg and sperm
cells meet

D: Implantation

Fertilized egg

your fallopian tube, in order to meet your newly ovulated egg. When sperm and egg meet (Step C), conception usually occurs, there in the fallopian tube. The newly formed embryo then takes from five to seven days to travel down the length of the tube and into the uterus, where it attaches itself to the spongy lining (Step D) and begins to grow.

To get pregnant fast: Make love between the time your temperature drops and the time it rises—a period of about twelve to twenty-four hours that usually occurs about thirteen to fifteen days after the start of your menstrual cycle.

Charting Your Five-Day Course to Pregnancy

Although you can increase your chance for a pregnancy if you make love during the five days before ovulation, unfortunately, there are no temperature changes that correlate to this time period.

However, unless you have a particularly erratic ovulation pattern, you should still be able to use the BBT to find your five most fertile days every month. How does this work?

By keeping very accurate BBT reading records for at least two to three months, you can ascertain the time in your cycle when you ovulate. For many women, it is twelve to fourteen days after their first day of bleeding. But whatever your pattern is, it's likely to be pretty consistent from month to month.

So, if after several months of BBT readings you determine that, for example, you ovulate on day twelve of your cycle, during the month you want to conceive, start counting on the first day of bleeding. Numbering this day as "one" use a calender to count ahead twelve days: Mark that day, then count backward five days. This is then the date you want to start making love, which you should continue for that entire week.

Method 2: Listen to Your Body

In addition to a temperature change, there is also another way your body lets you know when ovulation is approaching: through changes in the shape of your cervix and the amount of cervical mucus that is produced.

To check your cervical signs, gently insert your finger into your vagina every day. What are you looking for? Changes in the tactile feel of your cervical mucus as well as the shape of your cervix. Here's what to expect:

1. Start of the menstrual cycle

Mucus—dry. This is the relative condition of your vagina beginning several days after ovulation and continuing for up to nine days after the start of each menstrual cycle.

Corresponding cervical changes: During and right after menstru-

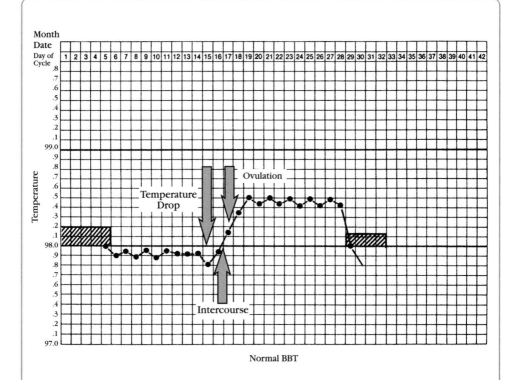

Normal BBT

The BBT or Basal Body Temperature Guide

Fluctuations in your basal body temperature (the temperature of your body upon waking) correlate with hormonal changes that can indicate your most fertile time.

To get pregnant fast: Always make love within the twelve- to twenty-four-hour period between the time your temperature drops (indicating ovulation is about to occur) and when it rises (indicating ovulation has occurred)—usually about twelve to fourteen days into your menstrual cycle.

By taking your BBT upon waking every morning (before you eat, drink, smoke, or get out of bed), and then recording your findings for two to three months' time, you can learn to chart your fertility curve, discovering when your most fertile time will occur in future cycles.

ation your cervix will be in a low position. It will feel firm and have a pointy shape, and it will be relatively easy to touch.

2. *Several days before ovulation*

Mucus: Creamy and wet. Mucus flow starts to increase about nine

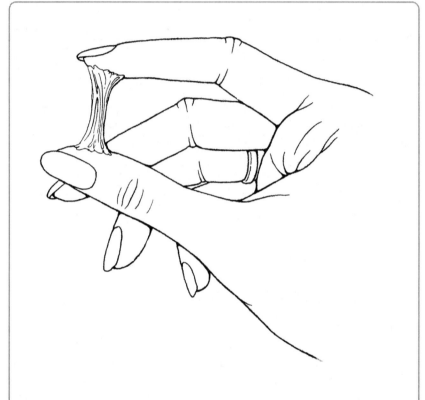

The Cervical Mucus Check

If you want to get pregnant, the best time to begin making love is when your mucus is creamy and wet. To test your mucus, gently insert your finger into your vagina. If mucus sticks easily to your finger and can be pulled between two fingers, much like raw egg white, it is likely you are ready to ovulate, in which case you have a very good chance of getting pregnant, provided you make love within 24 to 36 hours.

days after the start of your menstrual cycle. It has a smooth texture and a creamy white appearance.

3. *Approaching ovulation*

Mucus: Thin, slippery, stretchy, and clear. As you approach ovulation (approximately twelve to fourteen days into your cycle), your mucus takes on the appearance of egg white and has a slimy consistency. This allows it to transport sperm quickly through your vaginal canal and into your fallopian tubes.

Corresponding cervical changes: As you approach ovulation, your cervix will respond to rising estrogen levels by pulling slightly up and rotating forward. This places the opening in a better position for sperm passage. It might be slightly harder to reach; it will feel softer to the touch and be very wet. At this point cervical mucus is at its peak production.

Immediately following ovulation your mucus production takes a sharp decline. Whatever is left becomes gluelike and extremely sticky,

---

Important * Important * Important *

Do not attempt to ascertain your cervical mucus pattern while taking birth control pills, or for several weeks after you discontinue their use. The hormonal fluctuations associated both with pill use and with stoppage can cause wild variations in the quality and quantity of your mucus. Wait at least two months after discontinuing the pill before attempting to establish a mucus ovulation pattern.

Also important: Showering, bathing, and swimming can all temporarily alter the quality and quantity of your mucus, so be sure to check before these activities, or wait several hours afterward.

---

often resembling rubber cement. It remains at this consistency for two to three days, then becomes very dry again. Your cervix drops back down again, responding to a dip in estrogen levels. It will once again feel hard and pointy.

To get pregnant fast: Make love beginning when mucus is creamy and wet—about five days before ovulation is expected. Continue to make love every day until mucus production takes a sharp decline.

Method 3: How Your Saliva Can Help You Get Pregnant — the Newest Way to Chart Your Ovulation Patterns

One of the newest and possibly the most reliable ways to predict not only ovulation but a variety of hormonal activity is through saliva. How is this possible?

The latest research shows that many of the biochemical changes that occur in your reproductive hormones correspond to biochemical changes in saliva. By analyzing those changes, you can learn a great deal of information about not only your menstrual cycle but particularly your ovulation pattern. In fact, some saliva analysis can predict ovulation up to seven days before it occurs. In light of the new studies on the six-day window of conception opportunity, the saliva test may soon be one of the more valuable tools for couples trying to conceive.

Although there are a variety of systems available to analyze saliva, including a laboratory test and a home fertility "microscope," I believe the most reliable system is a product known as CUE II—introduced in its original form in the first edition of this book. So many couples wrote to tell me how well it worked to help them conceive, I was delighted when I learned that a less expensive and even more sensitive version is available now, one that helps predict ovulation a full seven days before it occurs!

How the CUE II Works

The basis of the system is a small, palm-sized box to which are connected two electronic probes—one that goes into the mouth and a second one for the vagina. The test begins by placing the oral probe into the mouth every morning. After a few seconds, a "saliva reading" is registered on a digital screen. A separate booklet tells you what the numbers mean in relation to your ovulation. You begin taking the oral test on the first day of your menstrual cycle and continue daily until the CUE II indicates you are within seven days of ovulation. Research results from the medical school of the University of Colorado Health Sciences Center, as well as other studies, show the CUE is more than 90 percent successful in predicting the most fertile days of the cycle.

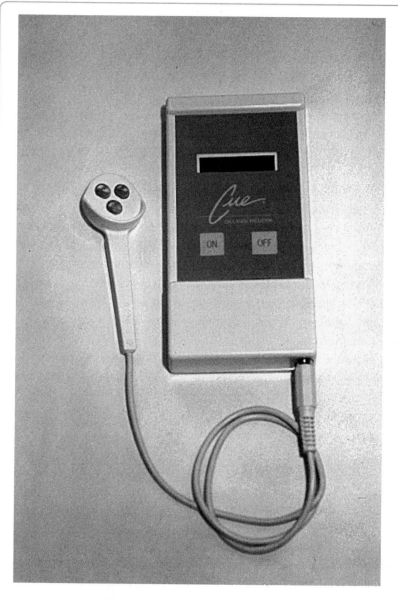

The CUE II Saliva Monitor

By measuring levels of electrolytes in your saliva (factors such as sodium and potassium) the CUE II ovulation predictor can tell when you will ovulate, up to six days before egg release occurs. The tiny saliva sensor (photo left) goes under the tongue, and the readings are registered on a very small handheld computer (photo right). The information is displayed on the digital screen.

To get pregnant fast: Begin having sex within twenty-four hours after the CUE II says you will ovulate within a week, and continue for the remaining six days. Usually intercourse every other day will be sufficient, but if your partner's sperm count is high, and he is in otherwise good health, feel free to make love every day during this valuable fertile time. You can also continue to monitor your saliva daily—it won't hurt you.

At the same time, however, you should also begin using the special CUE II vaginal sensor, a tiny probe that, in just a few short minutes, confirms when ovulation has occurred. If you use the vaginal probe every night during the seven days before ovulation, you will be able to pinpoint almost the exact time your egg left your ovary. If you don't conceive during that month, having this precise ovulation information can be very valuable in the coming months, as you go forward charting your most fertile time. It's also information that can be extremely useful to your doctor—and save you a lot of money as well—if you should seek professional fertility testing or treatment.

Currently, the price of the CUE II is about $385, but the company can rent you the base unit, for a nominal fee, in which case you pay only for your own set of sensors at a cost of about $85. This makes the CUE II quite comparable to other testing systems. (See the Resources section at the end of this book for information on how to purchase or rent the CUE II.)

Method 4: Ovulation Monitors and Predictor Kits

The discovery of some key hormones involved in the ovulation process—namely FSH and LH—opened a new world of biochemical technology, one which made tracking egg release markedly faster, easier, and more accurate. Thus, the concept of ovulation predictor kits was born.

Using a series of early morning urine samples, these kits measure levels of LH, the hormone released into your system in great abundance just before ovulation.

Although once considered the "gold standard" in terms of finding your most fertile time, in light of the new conception studies, the usefulness of ovulation predictor kits may be limited. Indeed, it now seems as if the only way these kits can be truly helpful is if they are used to "track" ovulation over a period of months, thus allowing you to better *predict* your six-day window of conception opportunity, or if you are certain to make love within no more than a few hours after your test shows positive for ovulation.

However, a brand-new twist on the traditional system may prove a lot more helpful. It's called the **Clear Plan Easy Fertility Monitor**, the first palm-sized electronic system to provide a woman with detailed, daily personal information about her fertility status. Based on a urine test, it helps to identify three subcycles in a monthly cycle: low, meaning chance of conception is small; high, meaning an increased chance of conception, typically one to five days before ovulation; and peak, meaning the highest chance of conception.

After the user stores personal information about her cycle in the tiny computerized device, it then calculates when she should perform a urine test and offers a digital reminder to do so. After reading the urine test, the computer classifies her fertility in one of the three above-mentioned categories. The monitor works by analyzing both estrogen and LH found in the urine. When used correctly it helps to predict ovulation about one to two days before it will occur. The cost is about two hundred dollars, with twenty urine test sticks. Thirty replacement sticks cost about fifty dollars. (See the Resources section for how to obtain free information on the Clear Plan Monitor.)

A WARNING ABOUT OVULATION PREDICTOR KITS

If you are over forty years of age and using either a commercial ovulation predictor kit or the new ovulation monitor, be aware that the onset of menopause can also cause elevated LH levels that do not signify ovulation. Although most women do not experience hormonal changes indicative of menopause until they approach their late forties, it is possible to get this type of high LH reading at an earlier age. For this reason, check with your doctor if your tests show elevated LH for longer than a day or two in midcycle.

> ### Important * Important *Important
>
> Some fertility drugs used to promote ovulation, such as Danocrine or Pergonal (read more about them in Part Three of this book), can affect the results of some ovulation predictor kits. If you are taking any fertility drugs, check with your doctor before using an ovulation predictor kit. One fertility drug that usually does not affect test results is Clomid.

Love, Sex, and Getting Pregnant: What You Need to Know

All he has to do is walk into the room and your heart begins to pound. Your breathing may become a little heavier, too, as you begin to feel your body tingle. Your face may feel a blush of heat, and if you are very aware, you may even notice a throbbing and a wetness in your genital area as your breasts become warm and hard, your nipples stiff and erect.

These are some of the signs of sexual stimulation, a complex emotional and biochemical reaction that can occur when a woman meets a man to whom she is sexually attracted.

Although research in this area is just beginning, there is considerable evidence that sexual arousal and fertility may be intimately entwined. Basing their theory on observations of animal behavior, in which the desire for mating is triggered only when the female ovulates, some researchers believe that, on an unconscious level, men and women respond somewhat the same.

While it is not consciously registered, men, for example, are thought to instinctively sense when a woman is entering the fertile phase of her monthly cycle. They respond to these silent signals with a series of biochemical changes of their own, some of which stimulate the desire for sex. A woman, in turn, can instinctively sense a man's stimulation and become stimulated as well. This encourages intercourse at the most fertile time, when conception odds are highest.

Some informal research among my own patient population seems to bear out this sex-fertility theory to some degree.

Women say . . . they feel their sexiest around the middle of their menstrual cycle when, not coincidentally, ovulation is occurring and hormones are in high gear. Needless to say, their fertility is also at its peak.

Their partners say . . . they often feel more sexually stimulated when their wives are ovulating, turned on most, they say, by subtle smells.

Other research has indicated that women who have a regular, satisfying sex life, with intercourse at least once a week, have more regular menstrual cycles and fewer fertility problems than those who don't.

Great Sex, Less Stress, More Babies!

In addition to stimulating hormone production, a satisfying sex life can also be a wonderful way to decrease physical tension—and thereby help encourage fertility. How? In much the same way that exercise reduces body tension that can interfere with hormone production, so can sex. Recent research has shown that the tension-releasing power of just one orgasm can be so great for some people that the effects are twenty times more powerful than the average dose of a tranquilizer like Valium or Xanax!

How Your Sexual Relationship Can Encourage Fertility

In addition to sexual desires, a loving, caring, emotionally supportive *friendship* with your mate may also have a profound positive effect on your fertility.

- Women who have not had a menstrual cycle for years can go into spontaneous ovulation when they fall in love.
- Even a chance meeting with Mr. Right can, in some women, have a biochemical effect that sets reproductive action in motion.

Whenever I think of this subject, I recall a particular patient, Marlene, who, for years, suffered from seemingly unexplained infertility. She and her husband were physically fine and a check back into their family and personal health backgrounds revealed no apparent problems, yet she could not conceive. Although she never fully revealed it, I had sensed that her marriage and her sex life were not happy or satisfying, and I suspected this might be behind her reproductive problems.

He Treated Her Badly — and Her Fertility Suffered

From the few occasions when Marlene did confide her feelings, I learned that her husband, Bob, was a chronic gambler who drank heavily and could be merciless at times in his verbal abuse of her. I also learned that she had been an abused child, and to escape her parents, she married Bob, her first boyfriend, right after high school. As a result, she never had the opportunity to develop much self-esteem.

The marriage lasted for ten years, but Bob eventually met another woman and left Marlene. For a long while she was devastated, but after some time had passed and she had begun to put the pieces of her life back together, Marlene discovered that her husband's departure had been the best thing that could have happened to her—and her fertility!

Good Sex Made the Difference

Not long after starting a new job in the real-estate business, Marlene met Roger, a warm, supportive, and very loving man who encouraged her in every possible way. Marlene blossomed. Not only did she return to school and acquire an advanced real-estate license, but she and Roger became partners in a real-estate business that began breaking sales records in their area. Two years later, they were married. The best news: just six months after that, Marlene was pregnant!

How Love Affects Fertility

Although no one can be completely sure that Marlene's body chemistry would not have changed on its own, there is growing evidence that when you feel happy, secure, and loved and have a fulfilling sex life, your fertility can prosper. How does this happen? As was explained more fully in Chapter 10, your hypothalamus gland, the command center for all your reproductive hormones, is an extremely sensitive barometer of your emotional climate. When you are happy and feel good, it works in peak order. When you are severely troubled, its functions can decrease, and in turn the biochemistry necessary for reproduction can suffer. Very often unexplained infertility is the result.

Will every romantic disagreement harm your fertility? Probably not. However, if your relationship is chronically stressful, you can experience serious hypothalamic changes, some of which may result in infertility.

Great Sex, Super Fertility—Here's Why!

In addition to keeping your hypothalamus in good working order, an emotionally and physically rewarding sexual relationship can yield yet another important benefit: an increase in your level of endorphins, the chemicals your body manufactures to dull your sense of pain and heighten your ability to experience pleasure.

Not only will this enable you to enjoy sex more, but high levels of endorphins have a beneficial effect on the hypothalamus gland, increasing the ability to communicate important reproductive signals to the pituitary gland. This can result in higher reproductive potential, enabling you to get pregnant faster and easier.

When Bad Sex Leads to Conception

Although Marlene's case is typical of hundreds I have seen over the years, it's important to note that not every woman's fertility is affected by the stress of bad sex. Just as being in a great relationship is no guarantee that you will get pregnant, being in a detrimental one is no promise that you won't. In fact, I have counseled many loving and caring couples who, despite their emotionally sound relationship, suffer from unexplained infertility. I have also seen some of the most disastrous relationships yield a pregnancy and take both the man and woman by complete surprise.

Practical Sex and Your Fertility

Later in this chapter you will learn how certain sexual positions can influence your ability to get pregnant. But there are also some practical aspects of sex that can affect your fertility as well. Here are some of the
things that can make a difference if you are trying to conceive.

ORAL SEX

Whether performed occasionally or frequently, oral sex by either partner
to either partner should have no long-term adverse effects on your reproductive health. However, because bacteria normally found in saliva
can have some degrading effects on sperm, they can reduce its ability to
fertilize an egg. For this reason you should avoid having oral sex performed by your partner on you at the time you are trying to conceive.

ANAL SEX

An increasingly popular sexual practice between men and women, when
done properly, anal sex can be highly erotic and extremely pleasurable
for both sexes. However, an important precaution must be taken. A man
must wash his penis with soap and water between acts of anal and vaginal intercourse. Otherwise, harmful bacteria that live in your anus can
be transferred into your reproductive tract via your partner's penis.
Should conception occur at this time, your newly fertilized egg may be
affected.

LUBRICANTS AND CREAMS: WHAT TO USE, WHAT TO AVOID

Many women find that using a lubricant during intercourse makes sex
more pleasurable. However, what you use can affect your ability to get
pregnant. Oil-based lubricants, such as petroleum jelly or massage oils,
can upset the natural pH level of your vagina and create a hostile envi-

ronment that can destroy sperm. In addition, some oil-based products can interfere with sperm's ability to swim through your reproductive system and sometimes can even block passage to your egg.

To encourage fertility, avoid all products containing a large amount of oil, opting instead for those that are **water**-based. (Read the ingredient label or look for the statement "Safe to Use with Condoms." Since oil can break down latex, these products are all water-based.)

How Hot Tubs Can Block Pregnancy

While hot tubs are popular for an extremely sensual form of intercourse, in terms of your fertility, the pleasure may not be worth the price: The high temperatures of hot tub waters may damage your "egg of the month" and interfere with conception.

When the temperature of a man's testicles is raised only a few degrees, his sperm count can suffer. Just one lovemaking session in a hot tub, or a soak just before intercourse, can damage a man's sperm count and hamper fertility for up to several weeks.

The solution? No hot tubs if you're trying to get pregnant.

CAN A VIBRATOR HARM YOUR FERTILITY?

If used properly (and not shared by others), a vibrator is not likely to have any effect on your fertility and generally is safe to use at the time of conception. However, it can harbor bacteria, particularly if it was used by anyone else who harbored an infection. The solution: Wash your vibrator in soap and water before using, but avoid getting water inside the mechanism.

Underwater Sex and Conception

Several years ago a patient came to see me after having returned from a relaxing vacation in the Caribbean. Although she and her husband had gone there for the purpose of conceiving a child, she was, understandably, upset when I informed her she was not pregnant. She had no fertility problems to speak of, and her ovulation timing was right on target with her trip. Still, nature simply did not comply.

Even with optimum biological and psychological conditions, pregnancy won't always occur, of course, but in Katrina's case, I somehow had the feeling there was another force working against her. Questioning her, I soon found out what it was. Katrina and Klaus had taken full advantage of the private pool in their lavish, exotic hotel suite and made love in the water several times a day. In fact, even when their sex occurred elsewhere, it almost always followed a nude dip in their private waters.

Although a sensual experience, making love underwater may not be advantageous for fertility. Not only can water cause a change in the vaginal mucus needed for proper sperm passage, the chlorine found in most pools can alter a woman's internal pH level (the amount of acid on the surface of tissue) and create an environment hostile to sperm.

The next time around, Katrina and Klaus stayed out of the pool—and they conceived almost immediately!

Douching and Your Fertility

Generally speaking, the vagina is a self-cleansing organ, with regular, normal secretions that provide a natural system of internal hygiene. It works as well after menstruation and intercourse as it does every day to help you remain healthy, clean, and odor-free. When odors do appear, they are generally the result of bacteria that reside on the outer portion of the vagina (called the labia) and can usually be eliminated via washing this area with soap and water. (Odors can also be caused by infections, which are generally treated with antibiotics).

So, unless recommended by your doctor for specific purposes (we'll tell you more about these in a moment), not only is regular douching **not necessary, it is also not recommended.** Indeed, some studies even suggest that it may harm your fertility. How?

Should any bacteria be present in your vagina—as the result of contracting an STD (see Chapter 5), or following an abortion or the insertion or removal of an IUD (see Chapter 2)—douching can quickly drive them into your reproductive tract, allowing faster and easier passage to your cervix and, ultimately, your fallopian tubes. This, in turn, can increase your risk of PID and its fertility-related consequences (see Chapter 2). The risk of contracting PID increases if you douche before, during, or right after menstruation, when your cervix is in a slightly more open position.

Because of its link to PID, there is some evidence that regular douching may also increase your risk of ectopic pregnancy (see Chapter 2). In at least one study, women who douched once a week had twice the incidence of ectopic pregnancy as those who did not douche at all. Even douching only once or twice a month can be harmful if it is done in the week following ovulation.

DOUCHING AND CONCEPTION: A NEW WARNING

When it is done just before or just after making love, douching can also disrupt your immediate ability to get pregnant. Why?

Much like the skin on your face and body, the lining of your vagina has a pH reading—the indication of the amount of acid on the surface. Under normal conditions, vaginal pH lies between 4.5 and 5.0, an environment that highly favors sperm. Douching, however, can cause your vagina to become either too acid or too alkaline. Either extreme can adversely affect sperm motility and survival. Unless your doctor diagnosed an abnormal pH balance (you'll learn what to do about that in a moment), douching just before attempting conception could adversely affect your ability to get pregnant.

Douching too soon after intercourse can also be a problem, simply because it washes sperm out of your body that may have made it to your fallopian tube. By cutting down on the number of sperm available for fertilization, you decrease your chance of conception. This can be especially crucial if your partner has even a marginally low sperm count or if your reproductive system contains barriers (such as endometriosis or scar tissue) that can slow down sperm travel.

In addition, I believe that should conception occur, douching too soon after making love, especially with high-pressure apparatus, may have adverse effects on your newly fertilized egg, possibly increasing your risk of miscarriage.

If you find it absolutely essential to douche after intercourse, make certain to wait at least two hours before doing so.

WHEN DOUCHING CAN HELP YOU

Sometimes, certain forms of vaginitis (especially a yeast infection) or other biochemical disturbances can alter the natural pH level of your vagina, making conception difficult. In such cases there are douches that can help.

If you are having trouble conceiving and your doctor diagnoses an abnormal vaginal pH level (either too low, meaning you have too much acid, or too high, indicating not enough acid is present), then one of two natural douches can be used to return the balance to normal.

- **To reduce vaginal acid:** Use a low-pressure douche of two tablespoons of baking soda in one quart of water just before intercourse.
- **To increase vaginal acid:** Use a low-pressure douche of two tablespoons of vinegar in one quart of water taken just before intercourse.

In addition, if you are having artificial insemination (see Part Three) in place of douching, your doctor may spray the inside of your vagina with a solution at the proper pH just before depositing the sperm. In some cases this may help to increase the rate of pregnancy.

Special note: Home-douching apparatus, especially the reusable type, can harbor potentially harmful bacteria that are literally sprayed into your body during the douching process. To avoid problems, properly cleanse all douching apparatus just before use, with lots of soap and hot water.

> ## *Douching Products: An Important Warning*
>
> Some commercially prepared douches contain ingredients that can harm a developing fetus when used during pregnancy. If you find that you must douche, before getting pregnant I suggest you also avoid these same products. Most are identified with a label that reads "Unsafe for Use During Pregnancy."

Sex and Conception: How to Make Love to Get Pregnant Fast

In addition to having intercourse during your most fertile time, how you make love can also influence the speed at which you get pregnant, and in some cases, whether you conceive at all.

In fact, the positions both you and your partner assume during and right after making love can significantly affect the passage of sperm from your vagina to your fallopian tube.

The Sexual Positions That Encourage Conception

Because individual anatomies and certain biological details are different for every couple, the sexual positions most effective for fertility can also vary. Generally, however, the following guidelines have proven to be helpful to many of my patients.

Male dominant or missionary style: This can be especially effective if a pillow is placed under your pelvic region, causing your vagina to tilt backward.

Knee to chest or rear entry style: This can help your partner deposit his sperm closer to your cervix and can be very effective for increasing the power of a marginal or even a low sperm count.

Lying on your side: Many of my patients report that this can be an especially important position if either partner suffers from back problems, or if the man is very overweight. By taking excess pressure off the delicate nerve endings that collect at the base of your spine, you may be able to relax more during intercourse, and that can help facilitate a speedy passage of sperm through your vagina.

How Not to Make Love

What are worst sexual positions for conception?

- Sitting
- Standing
- Female dominant (woman on top)
- Bending over

These positions discourage the rapid transport of sperm and can make conception more difficult.

Morning Sex and Your Fertility

Although there are no statistics to show that making love during any particular time of the day will increase conception odds, it is known that sperm count is generally highest in the morning, providing you have not made love the night before. Morning is also the time when male hormones are at their peak, which is why many men have their strongest sexual urges upon awakening. If sperm count is a deciding factor in your fertility, then morning love could make a difference.

How the Sun Can Help You Get Pregnant

Although research in this area is still considered new, at least one study has found that biological functions, including reproduction and the menstrual cycle, can be affected by exposure to natural light. The connection, it seems, is vitamin D, which we know is manufactured by the body in response to exposure to sunlight. According to research conducted at the Department of Cell Biology and Anatomy and the Department of Pharmacology at the University of North Carolina at Chapel Hill, vitamin D helps regulate reproduction by interacting with the hypothalamus and pituitary glands, as well as the uterus, the mammary glands, and the baby's placenta and fetal membranes.

On the basis of these studies, many researchers believe that, by helping your body manufacture and maintain adequate levels of vitamin D, spending time in the sun can increase your fertility. I have recommended the sunlight method to patients with unexplained infertility, so long as they were not extremely light sensitive. Several couples who had not been able to conceive did so after taking vacations in warm, sunny climates. Some of my patients even reported that the timing and regularity of their menstrual cycle improved after catching just a few extra hours of sunlight every week. And I have also seen patients develop temporary infertility when their jobs deprived them of their usual amount of sunlight.

Interestingly, newer studies have found that *minimal* exposure to natural light may also affect labor and delivery. According to researchers at Columbia Presbyterian–New York Cornell Medical Center, most deliveries made during winter months occurred around 5:00 P.M. As summer months approached, and the hours of available sunlight grew longer, delivery times shifted to earlier in the day. By summer, most women were delivering at lunchtime!

Can You Try Too Hard to Get Pregnant?

Nearly every couple who comes to me for fertility counseling knows at least one other couple who, after years of unsuccessfully trying to have a baby, finally conceived—but only after they had abandoned all hope. Thus, the notion of "trying too hard" continues to be perpetuated. Is it real?

Yes, but only when trying turns a natural, loving desire to have a baby into a demand filled with fear, worry, and anxiety, which are the real culprits that can block a pregnancy.

Can Sweat Make You More Fertile?

Although it has long been known that the scent of a fertile animal attracts a mate, new human studies have shown that the scent of a man's sweat, particularly when he's turned on, can not only turn a woman on, but actually increase her fertility by encouraging more regular menstrual cycles.

In reports presented to the American Chemical Society by the Monsell Chemical Senses Center in Philadelphia, it is suggested that these natural odors influence the secretion pattern of pituitary hormones, which may in turn affect the menstrual cycle. My hunch is that avoiding deodorant and perfumes designed to mask the natural scent of underarm secretions may well turn out to influence how fast you get pregnant.

Pheromones: Are They the Scent of Love?

Do you and your partner give off a subtle but powerful personal scent that encourages conception? Many scientists believe it's possible via pheromones, the "silent scent signal" that we have long known animals to use in order to communicate with each other in a purely instinctual way.

Now, however, new studies conducted at the University of Chicago reveal that humans also produce pheromones, and that we react to those produced by others, particularly in regard to fertility.

The new research, published in the journal *Nature*, reports that two distinct pheromones affect a woman's ability to ovulate—one that encourages eggs to be released and another that suppresses ovulation functions.

Although more study is needed before pheromones can be fully understood, doctors are hopeful that they may one day be used as both a natural fertility enhancement and a natural form of birth control.

Of course the factor that makes the concept of pheromones so difficult to research as well as understand is that the human nose is not capable of detecting their scent. Researchers, however, believe that sensitive nerve cells inside the nose respond to pheromones, even when we can't consciously smell them. It is these nerve cells that transmit impulses to the brain that ultimately affect, among other things, our reproductive biochemistry.

The Scent of a Woman:
Can Perfume Help You Conceive?

It has long been rumored that Cleopatra captivated Mark Antony via the use of precious, exotic oils—perfumes designed to stimulate the male psyche and encourage sexual desire. In more modern times, aromatherapy is often used to bring about similar results. Now some new science reveals the link between fragrance and desire may lie in this powerful network of nerve impulses inside the nose that help communicate important biochemical signals to the brain.

While I'm not certain that any one perfume will influence your ability to get pregnant faster, several of my patients have reported that at least two popular scents—Pheromone, by Marilyn Miglin (a Chicago-based company), and Tova Nights, by Beauty by Tova (a Beverly Hills company)—appear to have some encouraging results. A little research of my own has shown that both scents do contain natural fragrant oils that, according to aromatherapy sources, evoke physiological sexual responses that ultimately influence the production of some brain chemicals involved in reproduction.

While wearing a certain perfume certainly won't guarantee a pregnancy, it may be fun to give either of these two scents—or any that make you or your partner feel particularly romantic—a try.

Hypnosis and Pregnancy: Does It Work?

Although once considered as mystical as a crystal ball, important new research has given scientific credence to hypnotherapy and the role it can play in increasing fertility.

According to a British news report, the number of couples seeking this form of therapy in England has tripled over the past several years. One reason may be that the success rate is as high as 30 percent, as compared to just 1 percent for couples with unexplained infertility who seek no treatment.

Although there is no medical data to show how and why hypnosis works, many believe it helps reduce anxiety and stress, which in turn can help normalize hormone levels as well as reduce tubal spasms that can hurry a fertilized egg into the uterus before it is ready for implantation. Some scientific studies have also shown that hypnotherapy may reduce a woman's level of prolactin, a hormone that can suppress ovulation.

If you do consider using hypnotherapy to help you conceive, be certain to choose a therapist who is highly experienced, particularly in dealing with fertility issues. Usually, seeking out a practitioner who is also a licensed therapist, preferably with a Ph.D. in psychology or an M.D. in psychiatry, will help ensure that you receive qualified treatment.

One Dozen New and Time-Tested Ways to Encourage Conception

Although timing sex to coincide with ovulation is the easiest way to ensure conception, it isn't the only way. Here are twelve more suggestions that may help increase your odds even further.

1. Make Love with the Lights On

In addition to the role that sunlight can play in encouraging conception, other studies have shown that artificial light, such as a lamp, can affect your fertility, mainly by encouraging regular menstrual cycles and keeping ovulation on schedule. In one study, a woman was able to control the regularity of her menstrual cycle for three months by simply sleeping with the lights on, on the fourteenth, sixteenth, and seventeenth nights of her cycle. In addition, she could increase the length of her cycle according to the number of hours the light was turned off—half a night, as opposed to a whole night.

As a result of studies like these, some researchers believe that if you have sex and sleep with the lights on for several weeks, particularly if you use the new full-spectrum bulbs that mimic sunlight, you can help regulate your ovulation and that, in turn, can encourage conception.

2. Make Love Between October and March

According to reports in the *British Medical Journal,* making love from October to March can double your chances of pregnancy! Researchers speculate that egg quality as well as positive changes in the uterus can increase in direct relation to the changes in temperature, climate, and light that occur during these months.

The worst times to attempt conception? August and September. Although there are certainly many babies who were conceived during this time frame, according to research published in the *American Journal of Obstetrics and Gynecology,* births drop dramatically during April and May, indicating that August or September may not be the most fruitful months in which to attempt conception.

3. Make Love on Your Birthday

As reported in *Gynaekolge,* a respected Japanese medical journal, the fertility of some women may be season-sensitive, increasing around the time of their own birthday. According to the study, making love close to the day you were born may make conception faster and easier.

4. Be Turned On When You Make Love

Because being sexually stimulated can influence the flow of reproductive hormones, research indicates that couples who are very turned on when they try to conceive may have a faster, easier time getting pregnant. In addition, research has shown that the sperm count of men who ejaculate when they are turned on and making love is higher and more potent than when they masturbate. And don't forget the power that simple touching and caressing can have to boost your fertility. Studies show that just twenty to forty minutes of stimulating sexual caresses before intercourse can increase hormone levels and encourage fertility.

In short, whatever turns both of you on is a great conception booster.

5. Don't Make Love Under an Electric Blanket

Studies continue to show that the low-voltage emissions of electric blankets may adversely affect fertility. There is also evidence that conception that takes place under an electric blanket may yield a higher rate of certain birth defects and possibly miscarriage. So if you're trying to get pregnant, let your love keep you warm!

6. Make Love Close to the Time of Ovulation and Avoid Miscarriage

In a fertility study of 965 women, all of whom kept detailed records of sexual activity, it was shown that the likelihood of miscarriage decreased when conception took place at the time of ovulation. When fertilization occurred *after* ovulation, when eggs had already begun to disintegrate, not only was the chance for pregnancy very slim, the rate of miscarriage tripled.

7. Limit Movement After Intercourse

By remaining in bed for twenty to thirty minutes after intercourse, preferably on your back with a pillow under your pelvis, you can help encourage sperm to remain in your body and flow upward toward your fallopian tube. This, in turn, may facilitate a faster conception.

8. Use Fast Withdrawal

Research suggests that by withdrawing his penis immediately after releasing the first squirt of his ejaculation, your partner can increase sperm concentration and thereby improve chances for conception.

9. Retain Sperm in Your Vagina

Immediately after intercourse, lightly press the labia (lips) of your vagina together with your finger and hold for several minutes. This can help keep sperm inside your body and ensure that what has been deposited has the opportunity to swim toward your fallopian tube.

10. Avoid Alcohol and Drugs at the Time of Conception

Although some couples have grown accustomed to increasing sexual stimulation and enjoyment through the use of alcohol or drugs before making love, I cannot emphasize enough the importance of avoiding this practice, especially at the time of conception. Mounting evidence shows that alcohol in your bloodstream or your partner's at the time of conception can have some overwhelming negative effects not only on your fertility but on your baby as well.

11. Take Robitussin Cough Medicine

Robitussin, which contains the active ingredient guaifenesin and helps thin the mucus in your lungs, can also alter cervical mucus, making it thinner and better able to transport sperm. Many of my patients who were unable to conceive solved their own fertility problem by using this simple method. Take one to two teaspoons a day beginning three to four days before you want to conceive.

12. Make Love Often!

Although it was once believed that if man ejaculated too frequently, he might decrease his potency, new studies show that in fact the exact opposite may be true. Part of the new fertility study featured at the start of this chapter also found that making love as often as possible was among the best ways to encourage conception. Indeed, the couples who had intimate relations the most often had the greatest pregnancy rates.

It is my guess, however, that this is probably only true if the man's sperm count is high. If, however, sperm count is marginal (common for most men) or particularly if it is low, it's probably still a good idea to concentrate your lovemaking during the three days before ovulation and on the day of ovulation. This will help ensure that sperm count is at its maximum at the time when it's needed the most. You should also discourage your partner from masturbating during the time you want to get pregnant, since every ejaculation counts! Also be certain not to let more than seven days pass without intercourse if you are trying to conceive. Waiting too long between episodes of lovemaking could result in an abundance of dead sperm in your partner's ejaculate, which may result in a variety of conception problems.

A Final Word About Getting Pregnant

It is my hope that the suggestions in this chapter will help you obtain a fast and easy conception, but I don't want you to worry about accomplishing them. Feel calm and confident about your ability to get pregnant; feel happy and positive about being a parent. Maintaining the right emotional state is perhaps the best way to achieve a successful conception.

Relax . . . make love . . . enjoy!

Chapter Fourteen

Boy or Girl . . . Is There a Choice? The Latest News About Gender Selection

Most of my fertility patients are overjoyed at the prospect of simply being able to have a healthy child, and very few are concerned with gender.

Still, for some couples, there remains overwhelming desire to conceive either a boy or a girl. Sometimes, this can be driven by solid, medical reasoning—for example, when either parent harbors a defective gene that is gender specific. For others it can be a religious or ethnic decision. And for still others, having either a boy or a girl is simply the realization of their personal "dream family."

Regardless of the reason, however, if gender selection is what you want, there is no shortage of methods for you to try.

Of course, in some social and political arenas this entire topic is considered unethical. In others, however, it is deemed extremely acceptable.

Where you will stand on this issue will be entirely personal, and I wouldn't try to influence you in either direction.

What I will do right now, however, is help you explore some of the more popular methods of gender selection in use today and hope that this information will help you decide what's right for you and your family.

But before we begin I must remind you that your main goal should always be to have a healthy baby and to love and to cherish each and every child you conceive, regardless of gender.

How Gender Selection Works

Although there are various methods of gender selection to choose from, all are based on one simple fact: It is the sperm, and not the egg, that carries the genetic material (called chromosomes) that determines the sex of the child.

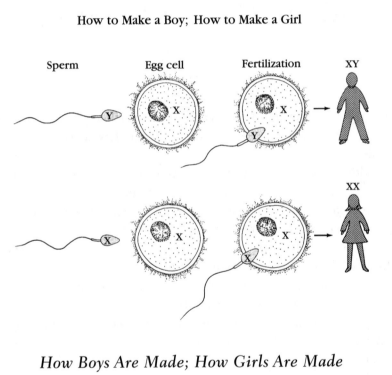

How to Make a Boy; How to Make a Girl

Sperm   Egg cell   Fertilization   XY

How Boys Are Made; How Girls Are Made

Top: Sperm carrying a "y" chromosome unites with egg, which always carries the "x" chromosome, to produce a boy.

Bottom: Sperm carrying an "x" chromosome units with egg, which also carries an "x" chromosome, to produce a girl.

More specifically, *sperm that carry the X chromosome produce a girl, while those that carry the Y produce a boy.*

In a single ejaculate your partner releases both, and some believe that it's just a matter of chance which type reaches the egg first and begins the fertilization process.

Many others, however, believe it's anything but a game of chance. Indeed, depending on whom you talk to, there can be a whole barrel full of factors affecting just which sperm, X or Y, begin the babymaking process. Gender selection techniques are, more or less, different ways of influencing those factors.

But do all the methods really work—and do they work equally well? Unfortunately, the answer depends largely on whom you ask. Certainly some have a scientific basis and the studies to back them up. Others claim tens of thousands of successful gender selection births, but in many instances, scientific studies have not been able to satisfactorily duplicate the results. In still other instances *only* anecdotal evidence exists, with virtually no scientific research available at all. So, often you will have to decide on your own which, if any, of these systems are worth a try.

Ovulation and Gender Selection

Regardless of which method of gender selection you may choose, in order to be successful, conception must be timed with ovulation. That is a must if you want to get pregnant.

The only exceptions, of course, are those methods that are used in conjunction with assisted reproductive technologies such as artificial insemination or in vitro fertilization. In these cases, your doctor will already be using various sophisticated medical tests (all described in Part Three of this book) to help determine when your eggs are ready for release.

Tried and True: The Shettles Method of Gender Selection

More than twenty years ago, a physician by the name of Landrum Shettles devised a method of gender selection that, since its inception, has reportedly worked for thousands of couples. Although scientific studies are scant, certainly, there is no shortage of parents who attest to its accuracy. Indeed, many of my own patients have verified that the Shettles method has proven effective.

The basis of his theory is that sperm that carries the X chromosome, needed for conception of a girl, swims slower and lives longer than sperm that carries the Y chromosome, necessary to conceive a boy. By manipulating the timing of when you have intercourse in relation to your ovulation (egg release), the Shettles method maintains that you can encourage conception with the sex-specific sperm.

So, if you want to conceive a boy, you should have intercourse as close to ovulation as possible. This will enable the faster, lighter, Y-carrying sperm to reach your egg first. If you want to conceive a girl, you should have intercourse three to five days before ovulation, and then abstain from sex. This will allow the faster but weaker Y male sperm to die off before your egg is available, thus leaving the path clear for the longer-lasting X female sperm to fertilize your egg as soon as it arrives.

Sex and Your Baby's Gender

In addition to when you make love, how you have intercourse can also influence your baby's gender. Why? Certain sexual positions, in conjunction with the depth of penetration and whether you achieve orgasm, can all be used to encourage either a Y sperm or an X sperm conception.

If you want a baby girl:

- Use shallow penetration in the "missionary" position (man on top) to allow your partner to deposit sperm at the mouth of your cervix. This is said to favor the slower-moving female sperm.

- Avoid orgasm. This will help keep your vaginal environment highly acidic, which helps kill off the male sperm before they reach your fallopian tube.

If you want a baby boy:

- Use deep penetration and the "rear entry" position, which will allow your partner to deposit sperm above the neck of your cervix, for fast entry into your uterus. Here the environment is also more alkaline, making it easier for male sperm to survive.
- Try to achieve orgasm at the same time your partner is ejaculating. This will also help foster a more alkaline environment that favors the Y male sperm.

Do Opposites Attract? The Whelan Method

In her book *Boy or Girl?*, medical expert Elizabeth Whelan, Sc.D., takes the opposite approach to Dr. Shettles in that she recommends intercourse at quite different times in the menstrual cycle.

To conceive a boy, Whelan advises intercourse four to six days before ovulation; to conceive a girl, abstain from sex until two to three days before egg release is expected. She claims her method is 68 percent successful when it comes to conceiving a boy, but just 56 percent successful in conceiving a girl.

Eat Chocolate — and Give Birth to a Baby Boy!

Can what you eat also influence the gender of your child? Some experts say yes. Specifically, a well-known European physician named Dr. Joseph Stolkowski conducted studies wherein he correlated a mother's prepregnancy diet with the sex of her baby.

The result: Women who ate foods rich in potassium and sodium (such as meat, fish, vegetables, chocolate, and salt) beginning at least six weeks before attempting conception were far more likely to conceive a boy.

Likewise, women who consumed foods high in calcium and magnesium, such as milk, cheese, nuts, beans, and cereals, during this same pre-conception period were more likely to give birth to a girl.

The premise behind his theories: Gender is influenced by what scientists call "ionic" factors—a type of natural electrical charge emitted by products of the earth, including such minerals as potassium, sodium, calcium, and magnesium. Stolkowski theorized that by manipulating her diet with the addition of certain mineral-rich (ion-charged) foods, a woman could alter her ovulation metabolism and thus influence whether her egg attracts the X or the Y sperm.

Although the initial study was small—just forty-seven French couples participated—the results were quite impressive. Thirty-nine of the couples were able to produce a child of the gender they wanted, simply by manipulating their diet.

The Electricity of Love: The SELNAS Method of Gender Selection

Although Dr. Stolkowski's studies were limited, there are many who believe that he was at the forefront of the most accurate system yet of safely choosing the sex of your child. I'm talking about the SELNAS method, one of the newest ways to control gender selection.

Using Dr. Stolkowski's research as his base, European biologist Patrick Schoun discovered that the membrane surrounding a human egg also emits ions, giving off a kind of electrical "charge" of its own. Reportedly, it is this energy that attracts either the X or Y sperm.

He also found that at specific times in a woman's monthly cycle, her egg is electrically "charged" to attract either the X or Y sperm exclusively. In addition, he also noted a clearly "neutral" time in the cycle when the electrical charge surrounding an egg is totally dependant upon environmental factors, including diet, which is one reason Dr. Stolkowski's food theories seemed to work so well.

In addition, Schoun also found that the time frame in which the egg is electrically charged one way or the other can range from one to ten days for each calender month and can change from month to month. So, for example, in January you may have ten consecutive days on which your egg is charged in a way that attracts the X sperm, while in February, you may have only three days when this can occur. So, by coordinating your most fertile time (the six days before ovulation) with the days when your egg is attracted to either the X or the Y sperm, you can plan sexual relations to coincide with the conception of either a boy or a girl.

How a Computer Came to the Rescue

While Dr. Schoun's theories were rapidly proving to be right, the individual calculations involved in determining the correct time to have sex were staggering. Indeed, it was nearly impossible for a couple to figure out the method on their own.

Finally, however, a group of French scientists found a way to enter all the necessary scientific data about the gender selection theory into a computer. They also included some personal information about the couple (including menstrual history, contraception use, and reproductive history), as well as their preference for either a boy or a girl. The end result was the development of the SELNAS method—a personalized, twelve-month gender selection calendar that clearly spelled out the days on which a particular egg would attract either the X or the Y sperm for an entire year.

Of course the SELNAS method does not predict ovulation—therefore it cannot help you *get* pregnant. What it can do, however, is point out on which days of the month you are most likely to conceive either a boy or a girl. Then, by using your personal ovulation chart to determine your most fertile time (five days before, and the day of, ovulation), you can use the calender to conceive a child of the gender of your choice.

If, in any given month, your gender selection days do not fall within your natural ovulation period, you will not get pregnant.

How well does this system work? A six-year study of 155 couples (1989–1994) yielded a success rate of 98.7 percent—153 of the 155 couples conceived the gender they desired. For the record, 81 of those couples wished to have a girl (52.3 percent) while 74 hoped for a boy (47.7 percent). As of 1999 approximately fifteen hundred parents have used SELNAS to select the sex of their baby, with accuracy remaining between 96 and 98 percent.

Additionally, 95 percent of the mothers (women who did not necessarily have fertility problems) who used the SELNAS calender in conjunction with their natural ovulation pattern conceived a child of the gender they desired within eight months, with most getting pregnant within four months. On rare occasions, when a woman's cycle is extremely irregular, or if her ovulation does not coincide with any SELNAS gender selection dates, French physicians often prescribe low-dose birth control pills (Loestrin 1/20-21) for one month, to help create ovulation on the desired days.

The SELNAS Natural Gender Selection Technique (including the personalized calender) is available in the United States (see Resources section at the end of this book), costing under $400. The company that prepares the computerized calenders (Laboratories Prokiad International, in France) offers a 100 percent money-back guarantee to any couple who follow the method and conceive a child of the opposite gender.

Finally, because the SELNAS method is not affected by miscarriage, if you should lose a pregnancy during a calender year, you can continue to use your specified dates for future conceptions in the remaining months—you won't need to purchase a new calender. Unfortunately, however, the SELNAS calender method does not appear to be as effective when fertility drugs are used to help achieve a pregnancy.

High-Tech Gender Selection: The New Methods

Since I know that many of you reading this book may come to rely, in some way, on the new fertility technologies to get pregnant, you should know there are also a variety of gender selection techniques designed to work with laboratory-assisted conceptions.

Among the most popular is a method developed to work with couples undergoing artificial insemination (see Chapter 20). Developed by California researcher Dr. Ronald Ericson more than twenty years ago, the technique involves forcing sperm samples to swim through a very thick concentration of human albumin (a component of blood). How can this help? Only the stronger, fast-moving "male" sperm (those carrying the Y chromosome) are able to swim through the solution and make it to the bottom of the test tube. The naturally more sluggish X female sperm (along with both male and female "dead" sperm) remain floating on top of the solution.

By performing this process several times, then collecting the sperm that consistently fall to the bottom of the test tube, doctors can be fairly certain they have a good concentration of Y male sperm, which is then placed directly into the uterus during the insemination process. Boy babies result about 80 percent of the time.

Unfortunately, however, since the Ericson method cannot determine the difference between the X female sperm and dead sperm that float up to the top of the albumin solution, the system is not helpful if you want a baby girl.

Star Wars and Your Baby's Sex: The Microsorting of Sperm

Imagine this: A system that uses laser beams and complicated DNA formulas to choose the sex of your baby! Sound futuristic? It's here now: Doctors at the Genetic and IVF Institute in Fairfax, Virginia, have come up with a way to identify gender-related DNA material inside each tiny sperm and to sort that sperm according to its genetic configuration.

And believe it or not, the basic theory that makes this complex scenario work is one of the most simple of all facts: The male-bearing Y sperm contain around 3 percent *less* genetic material than the female-bearing X sperm.

To help identify which is which, the sperm is stained with a special dye. A laser beam is then passed over the cells to activate the dye, which then allows sperm to be sorted according to the amount of genetic material they contain. Since, for example, the sperm carrying the X (female) chromosome has more DNA than the one carrying the Y (male) chromosome, more dye is activated, making them easier to identify.

When the sorting process is finished (the system is appropriately called Microsort), doctors ideally end up with a cache of both X and Y sperm and can then choose either for use in any number of reproductive technologies, including insemination or even in vitro fertilization (see Chapter 21).

Is Microsorting Safe?

Although the Microsort system may prove to be one of the most effective ways of performing gender selection, not everyone believes it is the safest method. I, in fact, become extremely concerned any time a procedure attempts to tamper with the DNA of a living cell, and I know many share this concern.

In this instance, we don't know, for example, if the dye used to stain the DNA has any long- or short-term effects, or if the lasers used to help sort the sperm can cause genetic damage. It's entirely possible that the most significant side effects of this procedure may not even appear until the child grows up or attempts to have children of his or her own. When we tinker with DNA we simply don't know the consequences.

Certainly, Microsort may prove to be a blessing for those who carry a genetic code for diseases that are clearly gender-specific, such as hemophilia. However, I firmly believe that all couples who choose to use Microsort, for any reason, must be told how much we don't know about the potential dangers of this system. Indeed, until further testing is done, and we have more verification of its relative safety in humans, I would advise you to think long and hard before agreeing to use Microsort.

The Ultimate Gender Selection Technique: And What You Need to Know

One of the most important fertility advances made in the 1990s was the development of preimplantation genetic diagnosis, or PGD—a system of identifying the presence of genetic diseases in embryos. Whether those embryos are formed in a laboratory, as part of the in vitro fertilization process (featured in Chapter 21), or conceived naturally in the body and then flushed from the uterus for testing, in PGD the tiny embryos are isolated and a single cell is removed. After examination under a high-powered microscope, doctors can determine whether the genes representing certain genetic diseases are present. They can also tell whether the embryo will yield a baby boy or a baby girl—and therein lies the link to gender selection.

Indeed, once the sex of the embryos is clearly identified, researchers can elect to transfer into the woman's uterus only those that match the parents' gender choice. The remaining embryos can then either be frozen for future use, given away to a couple who cannot conceive on their own, or discarded.

Although the procedure carries little likelihood of any long-term adverse effects, still, it has landed in a hotbed of controversy, particularly when embryos are discarded simply because they are not the desired gender. In fact, in many fertility centers the practice of using PGD strictly for sex selection of a nonmedical nature is greatly discouraged, and in some areas of the world it is against the law. In addition, PGD can also be expensive, and sometimes risky, particularly when embryos must be flushed from the uterus for testing.

As such, I urge you to have a serious discussion with your doctor about not only all the particulars involved in PGD, but also your reasons for wanting gender selection, as well as exploring your other sex selection options, before making a final decision on how you wish to proceed.

Gender Selection: A Final Thought

I don't think there is a parent-to-be who has not given at least *some* thought to whether they want a boy or a girl. From shopping for little pink dresses and bright blue blankets, to choosing wallpaper and nursery-room decor, to selecting names, I know that all of us have, in our hearts, a secret preference for how we want to build our family. And whether we have always envisioned our first to be a boy, or we look for a balance of boys and girls, or we plan for a whole slew of big brothers followed by a precious little sister, for many of us, our dreams become reality— whether we use one of the gender selection methods featured in this chapter or just Mother Nature's luck of the draw.

But as you continue on the road to parenthood, take care that the wonders of what you *can* accomplish do not blind you to what you set out to accomplish—the sharing of your life, your love, and your heart with a child.

Chapter Fifteen

Preventing Miscarriage: Now You Can

Some of the most exciting advances in reproductive medicine surround the breakthroughs in the prevention of chronic miscarriage. Today, there are many ways you and your doctor can protect your conception and reduce your risk of pregnancy loss, even if you have lost two, three, or even more pregnancies in the past. Among my own patients I have seen couples who have been plagued with the frustration of seemingly endless, unexplained recurring miscarriages conceive and deliver healthy babies, using the simplest of these new preventative measures.

Understanding Pregnancy Loss: The Latest News

Medically known as a "spontaneous abortion," for most couples a miscarriage normally happens only one time. The cause is usually an isolated chromosomal abnormality that occurs when fertilization involves a randomly defective egg or sperm. The condition, known as a blighted ovum, means the embryo is simply too weak to survive. When this type of conception occurs, all the usual hormonal activity associated with pregnancy takes place, causing the body to feel and act as if a normal gestation is in progress. But while the placenta begins to grow, making you "feel" pregnant, the defective embryo does not.

Usually, within the first twenty weeks after conception, the body recognizes that something is wrong. The placenta begins to shrink, which in turn causes a rise in prostaglandin, a body chemical linked to inflammation. When this occurs, cramping, staining, and bleeding, which are the classic signs of miscarriage, can also begin, and the pregnancy is lost.

While sometimes the now-useless placenta gets reabsorbed by the body, other times it remains an empty sac inside the uterus, in which case it must be removed, usually by D&C, a procedure that either scrapes the inside of the uterus or uses suction to "vacuum" out what remains of the placenta.

Under most circumstances, the next attempt at conception is healthy and normal. In fact, because reproductive hormones are often at their peak just before a miscarriage, I often advise my patients to try for another pregnancy as soon as one month following their loss. When they do, most find this second conception faster, easier, and healthy.

When Miscarriage Happens More Than Once

For some prospective parents, however, pregnancy loss is not an isolated event. A growing number of couples are continually plagued with what is medically called "habitual abortion," losing every conception that occurs. These couples are, in fact, considered to be infertile, unable to bring their pregnancy to term.

In the past, recurring miscarriage was thought to be caused by just one of two problems:

- Structural abnormalities within the mother's body, such as a blockage or deviation in the uterus, or weakness in the cervix
- Chromosomal abnormalities within either partner's body. Here, chronically defective genetic material present in either the egg or the sperm allows a pregnancy to occur, but ultimately results in miscarriage.

Now, however, much has changed. Although both structural and chromosomal abnormalities still account for a good number of recurring miscarriages, we now know there are also a significant number of other reasons why pregnancy loss occurs.

These include biological factors in the mother, such as:

- Hormone imbalance, particularly a shortage of progesterone
- Endometriosis
- Stress
- Diabetes
- Infection

Later in this chapter you will also read about certain biological factors in men, particularly sperm abnormalities, that also lead to miscarriage.

Additionally, the older you are when you get pregnant, the greater your risk of pregnancy loss. Women aged twenty to twenty-nine, for example, have a normal miscarriage rate of just 10 percent, while for those over age forty-five the risk can jump to nearly 50 percent. If you had difficulty conceiving, if you have a history of premature labor or premature birth, or if you have had four or more abortions, you might also be at higher risk for miscarriage. Other factors that increase your risk include a history of PID (pelvic inflammatory disease), repeated bouts with STDs (sexually transmitted diseases), recurring UTIs (urinary tract infections), or if your mother took DES when she was pregnant with you.

How Many Miscarriages Spell Trouble?

Most fertility experts now agree that having three or more consecutive pregnancy losses is a sign that a chronic malfunction may exist. I, however, have always believed that any pregnancy loss is a sign that a patient needs extra attention and treatment. In order to avoid future difficulties I urge you to seek at least preliminary fertility evaluation if you have miscarried even once.

Your Immune System and Miscarriage: What You Must Know

One of the newest, most advanced theories on the cause of pregnancy loss points to the immune system as the culprit.

Normally, this sophisticated biological defense system works much like a high-tech surveillance operation, continually scanning the body for harmful foreign invaders, such as bacteria and viruses. At the first sign that exposure has occurred, our immune system snaps to attention, manufacturing factors called antibodies to help protect us from disease (see Chapter 3).

So what does this have to do with pregnancy? In the past several years, new research has shown that a woman's immune system has still another job. It is also called into play during conception, as well as at the very early stages of pregnancy, to protect her baby when the threat of loss is the greatest. Some researchers have, in fact, shown that a mother's immune system continues to influence the development of her baby throughout the nine months of gestation.

In some women, however, a condition called "autoimmunity" develops. Here, the body begins to view its own tissues and organs as foreign invaders and thus produces antibodies against itself. When pregnancy occurs, this same "search and destroy" message is transferred to the baby. Viewing the conception as a dangerous foreign invader, the mother's immune system goes to work to destroy it. The end result: recurring miscarriage.

Could You Have an Immune System Problem?

You may want to consider an immunological treatment approach if you fall into any of the following categories:

- If you have lost more than two consecutive pregnancies and no cause can be found
- If you fail to get pregnant even after several laboratory-assisted cycles were considered successful (your eggs fertilized but the embryo failed to implant in your uterus)
- If you have a history of autoimmune disease such as lupus, or severe thyroid disorder. Because, comparatively speaking, laboratory assistance can be very expensive, some couples elect to eliminate all possible failure risks by testing for immunological problems before treatment.

Often, this chain of events can occur so soon after conception that many women believe they can't conceive. In reality, however, they are losing every conception before they even realize they are pregnant. Unfortunately, no one knows what causes a woman's immune system to malfunction in the first place. While some suspect a virus, others say stress or other medical conditions are involved. What we do know, however, is that some immunological factor appears to be responsible for up to 80 percent of all unexplained recurrent miscarriages.

Can Your Egg Be Allergic to Your Partner's Sperm?

The answer is yes. Although the problem is not particularly common, some controversial research has demonstrated situations in which the sperm and egg are thought to be so incompatible that they evoke a kind of allergic response within the mother's body, thus causing the pregnancy to destroy itself. The tests to determine this problem include a leukocyte antigen cross-match, levels of natural killer cells, and an embryo toxicity panel. Because they are such a sophisticated screening, they are currently performed in only a few select labs around the nation.

Four Powerful Immune Boosters to Save Your Pregnancy

Fortunately, researchers have discovered not only the ways in which immune system malfunctions can harm a pregnancy, but also the ways and means to stop that harm from occurring. If your doctor suspects your pregnancy losses are the result of immune deficiencies, one of the following treatments may help bring your next pregnancy to a successful completion.

Boost 1: Baby Aspirin

Immune problem: Your body attacks your baby's placenta and blood supply.

What happens: In order for your baby to receive the nutrients necessary to grow, your immune system must produce chemicals known as lipids and phospholipids. Acting as a kind of biological "glue," they aid in the formation of the placenta and blood vessels, both used to supply nutrients to your baby. When, however, something causes your immune system to go awry—including chronic pelvic inflammatory disease (PID), endometriosis, and pelvic adhesions—your body may begin to produce antibodies that work against these important lipids. Known as antiphospholipid antibodies, the result is the formation of blood clots in the blood vessels through which your body supplies nutrients to your developing baby. This not only limits your baby's development, but could do so to the point of starvation and, ultimately, pregnancy loss. Additionally, there is some research to suggest that these antibodies do the most damage in the pre-embryo state, before implantation can take place. This results in early miscarriage sometimes misinterpreted as inability to conceive.

Test: A screen for seven antiphospholipid antibodies is necessary. But because only a few centers, known as "reference laboratories," are capable of doing all seven screens, your doctor may recommend only testing for one or two antibodies. If this test comes out negative, however, be aware that the problem could still exist and the full panel of screening should then be considered.

Treatment: As complex as this problem sounds, treatment is relatively easy. It involves anticoagulant medication—drugs that work to stop the formation of the blood clots caused by the antibodies. This, in fact, can be accomplished by simply taking one baby aspirin (about one-quarter of an adult aspirin) a day throughout your pregnancy. In some instances, a low dose of the drug heparin, alone or in combination with the baby aspirin, can also help when used during the first twelve to twenty weeks of pregnancy.

What you should know: Because the molecules that make up heparin are relatively large, they cannot cross the placental barrier, which means the drug won't have any effect on your developing baby.

Women who do not respond to this treatment may want to consider the laboratory-assisted pregnancy treatment known as in vitro fertilization (IVF). Because the pre-embryo state takes place in a laboratory rather than a mother's body, studies show it may escape damage from antibodies.

Boost 2: Anti-inflammatory Drugs

Immune problem: Your body attacks your baby's cells.

What happens: The building blocks of all life are proteins, predominantly DNA and histones, which together help form the basis of each cell in our body. If, however, you have a history of inflammatory health problems, such as rheumatoid arthritis or lupus, your body is actively engaged in the manufacture of antibodies directed against these vital proteins. If you should get pregnant, these same antibodies can attack your uterus and your baby's placenta. This inflammation can make for an exceedingly hostile environment that ultimately can harm your baby's development, and result in miscarriage.

The test: Antinuclear antibody (ANA), anti-DNA, and antihistone antibody

The treatment: Since the inflammatory reaction in your body is the major threat to your baby, prescription anti-inflammatory drugs may help. These include corticosteroids such as oral prednisone, usually given in conjunction with the anticlotting drug heparin. For best results treatment is started before conception. Regular testing helps access the level of antibodies naturally building in your body. So, when the proper level is reached, treatment can be stopped. You are then free to attempt conception with, hopefully, far less risk of miscarriage.

What you should know: At least one study, conducted at the University of Toronto and published in the *New England Journal of Medicine,* revealed that prolonged prednisone therapy may increase the risk of premature birth as well as gestational diabetes and maternal hypertension in some women. Further, while it can be effective for many women, it may not work for all. For additional treatment options see Boost 4.

Boost 3: Your Partner

Immune problem: Failure to produce the blocking antibody, a biochemical that protects your baby from immune system destruction.

What happens: Because your baby is a combination of both your biology and your partner's, ordinarily your body would view your conception as a foreign object and try to destroy it. To keep this from happening, your developing baby actually sends out a kind of biochemical SOS, a signal that communicates the need to survive. Your body responds by manufacturing a substance called the "blocking antibody," a biochemical that, in simplest terms, turns "off" your immune system in relation to your pregnancy. Thus, your baby is free to grow without threat of destruction.

When, however, your tissue is very similar in structure to your partner's (something that occurs purely by chance and whose likelihood is not increased by similarities in ethnic background or race), your body does not read your baby's SOS. As a result, the blocking antibody is not made and your pregnancy is not likely to survive.

The test: A tissue typing test determines if your biology is similar to your partner's. If so, a second test, called flow cytometry, helps determine if your body can produce the blocking antibody in relation to your current partner.

The treatment: If, in fact, you cannot produce the blocking antibody, your partner's white blood cells become your treatment! How? A laboratory procedure separates his white blood cells from other blood parts and then concentrates them into a small vial of fluid. That fluid is then injected under the surface layer of your skin, and this procedure is repeated in four weeks. The goal: to flood your system with enough of your partner's biological remnants to trigger the production of the blocking antibody you will later need during pregnancy. Testing is done within two to four weeks after the second injection. If blocking antibodies are still in short supply, a third injection using double the amount of white blood cells is administered. In two to four weeks you are tested again. If you are still not producing enough blocking antibody, your partner's white blood cells will be mixed with those of a donor and you will be immunized once again. Eventually, you should produce enough of the blocking antibody to sustain a pregnancy, in which case you can conceive without fear of miscarriage. Important to note: White blood cells taken from either your partner or a donor undergo a rigorous preparation treatment that virtually eliminates all threat of disease transmission.

What you should know: It's important to realize that the problem of blocking antibodies should only be considered a possible cause of miscarriage if you have never carried a pregnancy to term with your current partner, or if you and your current partner appear to never have been pregnant.

Boost 4: Taming Your Internal Tiger

Immune problem: An overabundance of "killer" cells and an immune system that works overtime.

What happens: Using an intricate system of biochemical checks and balances, your immune system relies on both "killer" cells and "helper" cells in order to function properly. When, however, the killer cells outnumber the helper cells, your body loses its ability to judge what should be destroyed (such as developing tumors) and what should not be harmed (such as your developing baby). The end result: Your killer cells work overtime and your pregnancy becomes the target.

The test: A laboratory process called immunophenotype will identify five different types of killer cells and the levels of each, in relation to helper cells.

The treatment: Normally, having a strong army of killer cells is a good thing, particularly in regard to protection from cancer. This is not the case, however, if you are trying to get pregnant. In this instance, your doctor must work to "tame the tiger within" and essentially suppress some of your body's natural fighting instincts—at least enough to allow your baby a chance to thrive. One of the best treatments involves immunoglobulins, blood proteins that are normally part of the immune system. The treatment, called IVIG (intravenous immunoglobulin) consists of a three-hour infusion of highly purified immunoglobulin every twenty-eight days until pregnant, up to four months. After conception, treatment continues monthly for up to thirty-two weeks, or until delivery. Studies show IVIG works as a kind of fertility "sponge," absorbing the excess killer cells so they can't affect your baby, while enhancing your production of helper cells, which mediate and control what your immune system destroys and what it leaves alone.

Because IVIG can supply a broad spectrum of useful antibodies, the treatment may also be therapeutic in a number of situations wherein the immune system requires additional outside help, including increasing the production of blocking antibodies.

What you should know: Some women, primarily those with a low level of an antibody known as IGA, can have an allergic reaction to IVIG. Although the percentage affected is very small, because the reaction can be so serious, it is wise for all women to have IGA levels tested before any IVIG therapy. Side effects of IVIG are minimal and usually subside on their own. They can, however, include flushing, fever, dizziness, headache, nausea, muscle and joint pain, allergic skin reactions, and increased heart rate and blood pressure. Because this therapy is highly specialized and may not be widely available in your area, it can be expensive, and is not likely to be covered by insurance.

Men, Immunity, and Pregnancy: What You Must Know

When it comes to pregnancy, a woman's body is not the only immunological force to consider. Indeed, a man's immune system can also cause problems, primarily by producing a protein that literally floods his system with antibodies that attack sperm. This hampers their motility and ultimately reduces his ability to fertilize an egg. Most commonly this occurs after a vasectomy, which is why men who have a reversal of this procedure can't always regain their fertility. Ultimately, your doctor can test your partner's sperm for levels of antibodies. If they are present, treatment with the anti-inflammatory drug prednisone can help. A technique called "sperm washing" (you can read more about that in Chapters 20 and 21) can also work to isolate the antibodies from the sperm, thus increasing the chance for conception.

Preventing Pregnancy Loss: More Good News

In earlier chapters you learned about some of the lifestyle changes you can make to help ensure a healthier conception. Many of them can help

The New Immune Biopsy and a Brand-New Treatment Option

In addition to the ways already mentioned in which your immune system may interfere with a pregnancy, there is still one more problem that should be considered. According to the very newest research on the subject, studies conducted by Dr. Alan Beers of the Chicago Medical School, in a small but significant number of infertile women, certain destructive immune system cells (including macrophages, natural killer cells, and mast cells) are present in the uterus, where they work to damage the lining as well as the embryo. The end result is often recurrent pregnancy loss, either via natural conception, insemination, or through IVF and other implantation failures.

To accurately detect the problem, Dr. Beers recommends a uterine biopsy, a tissue sample of the uterus taken two to three days before a menstrual cycle is expected, or, at the latest, on the first day of bleeding during a cycle when pregnancy has not occurred. In addition, a biopsy can also be performed ten to fourteen days after an IVF transfer (see Chapter 21) that does not yield a pregnancy.

Specifically, the biopsy will look for evidence of inappropriate immune system cells in the uterine tissue. If a problem is discovered, a brand-new drug used to treat autoimmune disorders, called Enbrel, may help. Currently it is being tested for effectiveness in the uterus, and so far, results are promising.

You should consider this specialized endometrial biopsy if you have:

- A known autoimmune disease (such as lupus, fibromyalgia, rheumatoid arthritis, Crohn's Disease, thyroid disease, or any connective tissue disorder)
- A history of cervical dysplasia, carcinoma in-situ of the cervix, HPV (genital warts) infection, or endometriosis
- Two or more IVF failures, specifically with failed implantations, particularly if you experienced flulike symptoms after embryo transfer
- Repeated failed inseminations
- Experienced stabbing pelvic pain or intense cramping, or any strange symptom in your abdomen, pelvis, or legs following insemination or transfer (including cramping, jitteriness, jerking, or strange traveling sensations in the skin)

If this specialized biopsy is not available via a local laboratory, your doctor can take your tissue sample and send the specimen to one of the immune system laboratories listed in the Resources section of this book.

you avoid miscarriage as well. And, later in this chapter you will discover several more key things that you and your partner can do to help ensure your pregnancy. Self-help, however, is by no means the whole story. In addition to the immune system boosters we have already explored, what follows are a variety of other medical treatments that can help protect your pregnancy from harm.

Miscarriage Treatments: Mix and Match

Although the treatments listed in this section have been shown to work for the specific types of immune-related pregnancy loss problems as indicated, don't be surprised if your doctor suggests trying one or more of these treatments even if your problems don't quite fit into the categories we have described. Indeed, the area of reproductive immunology is so new, researchers are just beginning to understand the vast nature of these treatments and the number of problems that can be helped. This is particularly true for IVIG—the immunoglobulin infusions that are now being tried for a variety of different types of immunologic-related pregnancy loss.

Five Medical Breakthroughs That Can Save Your Pregnancy

Breakthrough 1: Natural Progesterone, the Hormone That Can Save Your Pregnancy

One of the most common causes of miscarriage is a faulty implantation. In this instance your conception was healthy and your baby is in good shape, but your embryo does not adequately attach to your uterus. This means your baby cannot be properly nourished, so it becomes impossible for it to thrive. In addition, if the implantation is exceptionally weak, normal movement by the mother is sometimes enough to shake it loose, causing miscarriage.

Although a number of factors can be responsible for implantation problems, one of the most common is a lack of progesterone, a hormone that is manufactured after ovulation. By softening and conditioning the lining of the uterus, it helps promote a healthier and stronger implantation. When however, progesterone is in short supply during the second half of the menstrual cycle (called a luteal phase defect), the uterine lining remains rigid. This can either prevent implantation from occurring or cause any that does occur to be weak. Ultimately, each pregnancy attempt can result in miscarriage.

How this treatment works: If blood tests or a uterine biopsy show progesterone is in short supply, taking supplements prior to conception will help build a lining that is strong enough to sustain a pregnancy. In addition, taking progesterone supplements right after conception can further prevent miscarriage by helping to keep the level of prostaglandins, a hormonelike substance, from rising too high. When elevated, prostaglandins cause uterine cramping similar to labor pains, which, in turn, can induce pregnancy loss.

Although this treatment is safe for you and your baby (no negative side effects have been reported), it's important that only *natural progesterone supplements* be used. Most synthetic forms (like the kind found in some birth control pills) will have no beneficial effects. However, some fertility clinics have reported success with hydroxyprogesterone caproate, a long-lasting synthetic progesterone.

Currently, natural progesterone treatment is usually administered as a vaginal suppository. At some point there was also an oil-based progesterone injection on the market, and it could return in the future.

And while studies show that it can be difficult to administer progesterone orally, mainly because it gets destroyed in the digestive system before it has a chance to work, a new oral form called Prometrium is said to overcome these problems. Made from wild yams, a potent source of natural progesterone that is suspended in peanut oil, Prometrium is currently approved only for the treatment of endometrial hyperplasia and in conjunction with hormone replacement therapy.

Although the package insert advises that it not be given to pregnant women, some doctors have found that it is as safe and effective as other forms of natural progesterone in treating a pregnancy-related progesterone deficiency. Your doctor can advise you whether Prometrium is right for you.

Finally, some pharmacists can now custom compound progesterone capsules in a way that overcomes at least part of the absorption problem. Although there are no formal studies available, clinical evidence has shown that these compounds can work. (See the Resources section at the end of this book for mail-order pharmacies offering this service.)

What you should know: If you are using progesterone in the vaginal suppository form, it should be administered three times a day. The reason: The most recent research suggests that the body is capable of absorbing only about 30 percent of the medication found in each suppository, and further, what is absorbed only remains in vaginal tissue for six to eight hours. So, in order to fully protect your pregnancy from loss, some experts believe you should use the progesterone suppositories three times daily. In addition, estrogen levels should be in a ratio of four to one with progesterone. If, in fact, the supplements cause estrogen levels to drop too low by comparison, your doctor may also prescribe supplements of this hormone to be used during the first six to eight weeks of your pregnancy.

A bonus: Studies show that if you use natural progesterone suppositories during the early part of your pregnancy, your baby may be more intelligent that those born to mothers who do not use this supplement.

You might need this treatment if:

- Blood tests or an endometrial biopsy indicate low progesterone levels during the last two weeks of any menstrual cycle
- Your body temperature does not rise after ovulation, or it fluctuates. Using the BBT guide in Chapter 13, you can help detect a progesterone deficiency by watching for a temperature increase of about one degree after ovulation. If this does not occur, progesterone may be deficient
- Your menstrual cycles are irregular. This can also indicate a hormone imbalance strong enough to affect your pregnancy

Breakthrough 2: Erythromycin, the Antibiotic That Can Prevent Miscarriage

In addition to causing infertility, certain types of bacterial infections can also cause miscarriage. They do so by affecting either the quality of your egg or your implantation, or by creating a hostile environment that debilitates sperm, causing a conception too weak to survive. The bacteria most likely to cause these problems are usually those associated with an STD, including:

- Chlamydia
- T-mycoplasma
- Gonorrhea
- Syphilis

Other maternal bacterial infections linked to miscarriage include *Ureaplasma urealyticum*, group B streptococci, and *Treponema pallidum*. Viruses known to cause miscarriage include rubella, cytomegalovirus, herpes, and Coxsackie virus.

Most recently, a bacteria known as listeria has also been linked to pregnancy loss. It often shows up in undercooked meat or poorly pasturized dairy products, as well as some raw vegetables. Another new bacteria, known as campylobacter—normally known to cause only gastroenteritis—is now thought to cause miscarriage as well. It too can result from undercooked meat.

How this treatment works: Ideally, all infections should be treated long before you get pregnant. Unfortunately, some of the bacteria responsible for pregnancy loss are difficult to detect, even with sophisticated laboratory tests. Additionally, some diseases, like chlamydia, may have no overt symptoms, so you may not even be aware that you are infected. For this reason, many fertility specialists now find it beneficial to routinely treat every couple who experiences unexplained recurring miscarriages with antibiotics, both before conception and for the first several weeks of pregnancy.

The medication of choice is usually erythromycin because it has been found safe for both Mom and baby. In fact, it is so safe and effective that many fertility clinics throughout the world now routinely prescribe erythromycin for any woman who has miscarried even once. I have found it to be one of the most beneficial treatments in preventing miscarriage and have used it time and again to help hundreds of patients overcome habitual pregnancy loss. The recommended dosage is 333 mg taken two to three times daily, beginning seven to ten days before you plan to get pregnant and continuing for six to eight weeks into the first trimester. Because bacteria linked to miscarriage can reside in your partner's body as well, as an extra measure of precaution he too must be treated, even if he tests negative for the infections in question.

You might need this treatment if:

- You or your partner are at high risk for STDs.
- You have experienced "unexplained" miscarriages in the past.
- Your last miscarriage was followed by a fever.
- You have difficulty conceiving and no reason can be found.

Because there are limited treatments available for viral infections and testing is difficult, your best bet here is to avoid contact with anyone you suspect may be infected during the time before you try to get pregnant and during the early stages of your pregnancy. Also, be sure to report any viruslike symptoms, including low-grade fever and fatigue, to your doctor before trying to conceive.

Breakthrough 3: Condoms — How They Prevent Sperm Allergy

In much the same way that you can be allergic to strawberries or roses, you can also be allergic to your partner's sperm. As a result, your body begins making sperm antibodies the moment he ejaculates into your vagina. Aimed at destroying what your body perceives as a deadly invader, the antibodies create an environment so hostile it becomes difficult or almost impossible for sperm to survive. And, in most cases, the sperm *does* die, and no pregnancy occurs. However, if your antibody reaction is mild to moderate, sperm may only be made defective. Fertilization is still possible, but the conception is usually too weak or too frail to survive, thus setting the miscarriage process in motion.

How this treatment works: As devastating as a sperm allergy can be, unvarying use of condoms for up to one year (or longer) can lessen your immune response to your partner's sperm. Working on the same principle used to treat food allergies, where abstinence can decrease sensitivity, by avoiding direct contact with your partner's sperm for as little as six to twelve months, you can gradually decrease your sensitivity. Condom therapy is usually accompanied by specific tests designed to measure your level of sperm antibodies at three-month intervals. When antibody production falls low enough, you are free to conceive without fear of miscarriage.

Additionally, you could also have an allergic reaction to your partner's seminal fluid, the ejaculate that carries sperm out of a man's body. When this is the case you can be treated via a procedure known as intravaginal rush desensitization. Administered on an outpatient basis, in your doctor's office or a hospital, the treatment involves an IV infusion of your partner's seminal fluid directly into your vagina. The semen is diluted to various strengths, with the infusion beginning with the weakest concentration. Every twenty minutes the strength of the fluid is increased until full-strength seminal fluid is tolerated. The desensitization procedure usually is completed in one session.

You might need these treatments if:

- You have unexplained miscarriages.
- You test positive for the presence of antisperm antibodies in your cervical mucus
- Your partner's sperm tests normal

Breakthrough 4: The Stitch Can Save Your Baby

Normally, tight bands of fibrous tissue surround your cervix, helping to keep it closed until just before you are about to deliver. When, however, due to a variety of factors (which can include disease, too many selective abortions, previous D&Cs, a genetic abnormality, or a multiple birth) these tissue bands weaken, they may not be able to adequately hold your baby within your uterus. If this does occur, problems can develop, usually some time in your second trimester, as your baby begins to gain weight and excess pressure develops within your stomach. As it does, your cervix will dilate, far too early, after which cramping can begin and a miscarriage occurs.

To keep this from happening, around the fourteenth week of pregnancy, your doctor can place a special stitch called Shirodkar suture (or cervical cerclage), around your cervix.

How this treatment can help: The goal of the stitch is to give your uterus the extra support it needs to hold your baby inside. I have personally found this treatment to be most effective for patients carrying twins or triplets, particularly following a laboratory-aided conception such as in vitro fertilization. Since fertility patients can be at a higher-than-average risk for pregnancy loss as well as premature labor, this treatment can increase the odds of pregnancy success by a tremendous margin. Because sometimes the stitch becomes loose, it's important to see your doctor regularly following this treatment, particularly in the first several weeks. If the stitch weakens, a second one can be put in place to increase the strength. Bed rest can also help take pressure off your cervix and give the stitch a chance to take hold.

In addition, one week out of each month your doctor may ask you to take an antibiotic to help prevent the risk of infection.

Your stitch will usually be removed, in your doctor's office, around two weeks before your due date, or during a Cesarean section. At this point your baby is fully developed, so labor would be welcome rather than discouraged. Having the stitch removed before labor can also ensure that no infection develops at birth, or that any that does occur has a chance to be eliminated before your birthing day. It is not unusual for you to see some bright, red blood following the removal of your stitch, and you could also go into labor within days or even hours.

You might need this treatment if:

- You are pregnant with more than one baby.
- You have had more than four induced abortions.
- A connective tissue disease has weakened your fibrous bands.
- Your doctor diagnoses a weak cervix for any reason.
- You have fibroid tumors or other uterine abnormalities.
- You have had several previous midtrimester pregnancy losses.
- Your mother took DES and as a result you have a divided or otherwise misshapen uterus.

Breakthrough 5: The New Medications That Prevent Miscarriage

Before we knew about all the many and varied factors that cause miscarriage, it was widely believed that any attempt by a fetus to leave the body before it's ready to be born should be regarded as a sign of an unhealthy pregnancy. Today, we know this is not true. Often, your baby *is* healthy, and the miscarriage is merely the result of some temporary physiological or biochemical problem in your body that can be fixed, thus allowing your pregnancy to continue.

Often that problem is premature uterine contractions. In this instance your uterus goes into spasms that, if not stopped, push your baby out too soon, thus resulting in miscarriage. Your baby isn't causing this to happen, so if the contractions can be stopped, your pregnancy can continue. The good news here: Over the past several years a variety of medications have become available that can help.

How this treatment works: Commonly known as labor inhibitors, the drugs that help stop premature labor are technically classified as tocolytics and include such medications as ritodrine hydrochloride, terbutaline, and magnesium sulfate. They work by relaxing the body's smooth muscles, the kind that line your uterus, so they stop the contractions that bring on premature labor. When administered at the onset of cramping, they can be extremely effective in preventing miscarriage.

Because, however, in high IV doses these drugs can also affect maternal blood pressure and pulse, strict medical supervision is necessary. Therefore, they are usually administered in a hospital, with your doctor present. Your blood pressure readings will be taken every twenty minutes for several hours after the IV drip begins. If no problems occur, therapy with terbutaline in tablet form or via an infusion pump can be continued at home. You will take this medication daily until approximately your thirty-seventh week of pregnancy, when your baby will likely be strong enough to be delivered.

You might need this treatment if:

- You have miscarried more than once in your second trimester or have had one or more premature births.
- You have experienced premature labor in the past.
- You are diagnosed with an incompetent cervix.
- You have uterine abnormalities or fibroid tumors, or were exposed to DES in your mother's womb.
- You have experienced repeated urinary tract infections.
- You have a multiple pregnancy.

Endometriosis and Miscarriage— an Important Connection

If you suffer from the menstrual-related disorder called endometriosis, studies show you are three times more likely to lose your pregnancy. Risks increase because endometrial lesions can block the fallopian tubes making egg passage difficult or impossible. When a fertilized egg remains inside your tube too long, it can simply die, or it can take root in the tube itself and start to grow. Known as ectopic pregnancy, when not diagnosed and treated early on, this condition is the leading cause of maternal death.

In addition, endometrial lesions emit high levels of a hormonelike substance known as prostaglandin, which can cause dramatic contractions within the uterus or fallopian tubes. This can force a fertilized egg from the body before it has adequate time to implant.

Finally, macrophage (immune cells that attack foreign bodies) are also found in greater abundance in the pelvis of endometriosis patients. Some studies show these cells may kill or maim sperm as they swim toward an egg, or destroy the embryo as it attempts to implant in the uterus.

Fortunately, treatment for endometriosis, including medication or laser surgery, can usually reduce the related risks of pregnancy loss (see Chapter 2).

Smoking and Miscarriage

While a variety of lifestyle factors can play a role in miscarriage, among the most serious is cigarettes. Indeed, research continues to show that rate of pregnancy loss is at least twenty times higher in women who smoke. Problems can also occur when your partner is a smoker, and you are constantly being bombarded with his secondhand smoke.

But how, exactly, does smoking affect your pregnancy? Each time you take a cigarette all its toxic components go directly into your baby's bloodstream, weakening his or her entire system. In addition, the nicotine in your body causes a constriction of veins and arteries, decreasing blood flow and consequently oxygen and other important nutrients to your baby. The more you smoke, the less nourishment and the more toxins your baby receives, until he or she can literally starve to death.

Later in your pregnancy smoking can lead to abruptio placentae, a condition wherein your baby's placenta deteriorates and pulls away from the wall of your uterus. Depending on when in your pregnancy this occurs, either a miscarriage or premature birth results. Fortunately, quitting smoking by the fourth month of pregnancy can eliminate your risk of this problem.

SMOKING BEFORE PREGNANCY: THE MISCARRIAGE LINK

If you smoke before conceiving and at the time of conception, your baby's placenta can attach too low in your womb. Called a placenta previa, this condition causes inadequate blood flow to your baby and contributes to miscarriage, premature birth, and fetal death.

The good news: On the positive side, avoiding cigarettes as well as secondhand smoke, at home and in your workplace, can significantly decrease your risk of pregnancy loss.

Coffee, Cigarettes, and Alcohol: The Miscarriage Connection

In addition to cigarettes, both alcohol and caffeine will have negative effects on your baby, and do increase the risk of miscarriage.

- Just two alcoholic drinks a day can significantly increase your risk of pregnancy loss.
- Consume more than 150 mg of caffeine daily (about two cups of coffee or three colas) and you are also more likely to experience a miscarriage.
- When cigarettes are combined with alcohol or coffee or both, the negative effects of all three are intensified.

So if you can't quit smoking, don't combine cigarettes with alcohol or caffeine, either before or after you get pregnant.

Dry-Cleaning, Nail Polish Remover, and Miscarriage: The New Links

It has long been suspected that certain environmental chemicals can increase the risk of pregnancy loss. Now, some of these suspicions have been confirmed. Indeed, a number of impressive studies have shown that otherwise healthy women exposed to a variety of common chemicals found in the workplace and at home can have quadruple the risk of miscarriage. These chemicals include xylene, trichloroethylene, and petroleum distillates, all found in solvents used to clean electronic components in many factories. In one study women making silicon chips in a factory where these chemicals were present had a miscarriage rate as high as 33 percent. Another risk chemical is acetone, frequently found in nail polish remover. According to studies at the University of Quebec, it also quadrupled the risk of miscarriage.

In addition, trichloroethylene and the chemical percholorethylene are both used in dry-cleaning. Living in close proximity to a dry-cleaner whose fumes are emitted into your living space presents the greatest risks, but even residues left in clothes after dry-cleaning can cause problems for some women. According to studies conducted at the School of Public Health at the University of California at Berkeley, exposure to these chemicals can increase the risk of pregnancy loss to nearly five times that of women who remain chemical-free. Of particular concern to me are the new at-home dry-cleaning systems—chemicals that are placed right inside your own washer-dryer unit to dry-clean your own clothes. Not only does this bring the exposure of dry-cleaning chemicals directly into your home environment, residues may also linger in your machine, contaminating other clothes with these chemicals.

Other consumer products that can increase the risk of pregnancy loss include paint thinners, paint strippers, and glycol ethers, an ingredient commonly found in some house paints.

The good news: If you can't avoid all chemical exposure, even reducing the amount you do inhale can help reduce the risk of pregnancy loss.

- Use only non-acetone nail polish removers.
- Air out dry-cleaning for at least forty-eight hours before wearing and avoid use of home dry-cleaning kits.

- Save the painting and other house repairs until after the baby is born or use only water-based latex paint or milk paint.
- Don't allow varnishing or staining of floors or furniture, even in the garage, while you are pregnant or trying to conceive.
- Talk to your boss about chemicals in your workplace; if they are present in your direct environment ask to be transferred to a different area of the building during your pregnancy (see Chapter 6).

Ovulation and Miscarriage: The New Link

British researchers have shown that LH, the hormone responsible for ovulation, may also be an important link to miscarriage.

The study, conducted by Dr. Lesley Regan, Dr. Elisabeth Owen, and Professor Howard Jacobs, all of the Rosie Maternity Hospital and University College of Medicine, Cambridge, England, involved 193 women all planning to get pregnant. After testing, researchers found those women with an elevated serum LH level before getting pregnant (they were tested on the seventh day of their menstrual cycle) had a miscarriage rate of 65 percent, as compared with 12 percent for those who had a normal LH reading.

Although the results, reported in the British medical journal *Lancet* are still considered inconclusive, they indicate that having your LH level tested before conceiving may alert you to the need for special precautions to avoid miscarriage.

Stress and Pregnancy Loss

There is no question that infertility of any kind, but particularly chronic pregnancy loss, is one of life's most stressful experiences. But can it also work in reverse, with high levels of stress increasing the risk of miscarriage? The question has become one of the great fertility debates of all time.

Recently, however, statistics have begun to mount showing that yes, stress does play a role in pregnancy loss as well as infertility, and moreover, that reducing stress can have some marvelous, positive effects on your entire reproductive system.

While doctors aren't sure exactly how, many believe it's hooked into your hypothalamus, the area of your brain that controls the ebb and flow of a number of reproductive hormones. Interestingly, the hypothalamus is also *very* sensitive to stress, so during times of increased tensions, you may not receive adequate amounts of the hormones necessary for a healthy implantation.

Other theories suggest undue or prolonged stress may also reduce the supply of blood to your baby, which in turn weakens the conception and can lead to miscarriage. Stress may also affect your fallopian tubes, sending them into spasms significant enough to move your fertilized egg into your uterus before it is ready for implantation. The end result here is also miscarriage.

Exercise and Miscarriage: What You Need to Know

For most women moderate exercise will not harm a pregnancy. In fact, unless your implantation is extremely weak, even direct injuries to your abdomen will likely do little harm. The key to a healthy fitness routine, however, is moderation. Conversely, overdo workouts while pregnant, and even a healthy implantation can suffer.

The connection is your body temperature, which is naturally higher when you are pregnant. *Extremely* vigorous workouts can quickly and easily bring body heat into the danger zone. When your body overheats your baby overheats as well—with one important difference. While *your* system allows excess heat to escape through your skin, your *baby* has no such opportunity to "cool down." So he or she remains hotter a lot longer. When the heat is excessive for a long enough period of time, as in an aerobic dance class lasting an hour or more, your baby can grow so hot that miscarriage spontaneously occurs.

To help guard against pregnancy loss, take the following precautions:

- Stop any vigorous exercise once you become pregnant. It is especially important to perform only *moderate to mild* workouts in your first trimester.

- Make certain all workout programs are preapproved by your doctor, especially after you conceive.
- If you show any signs of a weak implantation, including brown staining or bleeding *in any amount,* or if you are at high risk for miscarriage, refrain from *any* exercise during the first trimester of your pregnancy, or until your doctor says it's okay to resume working out.

Orgasm and Pregnancy Loss: Can Sex Cause a Miscarriage?

Patients who have miscarried often ask whether intercourse could have caused their pregnancy loss. One of my patients was so convinced that her husband's very active sex drive had somehow caused her miscarriage that she remained cold and sexually unresponsive to him for weeks. This, as you can imagine, is not a very advantageous situation for a couple trying to conceive their first child!

The truth is, if your body is normal and healthy, especially if you are young and your conception is strong, sex will not harm your pregnancy. However, if you are at high risk for miscarriage—if you are over age thirty, had endometriosis, or had difficulty conceiving—or if you have any of the high-risk factors mentioned earlier in this chapter, then yes, sex could cause problems, but usually only during the first few weeks of your pregnancy. If there are signs that your pregnancy is in jeopardy (such as staining or cramping) I would advise you to be exceptionally careful during your entire first trimester.

What sexual activities can harm your pregnancy the most?

- Heavy penile thrusting
- Intense pelvic activity, especially rocking
- Deep penetration
- Anal sex
- Repeated pounding on your uterus
- Use of vibrators

The motions that accompany all these activities can shake loose a weak implantation or force your fallopian tube or your uterus into a spasm that expels your fertilized egg. In addition, because sperm contains high levels of prostaglandin, the chemical that causes the painful uterine contractions of menstrual cramps, continued or frequent ejaculations into your vagina may induce dangerous tubal or uterine contractions that can expel any implantation that is even slightly weak.

Finally, orgasm, with or without penetration, can have a similar negative effect, but only if you are at very high risk.

Should you avoid sex during the start of your pregnancy? If your pregnancy is normal and your risk of miscarriage is low, sex won't harm your baby. If, however, you are at high risk for pregnancy loss, I would have to say you should avoid intercourse for the first eight weeks following your conception. If possible, you should also avoid intercourse for the first three to four months of your pregnancy.

How Water Beds Can Cause a Miscarriage

In a study of some seventeen hundred births by the University of Colorado Medical Center, it was found that the use of water beds during pregnancy can sharply increase the risk of miscarriage. The reason? Electrical fields present in the environment have been found to disturb fetal movement.

Is Bottled Water Linked to Miscarriage?

In a recent study by the California government it was learned that women who drank bottled water had a lower rate of miscarriage than those who drank tap water. Why? Some tap water has been found to contain dangerous levels of chemicals that can be toxic to a developing baby.

The Skin Treatment That Threatens Your Pregnancy

Derived from vitamin A and used to treat severe cases of acne, the medication acutane is one of the most harmful drugs connected to pregnancy problems. When taken during pregnancy it can contribute to miscarriage as well as cause an increase in the risk of birth defects. I strongly advise you never to use this medication unless you have completed your family. If you must use this drug, be certain to take all precautions necessary to keep from getting pregnant while this medication is in your system, and be certain to quit this medication and remain drug-free for a minimum of one year before trying to conceive.

Miscarriages and Men: How His Body Affects Your Pregnancy

Although sperm is extremely tiny (more than a million can fit on the head of a pin), each one contains enough genetic material to make a baby. When sperm quality is good, so too is the genetic material it contains, and that means your baby and your implantation are more likely to be healthy and strong. When, however, for any reason sperm is not perfect, the genetic material it contains can also be defective.

When an imperfect sperm fertilizes even the most perfect egg, the conceptus can be defective. When this happens your baby can be born with any number of birth defects, or your pregnancy can end in miscarriage. Indeed, recent studies show that partners of men with low sperm counts are up to six times more likely to miscarry—perhaps because there are fewer "perfect" sperm available for fertilization.

Since all men produce some defective sperm every day, there is no way to completely eliminate the threat of male-related miscarriages or birth defects.

However, because so many outside factors and individual health concerns are capable of affecting sperm quality, there are many things a man can do to promote a higher percentage of perfect sperm, including:

- Refrain from drinking alcohol at least forty-eight to seventy-two hours before conception.
- Increase his vitamin C intake to 1,000 mg daily and B-Complex to 100 mg daily for two weeks before conception.

- Be checked for STDs, especially T-mycoplasma.
- When possible, avoid contamination with environmental toxins, especially lead, ethyl alcohol, and organic solvents.
- Avoid X-rays.
- Quit smoking.
- Avoid drugs.

By taking a few simple precautions in the weeks and months before you want to conceive, your mate can help increase not only his potency but his ability to help you deliver a perfect child.

Twenty-One Super Easy Ways to Decrease Your Risk of Miscarriage Before and After You Conceive

What to Do Before You Get Pregnant

1. Take one to two prenatal vitamins (or two high-potency multivitamins with sufficient folic acid) daily, starting three months before conception.
2. Quit smoking.
3. Limit alcohol consumption: No more than three drinks per week in the month before getting pregnant. No alcohol forty-eight hours before conceiving.
4. Examine yourself frequently for any signs of STDs, especially unusual vaginal discharge with an unpleasant odor. Report any suspicious signs to your doctor and get treatment immediately.
5. Make certain your doctor checks you for the following medical conditions linked to miscarriage, just before you plan to conceive:

- Diabetes
- Hormone imbalance
- Chlamydia

- T-mycoplasma
- Thyroid malfunction
- Toxoplasmosis
- Rubella (German measles)

6. Make sure your partner is checked for:

- Low sperm count
- Sperm quality
- T-mycoplasma
- Chlamydia

7. Seek genetic counseling, particularly if you have had more than three miscarriages and no cause can be found.
8. Have a hysterosalpingogram, laparoscopy, or saline sonogram (methods of looking inside your uterus explained in Chapter 16) to determine if blockages or other abnormalities capable of causing a miscarriage exist.

What to Do After You Are Pregnant

9. Check with your doctor about taking 333 mg of erythromycin daily for six weeks to reduce the possibility of infections linked to miscarriage.
10. Take 1 mg of folic acid three times daily in conjunction with a high-potency multiple vitamin.
11. Stop all alcohol consumption.
12. Avoid use of any products containing caffeine.
13. Avoid as many sources of radiation as possible, including VDTs, electric blankets, heating pads, water beds, color TV (sit ten feet away from the front or back), microwave ovens, airport or other security X-rays, and medical X-rays.
14. Sleep on your left side to increase blood flow to your baby.
15. Avoid exceptionally strenuous exercise.

16. If your doctor determines you have an incompetent cervix, receive a Shirodkar suture no later than your fourteenth week of pregnancy.
17. Limit medication to those items absolutely necessary and avoid use of any recreational drugs.
18. With your doctor's permission, take one baby aspirin daily for the first eight to ten weeks of your pregnancy.
19. Avoid heavy lifting.
20. Avoid sex for at least six to eight weeks after conceiving.
21. Receive injections or use suppositories of natural progesterone for the first eight weeks of your pregnancy.

You Can Stop a Miscarriage

Studies show that in many instances of impending miscarriage the baby is healthy, so all possible steps must be taken to prevent pregnancy loss. The best place to start is by learning the warning signs of miscarriage and reporting them to your doctor immediately.

MISCARRIAGE: THE WARNING SIGNS

- Blood spotting (more than slight pink stain; brown stains are of special concern)
- Bleeding in any intensity
- Cramping, no matter how mild
- Dizziness
- Burning headache
- Swelling of joints
- Excessive nausea or vomiting
- Fever
- Extreme or sudden fatigue
- Fainting
- Severe or sudden backache
- Sudden loss of pregnancy symptoms
- Pelvic pain

What to Do When Symptoms Start

When any of the signs of miscarriage appear, you must call your doctor immediately. It is likely that he or she will ask you to come to the office or the hospital for an examination.

The first step is usually a pelvic exam to determine if your cervix is still closed. Next, a sonogram may be given to determine the exact environment of your uterus, and to see if your baby is healthy. Finally, you should be given a blood test to measure your levels of human chorionic gonadotropin (hCG), the hormonal indication that your pregnancy is progressing satisfactorily.

If You Do Miscarry: Treatments to Ensure You Conceive Again

To ensure healthy pregnancies in the future, make certain you receive the proper treatment and care after your miscarriage. Depending on the type of pregnancy loss you experience and when in your gestational term your loss occurs, your miscarriage will be classified in one of three distinct categories, each with its own treatment. Remember, in medical terminology, a miscarriage is known as a "spontaneous abortion." The following section uses that same terminology in describing what happens and the treatment that should follow.

The Complete Abortion (a "Total" Miscarriage)

When this occurs, the placenta has completely torn away from your uterine wall and your fetus is fully expelled into your vagina. Normally, bleeding will slow down and eventually stop, all pain will subside, and your uterus will begin contracting, returning to its normal shape and size. When this occurs there is usually no residual tissue left and your miscarriage is said to be complete. Although this determination must be made by your doctor, normally no further treatment is needed.

THE INCOMPLETE ABORTION (A "FRAGMENTED" MISCARRIAGE)

Although a miscarriage has occurred, your placenta may still be partly attached to your uterus, or remnants of fetal tissue may still be left inside. Because of this, your uterus cannot contract as it normally should and the blood flow resulting from the miscarriage process cannot be stopped. Seeing your doctor right away can help you avoid such complications as severe bleeding or infection, which can occur when fetal tissue is not completely discharged by the body. The remaining fetal tissue can also create blockages that can cause future fertility problems. The best way to avoid all these complications is via a suction evacuation followed by a D&C, which surgically scrapes your uterus and removes all remaining fetal tissue.

MISSED ABORTION (A "SILENT" MISCARRIAGE)

This occurs when your fetus dies some time before your twentieth week of pregnancy, but remains inside your body. There was likely no bleeding or pain, and your cervix was not dilated and remains closed. The first signs of a missed abortion are the absence of obvious pregnancy symptoms, along with a lack of weight gain, decrease in breast size, and a lack of fetal movement. A pregnancy blood test (hCG) and a sonogram will help confirm a missed abortion, which always requires a suction evacuation or D&C as soon as a diagnosis is made.

Warning: Never Diagnose Your Own Miscarriage

Because it is vital that your miscarriage be accurately categorized and treated, never try to diagnose your own pregnancy loss. Seek medical treatment whenever you believe your pregnancy is in jeopardy and get the proper follow-up care after a miscarriage occurs. This not only could help save your baby, it might preserve your future fertility as well.

Getting Pregnant Again

Even it if turns out that you do lose more than one pregnancy, don't give up hope. I recently treated a patient who had miscarried a total of twelve times but wouldn't give up her dream of motherhood. After no fewer than five doctors had told her it was hopeless, we discovered she was harboring a little-known (and hard-to-diagnose) parasite. Once the infection was cleared (it took just fourteen days of antibiotic treatment), she conceived naturally and delivered a full-term healthy baby!

As you have read in this chapter, there are a variety of new treatments to help overcome even chronic miscarriage, and newer treatments are still becoming available. And that means that no matter what your reason for recurring pregnancy loss, there is likely a treatment that's right for you.

What can also make a big difference, however, is getting the right medical treatment. And by "right" I mean finding a physician who is experienced in handling a high-risk pregnancy and, if possible, also experienced in treatments for chronic miscarriage. For some of you that may mean finding two separate doctors, a fertility specialist who can help you achieve a healthy pregnancy, and an OB/GYN able to help bring your pregnancy to term.

Part III

If You Don't Get Pregnant Right Away: How Science Can Help

Chapter Sixteen

Can I Have a Baby? How to Tell

Because much of the media attention on infertility focuses on situations involving older couples, many young men and women—in their thirties or even twenties—don't realize they too could have a problem.

In fact, how many times have you already heard the following statements from well-meaning friends and family, maybe even your own doctor?

- Late motherhood runs in the family. Just keep trying.
- You're too young to have fertility problems. Stop worrying and you'll get pregnant.
- You were pregnant once, you'll get pregnant again. There's nothing wrong.
- You can't rush nature. It has to take its time.

While it's true that not everyone's body works at the same speed, and some couples can take longer than others to conceive, still, when nature takes its course pregnancy should occur in less than a year. If you don't get pregnant within this time frame, it has been my experience that some factor requiring at least minor treatment probably exists.

How can you tell if you might have a problem? The best way to start is by listening to your own body.

How to Test Your Own Fertility

Because your monthly menstrual cycle is the core of all your reproductive functions, it can serve as one of the most effective barometers of your fertility. The length of your cycle, the amount you bleed, the days that elapse between periods, even the frequency and severity of any menstrual cramps all serve as clues to your reproductive health.

At the same time, knowing your cycle is "normal" is a good way to reassure you that, even if you don't get pregnant right away, it is, at least, possible.

What is a "normal" cycle? Here are some clues:

- Your period should fall anywhere between a twenty-six- and thirty-three-day time span, with twenty-eight days being the average.
- While occasional timing irregularities are normal, cycles should regulate back to normal within two months.
- Menstrual flow should start light and be sporadic on day one; increase intensity on day two; taper down by day three; end light by day four; taper off with light staining on days five and six.
- Blood flow should be smooth, even, and free of clots.

Fertility alert: You could have problems conceiving if these menstrual problems prevail for more than three months:

- Erratic periods with prolonged or significant changes in the length of time between periods
- The length of time between cycles is longer or shorter than what is considered normal, even if it's the same from month to month
- Lack of a menstrual cycle for more than three months
- Excessive bleeding, bleeding longer than six days, blood flow that is heavy for more than three days, or large volumes of blood loss
- Exceptionally scanty blood flow, or a period that ends abruptly after one or two days
- A flow that is watery or light in color or one that is thick and filled with clots

Menstrual Pain and Your Fertility

While every woman has an individual threshold of pain, you should feel only minimal discomfort when you are menstruating. If you experience undue abdominal cramping, nausea, vomiting, dizziness, backache, headaches, or any other significant physical or emotional symptom just before, during, or right after the onset of bleeding, you should see your doctor. Since pain and its accompanying symptoms can often be among the first signs of impending reproductive difficulties, early diagnosis is essential.

Ovulation: Another Important Fertility Sign

Although your menstrual cycle is a very good barometer of many reproductive functions, the one thing it cannot indicate is whether or not you are ovulating—making and releasing healthy eggs on a regular basis. That's because you can still get a relatively "normal" period even when your ovary does not release an egg.

Unfortunately, however, if your ovulation is extremely irregular, conception can be difficult. That's why it's extremely important to evaluate your ovulation potential as early as possible.

Can You Ovulate: How to Tell

To begin testing use the methods featured in Chapter 13, including the BBT temperature guide, the inspection of your cervical mucus, the saliva tests, and the ovulation monitors. You can also use an ovulation predictor kit; it won't necessarily help you *get* pregnant, but it can help determine if you are ovulating and if it's possible for you to conceive.

Be certain to record and keep track of test results, and to ensure accuracy, track ovulation for three consecutive months. Because it's possible to have some signs of ovulation without any egg release, for the most accurate reading you should use at least two methods simultaneously.

Should two or more prediction methods fail to indicate ovulation has occurred, then you may have a problem.

Other signs that you are *not* ovulating include:

- Few or no periods
- Irregular, prolonged or heavy periods
- Prolonged spotting during midcycle

Even if you do bleed normally, a lack of ovulation may be signaled by a decrease in some of the unpleasant symptoms that otherwise might occur during a cycle, such as breast soreness, menstrual cramps, or mood swings.

Regardless of your symptoms or the results of your personal ovulation testing, if more than twelve months of unprotected intercourse does not yield a pregnancy, ovulation failure should be checked along with other possible causes of infertility. As you will read later in this chapter, there are specific tests your doctor can do to help verify your personal findings.

Your Menstrual Enemies: What Blocks Ovulation

Although there are a variety of medical problems that can interfere with your ability to make and release healthy eggs, there are also a number of lifestyle factors that can cause problems. Fortunately, very often these are factors under your control. What affects ovulation most?

- Extreme exercise
- Emotional stress
- Dieting
- Poor nutrition, including a lack of B vitamins
- Extreme weight loss or weight gain
- Low body fat, high body fat
- Medications, recreational drugs, environmental toxins

How Your Family History Can Predict Your Fertility

As important as listening to your body is *listening to your mother*. What I mean is that often you can discover important information about your own reproductive potential when you look into your family's reproductive health history. While not all fertility-related problems are inherited (or inheritable), I have found that a significant number do run in families.

So, if you are having problems getting pregnant, or even if you're just thinking about conceiving and don't know if a problem could exist, it's a good idea to talk to your mother, grandmother, sisters, aunts, and cousins about whether they had any problems getting pregnant. I encourage all of my patients to speak to their family, and to try and discover a history of any fertility-related disorders that can be passed on, including:

- Endometriosis
- PMS
- Ovarian cysts
- Fibroid tumors

Important Questions to Ask Your Mother

It's a good idea to ask your mother (and if possible your grandmother) specific questions about her pregnancy history, including:

- How long it took her to conceive her first child
- If she had any miscarriages, and if so, how many
- If she ever experienced an ectopic or "tubal" pregnancy
- If she suffered with menstrual cramps or irregular cycles
- At what age she began menstruating, and, if applicable, the age she began menopause
- If she ever took DES (a synthetic female hormone widely used in the 1950s and 1960s to prevent miscarriage that has been linked to reproductive problems in offspring)

Take Charge of Your Fertility

One of the most important steps you can take to maximize your child-bearing potential is to seek the help of your doctor *as soon as you discover you might have a problem getting pregnant*. Certainly this should be your next step if testing shows your are not ovulating, or if more than twelve consecutive months of regular (three times weekly) intercourse does not result in pregnancy. Although it can take some couples longer than one year to conceive, even when everything is normal, if it turns out you do have a problem, the sooner you get help, the faster and easier it will be to get pregnant. Sadly, I have seen a number of patients who nearly lost all chance to conceive naturally, simply because they waited just *six months* too long before having something as simple as a silent STD diagnosed and treated. As a result, their reproductive systems suffered irreparable damage.

What should your doctor be looking for? A good place to start is by rechecking some of the factors included in your preconception exam, including:

- Chlamydia, T-mycoplasma, and other STDs
- Fibroid tumors
- Ovarian cysts
- Diabetes
- Thyroid malfunctions
- Endometriosis

Any of these conditions can develop in a relatively short time and affect your ability to conceive.

Providing your tests for the above-mentioned conditions do not reveal any major problems, your next step is some specific fertility testing. In many instances, this can be done by your gynecologist—but don't panic if your doctor suggests you need a fertility expert. The world of reproductive medicine is progressing at such a rapid pace that many OB/GYNs do not feel adequately versed on the latest tests and treatments, even those used for preliminary findings. If this turns out to be the case for you, don't be intimidated about seeking the help of an expert—either a reproductive endocrinologist or a gynecologist who specializes in infertility.

Later in this book you will find important information on how to select a specialist and learn what to look for in a treatment center. Right now, however, I want to explain some of the most important tests you should be receiving, regardless of where you seek treatment.

Your Basic Fertility Exam

Your basic workup should always begin with a review of your menstrual record. This includes the results of any basic tests your gynecologist may have performed, as well as an overview of some specifics about your personal menstrual cycle. (See "How to Test Your Own Fertility" earlier in this chapter for the type of things your doctor needs to know.)

Certainly, if you have used the BBT, alone or, ideally, in conjunction with other ovulation prediction methods, and have charted your results, bring them along.

Other things your doctor needs to know about you and your partner:

- If you have ever been pregnant and if you have had any children
- If your partner has ever fathered a child
- Any history of miscarriage, stillbirth or premature labor
- The age you began menstruating
- If your periods were ever abnormal, or if you were ever medically treated for menstrual irregularities or pain
- If you have any outstanding physical symptoms, particularly chronic backache, stomach pains, incontinence, fatigue, weakness, rashes, vaginal pain, or pain during intercourse, or if your partner experiences pain in his penis at any time
- If you or your partner have ever been medically treated for a sexually transmitted disease
- The age your mother, grandmother, and sister(s) began menopause (if applicable)

The Fertility Blood Tests: What You Need and Why

Approximately 40 percent of all female fertility problems are related to ovulation. Although your personal observations, such as cervical mucus patterns or your BBT, can provide important clues, your medical evaluation should still begin with specific tests to verify that you are making and releasing healthy eggs.

The best way to do that is with a number of tests designed to measure the brain chemicals and hormones involved in the egg-making process. These tests should include:

• **FSH:** This hormone gives your eggs the signal to develop and grow. If you are ovulating, FSH will drop as soon as your menstrual cycle begins. If it doesn't, you might be approaching menopause—a time when ovulation ceases. This test is especially important if you are over age thirty-five, since FSH levels normally rise and remain elevated just before the cessation of egg production.

The best time to take this test: Day one, two, or three of your menstrual cycle.

• **LH:** Secreted just before ovulation, a sudden surge of this hormone triggers egg release. Afterward, levels should drop. The initial "surge" can be tested via an ovulation predictor kit (which uses urine), while the subsequent fall, which should occur once your menstrual cycle begins, requires a blood test.

The best time to take this test: Using an ovulation predictor kit, start testing just before you think you will ovulate—approximately eleven to twelve days after the start of your previous menstrual cycle. The subsequent blood test should be performed by your doctor on day one, two, or three of your menstrual cycle.

• **Estrogen:** This is the hormone that rises as eggs develop and continues to remain high throughout your cycle, until your body verifies that you are not pregnant and your monthly period begins. It is also one of the hormones that helps build the spongy lining inside your uterus—the same lining that is shed as menstrual blood if a pregnancy does not occur. When tested at the correct point in your cycle, estrogen levels can

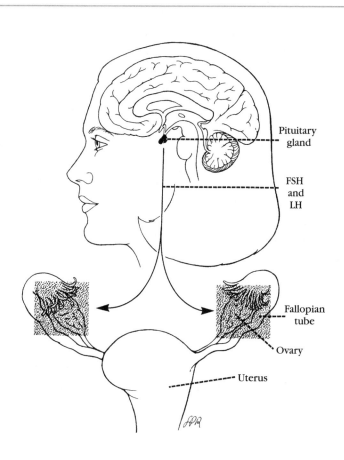

Pituitary gland

FSH and LH

Fallopian tube

Ovary

Uterus

The Brain Chemistry Linked to Conception

At the start of every menstrual cycle, FSH (follicle-stimulating hormone) is manufactured in the brain by the pituitary gland. After being released into the bloodstream, it heads straight for the ovaries, where it stimulates the follicles inside to begin growing. Once they reach maturity, a second message is sent back to the brain to manufacture LH (luteinizing hormone), which in turns helps trigger the release of your egg. By testing blood levels of FSH at various times in your cycle, your doctor can determine if you are making enough of this hormone to set the egg production cycle in motion.

reveal many things, including if you have ovulated, if the timing was correct, and if the normal amounts of hormone were secreted in the process.

The best time to take this test: Taken on day one, two, or three of your menstrual cycle, estrogen levels can tell if you have a hormone imbalance. Taken seven to ten days after an ovulation predictor test indicates a surge of LH, estrogen levels will reveal information about ovulation.

　　▪　**Progesterone:** After ovulation, the shell your egg leaves behind begins to manufacture the hormone progesterone, which, in turn, helps prepare your uterus for a healthy implantation. If a blood test shows progesterone is high in the second half of your cycle, then you have likely ovulated.

The best time to take this test: Seven to ten days after an ovulation predictor test indicates a surge of LH.

More Blood Tests That Can Help

Depending on the results of your workup thus far, your doctor may also suggest one or more of the following blood tests, some of which may be particularly revealing if your fertility problems are related to ovulation. Since these tests are not directly related to menstruation, they can be taken any time during your cycle.

- Prolactin pituitary hormone: Too much of the hormone prolactin works directly on the ovary to suppress the growth of your egg follicles.
- Thyroid hormone: The thyroid is the gland that secretes a hormone that governs metabolism, including the release of a variety of fertility biochemicals. When too much or too little thyroid hormone is secreted, ovulatory problems can result. In addition, a deficiency of thyroid hormone can also increase prolactin production.
- Adrenal androgens (DHEAs and testosterone): Typically known as "male" hormones, these substances are also found in minute amounts in the female body. When, however, levels surge out of control, it can initiate a variety of fertility problems, including PCOD—poly cystic ovarian disease

If You Don't Get a Period: The Tests You Need

For the majority of women with irregular menstrual cycles, or even no period at all, problems are usually hormonal in nature. In this instance, fertility medications, which you will read about later in this book, can often help.

However, for some a problem lies within the uterus itself. In short, these women are incapable of menstruating, so no amount of medication will help.

When this problem is suspected, your doctor may suggest a diagnostic exam known as the progesterone withdrawal test. It involves daily oral doses of the hormone progesterone over a five- to ten-day span, or one progesterone injection. If you are capable of menstruating, you should get a period within seven to twenty days after the progesterone is stopped.

If you do, you can be fairly certain that your ovaries are making enough estrogen to build your uterine lining and that your uterus is capable of responding to progesterone, which in turn suggests your fertility problem is probably hormonal in nature—usually a lack of progesterone.

If you *don't* get a period following progesterone therapy, your hormones could still be at fault—specifically you may not have enough estrogen to build a uterine lining. The next step is estrogen supplements, to give your system the boost it needs. This is followed by a second progesterone withdrawal test.

If you get a period following *this* test, then your fertility problem is likely a lack of estrogen, which could be a sign that menopause is approaching. In any event, you will probably respond well to a number of fertility medications.

However, should you fail to get a period within twenty days following your second progesterone/estrogen test, it could mean your uterus simply cannot respond to reproductive hormones. And that pinpoints the cause of your infertility as being uterine-related.

Reading Your Body Signals: Another Way to Test Your Fertility

As you read earlier, your cervical mucus plays an important role in helping you get pregnant, mostly by facilitating the movement of your partner's sperm through your reproductive system. During the first half of each menstrual cycle, your mucus is affected by estrogen. Taking a mucus sample some time between days ten and fourteen of your cycle will give some clue to whether sufficient amounts of this hormone are present, and if your eggs are being stimulated to grow. At the time of ovulation, extremely high levels of estrogen transform your mucus once again, this time making it thin and watery, which works to help transport sperm through your cervix to your fallopian tubes. Taking a test at this time

On the Horizon—Test That Can Predict Pregnancy Success

While testing hormone levels can provide some important clues concerning your ability to ovulate, some infinitely more sensitive screenings are now on the horizon. One of the most promising measures two proteins involved in egg production—follicular glycoprotein inhibit-B and insulin growth factor binding protein-3 (IGFBP-3). As a direct product of your ovaries, both help produce healthy eggs. Since this is such an essential aspect of getting pregnant, the measuring of these proteins may soon replace other, more complex tests to track fertility.

Other new tests under development will measure how well your ovaries respond to hormonal stimulation. Two of the most promising involve exogenous follicle-stimulating hormone (EFORT) and GRH agonists. Although they are currently considered fertility "markers," unfortunately, we still don't know enough about how they work in the body throughout a cycle to determine "normal" levels. And while this is likely to change in the near future, making these tests far more useful, today the information they provide is limited.

might help reveal if, indeed, sperm transport can be eliminated as one cause of your fertility problems.

Finally, after ovulation, the production of progesterone, which comes from the shell of your newly ovulated egg, balances the excess estrogen, so your mucus once again becomes thick. Testing your mucus in the last half of your cycle may help reveal if you have ovulated.

Generally, you can test your own mucus by gently inserting your finger into your vagina and examining it for the tactile feel and stretch-ability.

Or your doctor can perform a mucus test as well, with or without the addition of sperm (see below).

The Postcoital Test for Fertility Rhythm

This cervical exam offers a more precise way of measuring not only the quantity and quality of your cervical mucus, but more important, the way it interacts with your partner's sperm. Indeed, while you may have enough mucus, what you produce may be incompatible with your partner, creating a hostile vaginal environment that keeps you from getting pregnant. And this is where the postcoital test can help.

You can begin the exam at home, by using an ovulation prediction kit or the Cue II, starting two or three evenings before you expect to ovulate (see Chapter 13). When your test indicates ovulation is imminent, you should plan to have intercourse with your partner the very next morning. Call your doctor immediately afterward and make an appointment to go to the office within the next two hours. Be certain not to use any lubricants during intercourse, and do not bathe, douche, or use any perfumes or products in your genital area before visiting your doctor, since this could affect the quality of the second stage of your PC test. Once you arrive at your doctor's office, he or she will take a sample of your mucus, which should also contain your partner's sperm. By analyzing the mucus-sperm combination under a microscope, your doctor can tell a variety of things about the way in which your body and your partner's body are working together.

What is your doctor looking for?

- A "fern" pattern indicating healthy mucus
- Stretchability
- Cellular debris
- The number of sperm able to swim in the mucus and whether they move in circles or a straight line

Your doctor will also look for whether your mucus contains white blood cells that may be hostile to your partner's sperm, or sperm antibodies. All these things can provide important clues to why you are having a problem getting pregnant, and help in determining what, if any, fertility treatments are necessary.

Visualizing Your Fertility: The No-X-Ray Ultrasound Exam

One of the surest ways to determine a variety of important facts about your fertility is via ultrasound, the nonradiation way of imaging your reproductive organs. A look at your ovaries around the time of ovulation, for example, will indicate if there is a follicle present, or if ovulation has occurred. A scan of your uterus will reveal if it has received sufficient hormonal stimulation to build the spongy nest necessary for your developing baby to survive. In some instances, your doctor may also recommend a Doppler ultrasound, a test that not only visualizes your uterus but also measures blood flow patterns. As you will read later in this book, this can help determine important information about the success of your pregnancy. Finally, an MRI (magnetic resonance imaging) may be used to determine more specifics about uterine shape or form, or to identify specific obstructions seen on your ultrasound scan.

Under the Microscope: Your Fertility Biopsy

Because the lining of your uterus orchestrates such a vital role in preparing your body for pregnancy, sometimes your doctor may want a closer, more detailed look than an ultrasound scan provides. When this is the case, you may be asked to undergo an endometrial biopsy, a test that actually removes a tiny bit of tissue from your uterus for closer examination. What your doctor is looking for: signs that you have ovulated, most often evident in the presence of progesterone in your uterine tissue. For this reason the test should be performed in the second half of your menstrual cycle, close to the scheduled onset of bleeding.

The test is relatively simple and is usually performed in your doctor's office without the need for any general anesthesia. However, it can cause moderate cramping, both during the procedure and for several hours afterward, along with some slight spotting for a few days. Therefore, it's not a good idea to schedule any activities for twenty-four to forty-eight hours following this test.

Looking Inside Your Body: The Fertility X-Ray

In order to ensure that pregnancy is possible, your doctor must ascertain whether your fallopian tubes are open and will easily allow the passage of sperm to your egg, and later, your embryo to your uterus. And, of course, your uterus must also be healthy enough to provide a home in which your baby can develop and grow. It is also important that your entire reproductive system, especially your ovaries, is in the proper location and that all the parts are connected in the proper way.

The test that is most often used to determine all these factors is the hysterosalpingogram or HSG—in essence, a "fertility X-ray." Now, if you're thinking X-rays are dangerous to your reproductive health, you're generally right. However, the amount of radiation used in this test is so tiny (about 1 to 2 rads—the same as a chest X-ray) that you are in no danger of harming your organs. In fact, it would take upward of one thousand rads of radiation to approach the danger level.

The Fertility X-Ray: What You Need to Know

In order to take this test, you will be asked to lie on your back—similar to the position used during a Pap smear. The doctor will thread a thin tube through your vagina and cervix and into your uterus, as a harmless dye is injected. This dye flushes into the thin tubing and is released into your uterus, where it also flows into each fallopian tube. During this time various X-ray pictures are taken of the pattern made by the moving dye, particularly how it flows through the uterus and the fallopian tubes.

What will your doctor specifically be looking for:

- Structural abnormalities within your uterus, including fibroid tumors or polyps
- Adhesions or scar tissue, resulting from a molar pregnancy, an improperly performed Cesarean section, a myomectomy (fibroid removal), a diagnostic D&C, or a pregnancy termination
- A deviation in the shape or size of your uterus
- Tubal abnormalities, including scar tissue, resulting from endometriosis, PID, or a previous ectopic pregnancy, as well as a condition known as hydrosalpinx, a complete tubal blockage

For most women, this test produces only mild discomfort, and the results are well worth the effort. If, however, you are anxious about taking this test, talk to your doctor about medications that can help. I often suggest a mild pain reliever such as Motrin or Advil taken about one hour before the exam. Your doctor can also give you a mild tranquilizer such as Valium to relax your uterine muscles and prevent spasmodic cramping during the procedure. Finally, for the small percentage of patients who are very susceptible to pain, a medication such as Darvocet or Tylenol with codeine can help.

A necessary medication for all women undergoing this procedure, however, is a broad-spectrum antibiotic such as Vibromycin or Zithromax, beginning up to twenty-four hours before the test and continued for about three days afterward. Why? Sometimes, bacteria that safely reside only in your vagina and cervix can easily be passed into your uterus during this procedure, thus increasing your risk of PID. Taking the antibiotic, however, will help eliminate the threat of infection.

Red flag: If you have a history of pelvic inflammatory disease (PID), particularly more than one bout of infection, and there is any chance you have a current infection, this test should be avoided, and an alternative form of testing considered. If you have an allergy to shellfish, you should also avoid this test, since the dye used to help form the images is iodine-based—the same mineral that causes the shellfish allergy.

Underwater Vision: The New Ultrasound

A new twist on conventional ultrasound now allows your doctor to get a clearer, often more precise picture of your reproductive organs as well as your potential to get pregnant. The procedure is called an ultrasound HSG and like an ordinary sonogram it uses sound waves that bounce off your organs to form a picture on a computerized screen. The new twist, however, involves first flooding your uterine cavity and tubes with a harmless saline solution. Then, by watching the path the fluid takes, the sonogram may diagnose the same types of problems as a hysterosalpingogram, and may be more comfortable for you to endure. Since this test does not require the use of dyes, it may be helpful for those with allergies. Additionally, pictures formed by the new ultrasound are usually in 3D rather than the 2D type offered by the standard HSG exam, so a more detailed picture is often possible. For you that means a better, more accurate diagnosis of your fertility problems.

Although this procedure is one of the newest weapons in the arsenal of fertility testing, studies published in the *International Journal of Gynecology and Obstetrics* have already revealed that, if performed correctly, it is as accurate in predicting uterine and tubal abnormalities as an HSG.

Where Do We Go from Here?

Depending on what your basic fertility workup reveals, other, more complex diagnostic procedures may become necessary. In many instances, these same procedures will be able to treat and solve your fertility problems at the same time they are diagnosed.

In the next chapter you will find the newest, most important of these diagnostic treatments, with the latest information on how they can help you conceive.

In the meantime, however, **don't forget your partner!** At the same time you are taking the tests featured in this chapter, he should be tested as well. His preliminary workup should include, at the very least, a sperm count and bacterial culture, particularly for STDs. In most cases your doctor can send your partner to a laboratory for testing, or to a specialist. In either case, I can't emphasize enough the importance of male testing *before* you are subjected to any highly invasive fertility tests or treatments. Up to 50 percent of all infertility problems are male-related and your partner must rule out at least the most basic causes before asking you to complete another round of tests.

Seeing a Fertility Expert

If and when you do decide to see a fertility expert, be certain to bring the results of any tests your gynecologist has taken, including all X-rays and scans. If tests have been performed within six months, there is no need to repeat them. Any doctor who refuses to look at previous test results and *insists* on repeating *all* procedures should be viewed with a skeptical eye.

Likewise, if your fertility expert dismisses you after an exceptionally short visit, particularly if he or she has not examined you, claiming nothing more can be done to help—don't get discouraged. Instead, **look for another doctor.** I can't tell you the number of patients I have successfully treated after not one, but two, three, sometimes four doctors have told them there is no hope. In one instance, a patient of mine—a forty-

Infertility at a Glance: Causes and Treatments

Problem: Ovulation malfunction or failure
Major sign: Menstrual irregularities
What can help you get pregnant: Fertility medications (see Chapter 19) and, if FSH is elevated, also egg donation (see Chapter 23)

Problem: Poly cystic ovarian disease (PCOD)
Major sign: Abnormal estrogen (E2) and LH test results
What can help you get pregnant: The fertility drug clomiphene or gonadotropin (see Chapter 19)

Problem: Pituitary malfunction
Major sign: Elevated prolactin levels
What can help you get pregnant: The medications bromocriptine or carbergoline (see Chapter 19)

Problem: Hypothalamus-related menstrual irregularities
Major sign: Menstrual irregularity with abnormal FSH and LH test results
What can help you get pregnant: Fertility drugs clomiphene or gonadotropin (see Chapter 19) or donor eggs (see Chapter 23)

Problem: Premature ovarian failure
Major symptom: Elevated FSH levels
What can help you get pregnant: Donor eggs (see Chapter 23)

Problem: Anatomic uterine abnormalities
Major signs: Adhesions; misshapen uterus, tubal obstruction, endometriosis, fibroid tumors, ovarian cysts; abnormal hysterosalpingogram
What can help you get pregnant: Surgeries to correct the abnormalities (including laparoscopy, myomectomy, or hysteroscopy—see Chapter 17); also in vitro fertilization; GIFT, ZIFT (see Chapters 21 and 22)

Problem: Cervical mucus abnormalities
Major signs: Abnormal postcoital test
What can help you get pregnant: Intrauterine insemination (see Chapter 20)

five-year-old college professor—was told by a half-dozen so-called experts that there was no way she could ever get pregnant. I am happy to report she is now the mother of a beautiful baby girl, whom she conceived *naturally*. Her only fertility treatment: She followed the fertility diet and vitamin plan featured in Part Two of this book.

The point to remember is this: Don't give up on your motherhood dreams without first learning about *all* your fertility options. If you know in your heart that you want to be a mother, don't take "no" for an answer—not from your gynecologist, your fertility expert, or even your husband or family. Remember to, that if a problem *is* discovered, a plethora of new, fast, and easy treatments are available to help.

So don't be afraid to question your fertility, and don't waste time wondering about it. Instead, take charge—and the baby you were destined to have will be yours!

Chapter Seventeen

The New Fertility Surgeries:

Natural Conception Made Fast and Easy

As recently as the 1980s, treating many fertility problems required traumatic procedures and often costly hospital stays. Today, new surgical techniques and instruments, particularly laser technologies, combined with lighter, faster-acting anesthesia and new postoperative medicines are enabling doctors to quickly and easily perform even the most complex fertility procedures, often right in their offices. In fact, many fertility-restoring treatments are now so simple, you can be back to your normal routine in just twenty-four to forty-eight hours. In many instances you will be able to conceive naturally, in just a matter of weeks.

Can Fertility Surgery Help You? How to Tell

Although new medications are making some fertility procedures unnecessary, I have found that for many of my patients, surgery is still the fastest, easiest route to a natural conception. It can be particularly helpful if your doctor diagnoses one or more of the following conditions:

- **Cervical and vaginal abnormalities:** These include structural problems within your cervix or vagina, including congenital malformations, and obstructions such as cysts, tumors, and adhesions (scar tissue), all of which can keep sperm from reaching your fallopian tubes.

- **Uterine abnormalities:** This category covers congenital malformations affecting the shape and size of your uterus, including uterine

septum, where an excess wall of tissue partially divides this organ, sometimes resulting in the development of a double uterus. Also included in
this category are submucus-type fibroid tumors (which grow inside the
uterus) and adhesions from previous gynecological procedures or PID.
These problems normally cause infertility by interfering with a healthy
implantation or subsequent growth and development of your baby. Problems in the uterus can also increase your risk of miscarriage.

- **Fallopian tube abnormalities:** These include blockages inside
the tube (resulting from infection, ectopic pregnancies, or endometriosis) as well as damaged fimbria (tubal ends) and internal tubal adhesions.
All these problems can keep sperm from reaching your egg, or an egg that
has been fertilized may not be able to reach your uterus, possibly resulting in an ectopic pregnancy.

- **Ovarian abnormalities:** The most common problem here is cyst
formation, especially those caused by endometriosis. In other instances,
scar tissue from previous PID or endometriosis can completely encase
the ovary. Either condition can interfere with egg production and ovulation.

Time-Saving, Money-Saving Ways to Save Your Fertility

If your fertility blood tests and your pelvic exam do not provide a reason
why you can't get pregnant, the possibility of structural problems should
be investigated. The quickest, easiest method is via endoscopy—a diagnostic technique that uses various telescopelike devices to view your internal organs, and in many instances render treatment at the same time.
This can save you not only the trauma of a second operation but also the
expense and the recovery time of multiple procedures, which is something my patients have always appreciated.

In addition, sometimes videos can be taken through the endoscopic
instruments, providing a record of everything your doctor sees. This can
also save time and money if you seek a second opinion or if you need to
see additional specialists.

The Procedures—and How They Can Help

The three basic endoscopic procedures used in conjunction with fertility problems are culdoscopy, hysteroscopy, and laparoscopy. The newest is called falloscopy and is used to diagnose and treat problems within the fallopian tubes. I have used all four methods in my practice and found great success with each of them. To help you understand a little more about each one, I've prepared the following guide.

Procedure: Culdoscopy

Used primarily to study your uterus, fallopian tubes, and ovaries, culdoscopy helps determine abnormalities in shape or size and identifies the presence of endometriosis or adhesions. It also detects early signs of ovarian disease, including cysts and tumors.

Because its surgical applications are limited, culdoscopy is not used today as often as in the past. However, it can still be an effective means of removing small amounts of scar tissue and adhesions and performing ovarian biopsies.

How it's done: First you are sedated and positioned on a procedure table. Your head is placed sideways on a pillow, and your arms are folded under your chest. Your knees are drawn up so that you are in a semi-kneeling position. This helps place your vagina in a backward position, which increases test accuracy.

Once the position has been assumed, your doctor places a speculum inside your vagina to hold it open, makes a small internal incision just above your cervix, and inserts an instrument called a culdoscope—a type of telescopic device that allows a study of the back surface of your uterus, fallopian tubes, and ovaries. By inserting several types of instruments next to the culdoscope, several surgical procedures can be performed.

Precautions: A culdoscopy should never be performed when you have any of the following conditions:

- Peritonitis
- PID
- Intestinal obstructions
- Unstable cardiovascular system
- Severe endometriosis
- Previous myomectomy or extensive pelvic surgery

Complications can include infection and bleeding at the puncture site.

Procedure: Hysteroscopy

First developed during the 1980s, this procedure detects abnormalities in the shape and structure of your uterus. This includes congenital abnormalities (such as misshapen, divided, or even a missing uterus) that may be present from birth, as well as uterine abnormalities that can develop during the reproductive years, such as fibroid tumors. In fact, fibroid tumors smaller than three millimeters can actually be removed during this procedure. It can also diagnose, and if necessary remove, adhesions resulting from previous procedures such as a D&C (a surgical scraping of the uterus) or abortions, or from infections, or even from IUD use.

Finally, a hysteroscopy can also be used alone or in combination with a falloscope (see below) to evaluate your fallopian tubes, and to help determine the existence of any obstructions.

How it's done: After placing you under a light anesthetic or sedative, your doctor will dilate your cervix and then insert a thin, fiberoptic telescoping rod into your vagina, through your cervical canal, and up into your uterus. Your uterine cavity will be expanded by injecting a harmless gas such as carbon dioxide or a liquid solution. Both work to push the walls of your uterus apart allowing for a better view. By inserting additional instruments through the hysteroscope, your doctor can perform a number of surgical procedures.

Precautions: When performed for fertility purposes, this procedure is best done immediately after your menstrual period ends and before ovulation. Still, a hysteroscopy should not be done during your menstrual period or if any of the following conditions exist:

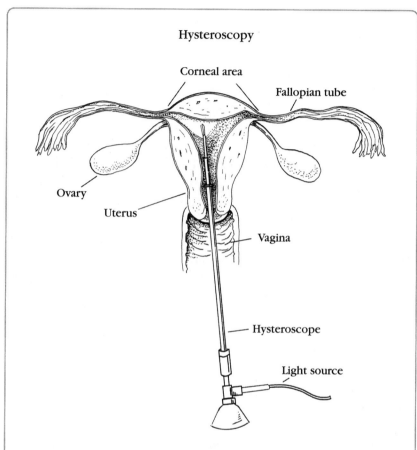

Hysteroscopy

Corneal area

Fallopian tube

Ovary

Uterus

Vagina

Hysteroscope

Light source

Hysteroscopy: *The Diagnostic Procedure That Can Help You Get Pregnant*

After dilating your cervix, your doctor will insert a thin, fiberoptic tube attached to a light source into your vagina, through your cervix, and ultimately into your uterus. The inside of your uterus is expanded slightly using a harmless gas, which enables your doctor to get a clear picture of the inside of your reproductive tract, including your fallopian tubes. If any minor abnormalities are found, such as tiny fibroid tumors or bits of scar tissue, additional instruments can be inserted through the hysteroscope and the blockages removed.

- An infection anywhere in your reproductive tract
- Profuse uterine bleeding, of any cause
- Pregnancy
- A recent uterine perforation—often the result of a medical procedure
- Known cervical or uterine cancer

Additionally, your doctor can reduce the complications associated with a non-emergency hysteroscopy with a fertility medication known as gonadotropin-releasing hormone (GnRH), which you'll read about later in the book. Essentially, however, it works to prevent a thickening of the uterine lining that normally occurs during each menstrual cycle. By keeping the lining thin, your doctor may be able to better see inside your reproductive system. And because your uterine lining is thinner, the procedure will also be shorter and cause less blood loss. In research presented to the American Association of Gynecologic Laparoscopists, it was shown that when used for six to twelve weeks before a hysteroscopy, GnRH (Lupron) not only decreased risk factors associated with this procedure, but also increased effectiveness.

Procedure: Falloscopy

One of the newest forms of endoscopic examination, this procedure was developed specifically to look inside the fallopian tubes and diagnose a number of abnormalities capable of blocking the route from sperm to egg, or embryo to uterus. Because of their location, fallopian tubes can be difficult to reach, particularly because they are delicate and very narrow. This new procedure, which makes use of one of several new types of devices designed to go directly inside the tube, makes diagnosis safer, easier, and ultimately more accurate.

How it's done: Using a catheter-based system, your doctor will insert a flexible tube through your vagina and cervix, threading it into one of your fallopian tubes. Containing some three thousand imaging fibers, the catheter is slowly pulled through the tube, which in turn illuminates the inside, thus allowing your doctor to visualize the tubal wall and note whether it is healthy or if any obstructions exist. In studies comparing falloscopy to hysterosalpingogram, another common method of visualizing fallopian tubes (see Chapter 16), this new technology corrected false information or provided additional, important clinical data in nearly 70 percent of cases.

Precautions: Studies show the rate of complications as a result of falloscopy averages less than 4 percent. This can be reduced further with additional training and the use of antibiotics.

Procedure: Laparoscopy

By far the most common, most useful, and best of all endoscopic procedures is a laparoscopy—a procedure that allows a direct view of all your pelvic organs, including uterus, ovaries, and a portion of your fallopian tubes. It also offers the opportunity to perform a number of important surgical procedures. Laparoscopy is most often used for:

- Evaluation of ovarian disease, possible genital abnormalities and tubal patency, and other conditions affecting egg transport.
- Evaluation of pelvic pain or pelvic inflammatory disease (PID)
- Differentiating between a fibroid tumor and a cyst
- Classification and removal of endometriosis
- A second look at previous fertility surgery
- Evaluation of a uterine perforation that may have resulted from an abortion
- Biopsies of tubes, ovary, and uterus
- Removal of adhesions
- Aspiration (deflating) and removal of ovarian cysts
- Removal of ectopic pregnancy
- Repairing some types of damage to fallopian tubes
- Diagnosis and removal of some types of fibroid tumors
- Performing some types of hysterectomies

This procedure is also used in conjunction with certain steps involved in various forms of IVF (in vitro fertilization), which are explained in detail in Chapters 21 and 22.

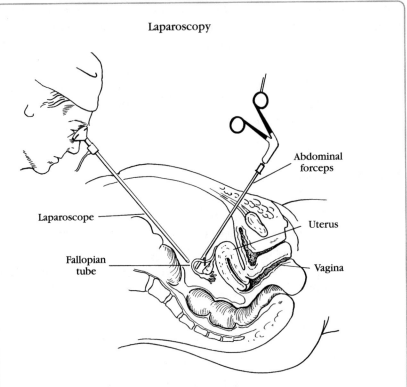

Laparoscopy

Laparoscopy: The Most Useful Fertility Surgery

During this procedure your doctor will make one tiny incision into your belly button and insert a long, thin viewing tube. This enables a clear view inside your entire reproductive system. If treatment becomes necessary, one or two additional small incisions are made near your bikini line, where surgical instruments, including a laser, can be inserted. Then, looking through the eyepiece, your doctor can perform the necessary surgery. Just one or two stitches close the incisions, which normally heal quite quickly, without a scar.

How it's done: After sedating you with a mild anesthetic, your doctor will make a tiny incision into your belly button—one that will leave no scar. Often, a tiny video camera attached to a long, thin tube will be inserted into the incision and threaded through your abdominal cavity.

To help your doctor to better see all your organs, your abdominal cavity is filled with carbon dioxide gas, which is pumped through the incision. At this point your doctor can view your organs either via the laparoscope (a tiny microscope inserted into the incision) or by looking at a computer screen that holds the image relayed from the tiny video camera inserted at the start of your procedure.

If treatment becomes necessary your doctor will make one or two additional small incisions (about the size of a pencil eraser) into your abdomen, usually right at the bikini line, so no scar can be seen. Long, ultrathin instruments—including certain types of laser equipment—are then inserted into the incisions. Watching the image on the video monitor or through the laparoscope, your doctor will then grasp, hold, cut, burn, vaporize, or otherwise treat a number of abnormalities on the spot, thus saving you the trauma and expense of additional surgery.

Precautions: For the most part, laparoscopy is a safe and uncomplicated procedure, providing it is done by an experienced doctor who performs this operation on a regular basis. In the hands of an inexperienced physician, however, it can result in several problems, including

The Gasless Laparoscopy

For most patients, the carbon dioxide gas used in a laparoscopy poses no problems. For some, however, particularly those with one of several types of cardiac conditions, it can create undue pressure on the heart, increasing the risk of problems.

In an attempt to remedy this situation, several new devices are under development to allow for a "gasless" procedure. One such instrument, called the Laparolift, works to lift and separate uterine tissue, making it easier for your doctor to see your internal organs without having to expand your uterine cavity with gas. Although studies show the gasless laparoscopy can be beneficial if you have a heart condition, the surgery is still technically more difficult to execute. Further, compromised visualization (the site is still clearer when gas is used) may reduce accuracy and increase operative times. All this means that, right now, the gasless laparoscopy should only be used under extraordinary circumstances.

damage to the intestines (occurring while putting in the gas to expand the abdomen), blood vessels, bladder, or kidney. In some instances it may also cause scarring or damage to the reproductive organs, which, in turn, may increase fertility problems. Fortunately, all these risks can be greatly minimized by making sure your doctor is experienced in this procedure.

In many instances, a laparoscopy is an outpatient procedure that doctors can perform in their own office or clinic. Depending on the type of anesthesia you receive, you are usually able to go home within one to four hours. You may feel some discomfort afterward, including shoulder pain, which results from pressure in your abdomen caused by the gas used in this procedure. Some of this discomfort can be avoided if your doctor gently presses on your abdomen after the procedure is completed, which will help release the gas.

Still, you may also experience some dull or even sharp pains near the incision as the healing process takes place. Medication; warm, moist heat; and rest can help. In most instances you will be advised to avoid driving, exercise, sex, heavy lifting, or strenuous housework for one to two weeks following a laparoscopy.

You can also play a role in ensuring the success of your surgery by immediately reporting any of these postsurgical symptoms to your doctor:

- An expanding bruise under or near your incision(s), which could indicate the presence of a blood clot
- Recurring vomiting, fever, or abdominal swelling
- Heavy vaginal bleeding (spotting and slight bleeding is okay)
- Intense pain that worsens with medication
- Kidney pain or pain in the small of your back

Tubal Surgery: More Ways to Help You Get Pregnant Fast

While endoscopy can help a great many fertility problems, sometimes a slightly more complex, tubal surgery is needed. This is particularly true when you have extensive fallopian tube damage resulting from either pelvic inflammatory disease or one of several STDs, or if you want to reverse a tubal ligation, the operation that "tied your tubes" to prevent pregnancy.

What Microsurgery Is—and How It Can Restore Your Fertility

In the simplest terms, microsurgery is a procedure that uses extremely small incisions, made possible by the development of extremely fine-gauge medical instruments. The goal here is to minimize trauma to your tissues, which in turn will reduce the risk of postoperative scarring and the formation of scar tissue.

In many ways, microsurgery also allows your doctor to visualize and consequently treat more types of problems, particularly those involving very tiny blood vessels. This is because most often the entire surgery is performed under a microscope or medical magnifying glasses—particularly important if, for example, your doctor is trying to separate normal tissue from scar tissue.

Microsurgeons are also specially trained to handle tissue in an extremely gentle manner and to operate with minimal blood loss. This further helps reduce scar tissue formation.

From a fertility standpoint, getting pregnant after microsurgery is far more likely than after traditional surgery.

While at one time any problem involving fallopian tubes was considered irreversible, today this is no longer the case. Thanks to the advent of microsurgery (see the box above) as well as laser surgery (a nearly bloodless form of operating), a number of these procedures are now safely and easily performed.

If your doctor suspects fallopian tube damage, surgery should, however, only be considered after one or more diagnostic tests (including a hysterosalpingogram) confirm that at least one of your tubes is blocked. When this is the case, one of the following surgeries can help.

- **Salpingostomy:** Most often performed to remove *significant* blockages in your fallopian tubes, such as those caused by *extensive* adhesions (scar tissue) as a result of PID. During this procedure, your doctor will make an incision near the fimbriated fingerlike end of the tube, so that the blockages or damaged tissue can be removed.

- **Fimbrioplasty:** This procedure is used to correct mild to moderate damage to your fimbria. Severe damage that completely closes the tube (a condition called hydrosalpinx) should be left alone; conception in such a case is best achieved via a laboratory procedure, such as in vitro fertilization (IVF—see Chapter 21).

- **Reanastomosis:** This procedure was developed to reverse a voluntary tubal ligation, the procedure that "ties" the fallopian tubes to prevent pregnancy. It can also help repair some congenital malformations, remove remnants of an ectopic pregnancy, or remove a cyst or tumor from inside your tube.

- **Tubal reimplantation:** In this procedure your fallopian tube will be detached from your uterus, the damaged portion removed or cut away, and the remaining healthy section reconnected to your uterine wall. This is normally done to correct a condition wherein a portion of your fallopian tube closest to your uterus is blocked and cannot be surgically opened.

News Flash: Untying the Birth Control Knot

New studies have shown that it may no longer be necessary to perform traditional surgery to reverse tubal ligation. Indeed, prize-winning research presented to the World Congress on Infertility in fall 1998 revealed that laparoscopic *microsurgery* is, in some cases, as effective as traditional reanastomosis, while being less invasive and easier for the patient to endure. Of the nearly two hundred patients who agreed to try laparoscopy to reverse tubal ligation, more than 80 percent were able to get pregnant, most within four months following their surgery. It is likely that in the near future, laparoscopy may become the procedure of choice for most types of tubal surgery.

A Word of Advice About Tubal Surgery

Although advances in tubal surgery are now making it possible to correct a great many fertility problems, still, you should approach these treatments with some caution and concern. Because fallopian tubes are composed of such delicate tissue, often you may be far better off turning to a laboratory-aided conception, such as in vitro fertilization (IVF). As you will read in Chapter 21, this procedure was designed to bypass the fallopian tubes entirely, so pregnancy is likely to be faster and easier than it would be even if your tubes were fully repaired.

Indeed, the average amount of time between tubal surgery and pregnancy is at least ten months—and in many instances, no pregnancy results at all. Additionally, no matter how successful your tubal surgery may be, your risk of ectopic pregnancy remains high—up to 40 percent in some instances.

A good rule of thumb: The more extensive your tubal damage, and the more drastic your surgery needs to be, the better off you will be bypassing the operation and moving ahead directly to IVF.

That said, you should still consider tubal surgery, particularly if you are very insistent upon achieving pregnancy in a totally natural manner. However, to be certain you fully understand all your options and the relatively low success rate of certain types of tubal surgery, definitely consult at least two specialists before deciding whether to proceed.

The Nonsurgical Ways to Save Your Fallopian Tubes

Depending on the extent and the type of blockage in your fallopian tube, two new methods of treatment—both similar to those used to open passages to the heart and brain—can help.

The Tubal "Roto-Rooter"

In much the same way doctors can now insert a kind of medical "roto-rooter" to clear arterial debris blocking blood flow to the heart, so too does a similar procedure work to clear out your fallopian tubes.

Known as a "tubal recannulization," this procedure uses a series of small guide wires to move ultrathin plastic tubes through your cervix, into your uterine cavity, to your fallopian tubes. Once they are in place, fluid is flushed through the catheters into your tubes. If the tubes open, and the liquid goes through, then your problem was likely a spasm and not a true blockage. If, however, the fluid does not pass, an ultrathin wire is inserted into the tube. Using a gentle "roto-rooter" action, the wire dislodges the debris and small blockages, particularly those caused by protein buildup. An outpatient procedure, done alone or in combination with laparoscopy, this treatment is painless thanks to local anesthetic, and it is successful for up to 50 percent of women whose fallopian obstruction is located in the proximal portion of their tube (the section that connects directly to the uterus). Indeed, this procedure is now considered the first line of defense for this type of tubal blockage. If, however, you don't get pregnant within a few months, the obstruction may close again.

Most often tubal recannulization is performed by a radiologist, and can be done at the time you are receiving your hysterosalpingogram. In rare instances, a blockage may not be verifiable without a laparoscopy, in which case the recannulization must be rescheduled as an independent procedure.

How a Balloon Can Save Your Fertility

Taking its cue from still another cardiac treatment is a procedure known as "transcervical balloon tuboplasty," a kind of "angioplasty" of the reproductive system. Developed in Chicago by Dr. Edmund Corfino, the treatment begins with a thin, plastic catheter into which a tiny guide wire has been placed. At the tip of the catheter is a collapsed balloon. With the cardiac procedure the catheter is placed into a blood vessel, while in the tubal version it is threaded through your abdomen to your tube, via a tiny incision. In either instance, once the wire reaches the obstructed portion, the balloon is inflated, which expands and opens the blockage. When this procedure is performed on the fallopian tubes, the balloon is inflated again and the procedure repeated as many times as necessary to clear a passageway inside. Unfortunately there are no formal statistics on how long the tube remains open, or the rate of pregnancy following the procedure. Still, the results thus far look promising.

The Fibroid Surgery That Preserves Your Fertility

As you read earlier in this book, fibroid tumors can be a major source of fertility problems, decreasing your chances for a healthy implantation and increasing your risk of miscarriage by a significant margin (see Chapter 2). As recently as the 1980s the general treatment for fibroid tumors was often hysterectomy—the removal of all the reproductive organs that brings an obvious close to the reproductive years. And some doctors still insist on this procedure today.

However, the most modern and progressive surgeons know that for the most part, only the tumors need to be removed, leaving your uterus totally intact. The operation that can accomplish this is called a myomectomy, and it should always be the procedure of choice when you want to retain your childbearing options.

How a Myomectomy Is Performed

This operation requires only one thin bikini incision right above your pubic bone and leaves only a minimal scar. Once inside, your surgeon makes a tiny slit in your uterus, lifts back the tissue, exposes your fibroid growths, and removes them at their base. Your incision is then stitched and the operation is complete. Recovery time is four to five hospital days and four to six weeks of home care.

A Safer Myomectomy: What Your Doctor Should Do

Your doctor can help ensure the success of your traditional surgical myomectomy, as well as your safety, by taking the following precautions:

- A laser or electro cautery knife should be used to "seal" cut blood vessels. This minimizes bleeding.

- A tourniquet should be placed around your uterus during the operation. This also significantly cuts blood loss.

- The drug petressin should be injected into the uterus, and an intravenous solution of the drug oxytocin should be used during the operation to minimize bleeding.

- Dextran 70, a highly viscous solution, should be injected into the abdomen, and the medication hydrocortisone should be given both intra-abdominally during the operation and intravenously for a few days following surgery to prevent the formation of abdominal adhesions—scar tissue that can cause infertility.

- Antibiotics should be administered after surgery to guard against postoperative infection.

- Uterine suspension (pulling the uterus upward during surgery) can be done to decrease adhesions and enhance fertility.

Hysterectomy Versus Myomectomy: It Should Be Your Choice

As beneficial as myomectomies can be, not all doctors are qualified to perform them. For this reason, many physicians may not even inform you about this procedure. Some may try to scare you into having a hysterectomy by telling you that a myomectomy is a very bloody or risky operation. In my opinion this is absolutely unfounded. I have performed over a thousand myomectomies and on only one occasion did a patient require a blood transfusion. Other fertility specialists who routinely perform this operation have had similar results. In fact, when done properly by an experienced myomectomy surgeon the operation is one of the safest, most effective fertility-preserving procedures being performed today, and you should give it prime consideration if you are diagnosed as having fibroid tumors that cannot be treated with medication.

A New Fibroid Surgery: What You Should Know

As advances in laparoscopic surgery continue, new studies show that it may, in fact, play a role in removing certain types of fibroid tumors. Known as the "laparoscopic myoma coagulation," or "myolysis," the procedure uses the customary tiny abdominal incision, into which your doctor will place special laser equipment that works to destroy the blood supply of your tumor. And that in turn means the fibroid will disintegrate on its own. A second alternative uses a set of needles attached to other laparoscopic instruments to inject the fibroid, which also destroys the blood supply.

To make treatment even easier, drugs such as leuprolide can be taken for three to five months before surgery. This will help temporarily shrink the tumors, making the laparoscopic myomectomy even more likely to succeed. Compared to a standard hysterectomy, which requires up to six weeks of recovery, myolysis is an outpatient procedure that allows you to return to work within five days.

Currently, however, these new procedures are used primarily on women who have completed their families and are diagnosed with serosa or subserosal (see Chapter 2) tumors measuring 10 cm or less. However, it's likely that in the near future these new procedures may also prove effective for women who want to preserve their reproductive health.

The Surgery That Saves Your Fertility — Even After Cancer

In the past, a diagnosis of cervical cancer sometimes demanded a hysterectomy, putting an obvious end to your reproductive potential. Now, however, important new studies show that removing only the cervix (a procedure known as "radical trachelectomy," or RT) and leaving your uterus intact can be an optional treatment for noninvasive cervical cancer and one that also preserves fertility. In research conducted by Dr. Michael Roy at Laval University in Quebec City, Canada, of twenty-six young women who underwent the RT procedure, five were able to get pregnant afterward, with more pregnancies expected from the group. Because the procedure is still considered experimental in the United States, all births must be delivered via Cesarean section and patients must be counseled to wait at least six months after their surgery before attempting conception.

At this time, however, most physicians in the United States will bypass a hysterectomy when possible, and instead perform a large cone biopsy (removal of the inner cone portion of the cervix where the cancer usually grows), another worthy treatment for very early stage cervical cancer.

If You Decide on Fertility Surgery: What You Need to Know

If your doctor suggests that fertility surgery will help you, *you* must play an active, aggressive role in making that decision. The best way to do that is not only to find out as much as you can about your specific problem, but also to familiarize yourself with some of the specifics of the operation, as well as with some of the practical aspects of fertility surgery in general. Remember to solicit the following information from your doctor *well before* you schedule a surgery.

1. The *complete recovery time of your operation:* This includes any time spent in the hospital or office as well as convalescing time at home.

2. *The rate of pregnancy after surgery:* While some fertility operations are genuinely worthwhile, others produce no significant results. Here are the success rates for pregnancy following some of the most common surgeries:

   - Salpingnostomy: Up to 39 percent
   - Fimbrioplasty: Up to 67 percent
   - Tubal reimplantation: Up to 32 percent
   - Anastomosis: Up to 64 percent

3. *Your doctor's surgical qualifications:*

- How long has your doctor has been performing fertility surgery?
- How many fertility-related procedures has your physician performed, and particularly how many of the one he or she will be administering to you?
- What precautions does your doctor plan to take to minimize the threat of postoperative complications and hasten recovery time?
- What has been your doctor's personal success rate for pregnancies resulting from his fertility operations?

     You have every right to know the answers to these questions, and if your doctor refuses to provide you with this information, seek help elsewhere.

4. *The total cost of your operation, including follow-up visit and how much your insurance will cover:* Insurance plans vary greatly so don't assume that every medical procedure is automatically covered by your policy. Some fertility treatments are not covered at all while others are covered in full. Your doctor should have this information. If he or she does not, contact your insurance company and get its reply in writing.

5. *Where the surgery will be performed and the type of staff that will be caring for you:* This is vitally important if your doctor will be performing your surgery on an outpatient basis. Since all surgery requires at least two to three hours' recovery time in the office or clinic in which it was performed, you need to know the following:

- Are there qualified surgical and recovery room personnel who are experienced, trained, and certified—including certified anesthesiologists and nurses?
- Is the recovery room equipped to handle any medical emergencies that might arise from your operation?
- Does the clinic or hospital your doctor uses have a safe reputation? Ask for the names of patients who have had similar operations in the same facility and question them on the care they received.

Some Final Advice: Know All Your Options

Fertility surgery has come a long way in just the past five years. But, as beneficial as these operations can be, they are not right for every woman. Sometimes surgery causes extensive scar tissue that ultimately causes you more fertility problems *after* your operation. A number of patients have come to me, frustrated and angry, as well as infertile, because their previous doctors had talked them into operations they never should have had.

When Should You Think Twice About Fertility Surgery?

If any of these conditions exist, an operation might not help you:

- Fallopian tubes that are severely blocked or damaged, due either to a severe case of PID or to the occurrence of several infections over time
- Deeply embedded scar tissue or adhesions on your ovaries or especially your fallopian tubes
- Extensive endometriosis that has caused severe tubal or other organ damage, as well as excessive adhesions, all of which would be too difficult to repair surgically
- Extensive tubal or uterine damage due to previous surgery
- Tubal damage due to ectopic pregnancy

When surgery is absolutely necessary, when possible, choose a less invasive laparoscopy over the traditional surgical laparotomy. If you must have a laparotomy, make certain your doctor uses microsurgical techniques and instruments.

Be Prudent, But Don't Lose Hope

I tell you all this not to scare or dissuade you, only to help you decide wisely. Always get a second opinion—and if need be a third—before making up your mind about having an operation. Today, there are often many options from which to choose, and it's important that you know all your alternatives before making a decision.

In addition, keep in mind that there are also many options to help you conceive, including the full array of laboratory-aided conceptions such as IVF, GIFT, or ZIFT, all described in the final chapters of this book. Sometimes they can be a faster, easier, and even safer way to get pregnant than undergoing one or more of these operations.

Chapter Eighteen

When He's the Reason You Can't Conceive:

The Newest Treatments for Male Infertility

Statistics now confirm what many fertility specialists have known for a long time—that almost half of all couples' fertility problems are male-related. I have certainly found this to be true in my own practice, where the number of female patients whose partners have reproductive problems has risen significantly in just the past few years.

The good news is that medicine has made great strides in this area, particularly in recent years. Today, the technology behind male reproductive health is so advanced that even men who have zero sperm count are still capable of making a baby!

But before I explain what these new technologies are all about, it's important that we go back to the very basis of male fertility—his sperm. Although technology today is such that essentially all sperm problems can be overcome, it's important that you and your partner understand what can go wrong.

Understanding Male Fertility: What You Need to Know

Although there are a variety of different factors capable of affecting a man's fertility, the underlying cause is always sperm-related. For this reason, the very best and fastest way to determine if your partner has a fertility problem is for him to have a sperm count, which is actually an analysis of *several* factors related to fertility.

- **Number of sperm:** The fewer sperm your partner has, the less his chances of naturally fertilizing your egg. If the amount your partner manufactures is under 20 million sperm per milliliter of ejaculate, then chances for natural conception, as well as some forms of laboratory-assisted conception, drop dramatically.

- **Sperm quality:** This refers to the percentage of *good* sperm your partner manufactures. A high sperm count means nothing if the percentage of healthy sperm is not also high. Unhealthy sperm (those that are deformed as a result of disease, in the manufacturing process, or because of a chromosomal abnormality) are usually too weak to either fertilize an egg or bring about a successful conception.

- **Sperm motility:** This describes the ability of sperm to reach your egg. If sperm motility is poor, it means it does not have the "energy" to swim to an egg. This condition often coexists with poor sperm quality.

Important note: Because all three of these factors can easily be influenced by bacterial infections, cultures should always be taken at the same time as a sperm count. This includes a check for infections to which your partner knows he has been exposed or those for which he is experiencing symptoms. He should also be tested for the silent infections linked to infertility, such as chlamydia or T-mycoplasma.

If any infections are found, you, as well as your partner, must receive immediate treatment with antibiotics, as described in Chapter 5. Then, sperm must be retested after you are both shown to be infection-free.

Good Sperm – Bad Sperm: What Does It Mean?

Although in some instances the results of a sperm count will be conclusive, at other times results may not be so easy to interpret. I have found that sometimes even two men with *identical* test results may not have equal success in conceiving a child. Why? Most often, a man's fertility is also dependent on factors present in his partner's body. As such, what's going on inside you can also affect your partner's ability to naturally father a child.

If your reproductive system is *very* healthy and your partner has a borderline or low sperm count, natural conception can still occur. Because your system has no barriers, the few good sperm he has have a very good chance of reaching your egg.

If, however, you have even a slight defect in your reproductive system (such as irregular ovulation, mild endometriosis, or a hostile vaginal environment caused by an infection or a sperm allergy), then even a moderate sperm count can be too deficient to bring about a conception.

Indeed, the status of each partner's individual fertility is so interdependent that most conception problems actually rest with the man *and* woman simultaneously. For this reason it's vital that your partner's sperm be analyzed *not just independently* but also in conjunction with *your* fertility.

If Sperm Is Bad: The Next Step

A preliminary sperm count and bacterial culture can usually be taken by the same fertility specialist or clinic treating you. However, if the results indicate a problem, your partner should consider further testing with one of two types of male fertility specialists:

Urologist: The male counterpart of your gynecologist, this specialist should be board-certified in urology (a broad category that covers disorders of the kidney, urinary tract, bladder, and male reproductive organs). Additional training in reproductive endocrinology is a plus.

Andrologist: These are researchers who study male reproduction. Most often they have a Ph.D. rather than an M.D. degree, with a specialty in biochemistry, endocrinology, or physiology. Frequently andrologists or embryologists are the laboratory specialists who direct sperm procedures for fertility centers.

When Low Sperm Count Is Only Temporary

Sometimes a low sperm count is temporary, brought on by any number of passing factors in a man's life, including:

- Colds, the flu, a virus
- Any infection causing white blood cell count to rise, such as an abscessed tooth or an infected finger or toe
- Poor nutrition, particularly a deficiency of zinc, vitamin C, and the B-Complex vitamins
- Overuse of cigarettes or alcohol, or any use of street drugs
- Certain medications, especially those used to treat high blood pressure or ulcers
- Stress
- Lack of sleep

If any of these conditions exist at the time a man has his sperm checked, he should notify his doctor. Before seeking further fertility treatment, he should have at least one more sperm count taken when these conditions have cleared.

The Male Fertility Exam

Assuming sperm analysis and bacterial cultures have been completed, your partner's expanded fertility exam should include all the organs of his reproductive system, including the penis, testicles, scrotal sac, vas deferens (where sperm is transported), and rectum (see Chapter 4). The doctor will be looking for abnormalities in shape, size, or feel of the organs, as well as skin eruptions, discolorations, or discharges. Most important, he or she will try to ascertain if there are any blockages anywhere in the reproductive tract, including any lumps, tumors, or cysts.

Providing no gross abnormalities are found during this exam, the next step is to begin a closer examination of your partner's sperm, specifically its ability to fuse with your egg. Indeed, in order to create a child, sperm must not only penetrate your egg's shell but also fuse with the genetic material inside.

For many years the only way to know for certain if this was possible was to retrieve your eggs and combine them with your partner's sperm in a laboratory setting. Because of all that's involved in stimulating and retrieving your eggs, however, this method of testing was not only impractical, it can be medically irresponsible.

Researchers, however, soon found a way around the situation. They theorized that if they could remove the outside shell of an animal egg and pair it with human sperm, they could see if fusion was possible. Since hamster eggs are very close, physiologically, to human eggs, they were chosen to test the theory—which ultimately turned out to be correct. As a result, the hamster penetration assay (HPA) was born.

Can He Make a Baby? How to Find Out Fast

As the HPA test begins, your partner will give a sperm sample, which in turn will be placed into a test tube with the hamster eggs. If, after twenty-four hours, they do not fuse, fertilization of human eggs may be difficult or impossible.

It is important to note, however, that up to 10 percent of men whose sperm cannot fuse with a hamster egg can still fertilize a human egg during laboratory-aided conceptions. Conversely, a small percentage of men who can fuse with the hamster egg cannot fertilize a human egg under any circumstances.

Additionally, you should also know that sometimes the medium (fluids) used in the HPA test can vary from lab to lab, and that can also affect test results, even when the same sperm is used. One way to avoid a false test result is to make certain the laboratory also uses "donor control sperm" to perform the same test using the same eggs and culture medium used to test your partner's sperm. If the donor sperm fuses with the hamster egg and your partner's sperm does not, then you can be fairly sure the results are not a laboratory mistake.

Finally, because sperm penetration rates can also be variable, changing from day to day, the hamster test is in no way considered a conclusive diagnostic technique.

I Hearing You Knocking: Getting in the Fertility Door

Although it's vital for sperm to fuse with an egg, before that can happen, it must penetrate the multilayered coating of the outer shell. In order to accomplish this the head of each sperm (called the acrosome) contains a packet of shell-dissolving enzymes—released when contact with the egg is made.

To see if enzyme activity is adequate to complete this step, your partner will need a test known as the hemizona assay.

Developed in the late 1980s at the Jones Institute in Virginia, this test uses frozen donor eggs (collected but never used in an IVF procedure) to directly test the fertilization potential of sperm. In effect, it is really the "human" version of the hamster test mentioned earlier. The eggs are thawed, cut in half, and placed into a culture fluid similar to what is used during IVF fertilization. Then, two sets of sperm are placed alongside the egg halves—one from a donor with a proven fertility track record, the other from your partner's sperm, the fertility potential of which remains unknown. If the donor sperm penetrates the outside zona membrane of the test egg—indicating fertilization is possible—then your partner's should as well. If it doesn't, then it's clear his sperm has some type of deficiency in this area. Although this test is a great way to judge sperm's ability to get through an egg membrane, because that egg is essentially dead (they often can't survive the freezing process), it can't tell you if it's possible to make the kind of connection inside the shell necessary for fertilization to occur. For that, you still need the hamster test, which uses fresh, not frozen eggs.

As such, these two procedures are often done simultaneously—the human egg test to predict sperm's ability to penetrate the outer shell, and the hamster test to determine whether the sperm can fuse with a living egg.

Other Tests for Male Fertility

- **The mucus penetration test:** A kind of reproductive "obstacle course" for male fertility, this test determines if sperm can negotiate its way through cervical mucus. And, in fact, it is conducted by placing sperm into a tube containing mucus, which is then examined under a microscope. Your doctor is looking for the percentage of sperm that are alive, and how many have made their way through the entire length of the tube. While this test will help demonstrate sperm survival and motility, even if your partner wins the conception Olympics for speed, there is still no guarantee he will be able to fertilize your egg.

   • **Electron microscopy:** This test is best used to unravel complex congenital sperm defects after more generalized testing indicates that a problem exists. It involves subjecting sperm samples to a highly powerful microscopic examination—with power to magnify up to one hundred thousand times what the normal eye can see. So, for example, if your partner's sperm is identified as having motility problems, this test will allow his doctor to see if, in fact, there is any defect within the sperm itself that might account for the slow movement. While this is a helpful test for some men, it should never be used as a first-line fertility workup.

Sugar and Male Fertility: The Lazy Sperm Test

Sometimes finding the cause of fertility problems takes years of investigation and research. Other times, the answer is right under your nose. That's exactly what a group of University of California researchers found out when they came upon a test for male fertility so simple, it's practically right out of a high-school biology lab. The new, ultra-low-tech test helps determine the difference between "lazy sperm," that which is alive and just not moving, and "dead sperm," which cannot fertilize an egg.

It involves the basic principal of osmosis: Simply put, live tissue will soak up fluid, while dead tissue will not. To put the theory to the test researchers soaked the sperm sample in sugar water, and sure enough, some sperm swelled, while others did not. The researchers then gently prodded the swollen sperm, and they did indeed prove to be alive.

Once "live" sperm are identified, they can then be used for a variety of assisted reproductive techniques, from simple inseminations to complex in vitro fertilizations.

The Fertility Blood Tests: What Your Partner Needs

In addition to direct examination of your partner's sperm, he will also need a series of blood tests designed to tell him additional facts about his reproductive health. The most common of these tests include:

- **T3 and T4 thyroid function tests:** When thyroid function is low (hypothyroidism), sperm production can become so sluggish that it nearly comes to a complete halt. In most instances, thyroid medication can restore the function of this important gland and in the process help return sperm production and count to normal.

- **FSH and LH:** The same brain hormones that affect egg production in a woman also affect sperm production in a man. If hormone levels drop low enough, a sperm deficiency can develop. Fortunately, when this is the case, treatment with a variety of fertility medications (see below) can help.

- **Testosterone:** Deficiencies in this hormone can be an indication of a biochemical imbalance or problems within the testicles themselves. If testosterone is low, additional diagnostic procedures, including a testicle biopsy (which you'll read about in a moment), may be necessary.

- **Prolactin:** When prolactin levels are low, levels of both FSH and LH can drop off as well. By correcting any deficiency here, your partner may be able to get other important reproductive hormones back on track.

Male Fertility Drugs: What Might Help

In much the same way that certain fertility medications can increase a woman's chances for pregnancy success (see Chapter 19), there is some evidence that some of these same drugs can work for men. This can be particularly true when tests indicate your partner has a marked decrease in either FSH or LH.

In other instances, medications with a direct effect on specific male physiology, such as testosterone, may also help to increase sperm production and, ultimately, fertility.

Although none of these medications is considered a "cure" for male infertility, in some instances they may provide the boost a man's body needs to bring about conception.

Which drugs can help your partner increase sperm production?

- **Clomiphene citrate (Clomid)**: 25 to 50 mg taken on a regular basis (either daily or every other day) can improve pituitary function, which in turn increases production of FSH and LH. This regimen is normally prescribed for men with a mild deficiency of these hormones.

- **Metrodin or Pergonal**: 150 IUs of either of these drugs three times a week has been successful in treating men with moderate to severe FSH or LH deficiencies. When used for three to six months on a regular basis these medications can even restore severely compromised sperm production.

- **HCG**: Injections of this fertility drug given twice a week have been shown to stimulate the production of cells within the testicles that produce testosterone. This in turn helps increase sperm production.

- **Parlodel**: The same drug used to help reduce prolactin levels in women can do the same for men. When this hormone returns to normal, testosterone production may increase.

- **Aromatase inhibitors**: These drugs block the conversion of testosterone to estrogen, which ultimately stimulates the testicles to produce more sperm. However, it remains to be seen whether this also results in a higher pregnancy rate.

- **Kallikrein**: This protein exerts an anti-inflammatory response that some studies have shown can regulate sperm motility, and in the process double pregnancy rates. This medication should not be used if a preexisting inflammation exists in either the epididymis or the prostate gland.

- Indomethacin: A medication that works to inhibit the production of prostaglandin, a chemical made by the body in response to inflammation, which also affects sperm motility and concentration. At least one study showed treatment with 75 mg a day of indomethacin increased pregnancy rates by some 35 percent.

Before your partner consents to using any of these fertility medications, you should both know there is limited evidence that these drugs work on men. At best, they provide a temporary change in the condition of sperm, which, in fact, can be hard to separate from the natural variations in motility and morphology that sperm goes through every day on its own. And, since fertility drugs are both expensive and fraught with side effects (which, depending on the drug, can include vision disturbances, weight gain or loss, changes in libido, gastrointestinal or neurological disturbances, skin problems, and mood changes), their use should never be taken lightly. While there are definitely certain circumstances under which these medications may be extremely helpful to your partner, he should have an open discussion with his doctor first, concerning what the drugs will and won't accomplish.

Additionally, if his tests show consistently elevated levels of FSH and LH, fertility drugs will not help. Most often, high levels of these hormones indicate testicular failure, meaning no testosterone is being made. This can be the result of end-stage reproductive infections, or trauma to the genitals themselves. In either case, when no testosterone is being made, no amount of fertility medication is capable of triggering sperm production.

Hot Testicles and Infertility: What You Need to Know

One of the most common genital conditions found in men is called varicocele, which results when a vein outside the scrotum becomes dilated and enlarged, similar to varicose veins in the legs. This slows the flow of blood around the testicles, which in turn causes their temperature to rise and remain elevated—and therein lies the link to infertility. In nearly half the men who have varicocele, sperm formation and motility can be dramatically affected. While it can begin as early as puberty, many men do not experience the total reproductive impact until well into their thirties or forties. Some have already fathered one or more children. However, it's also important to note that up to 15 percent of *all* men have varicocele and many do not suffer its fertility-related consequences.

Although a very large varicocele can often be felt upon examination—and a check for this condition should definitely be part of your partner's fertility physical—when smaller veins are involved problems can only be detected via a Doppler stethoscope, a device that allows a urologist to listen for the blood flow patterns that are consistent with dilated veins.

From Zero Sperm to Fatherhood in Less Than Sixty Minutes

Fortunately, even if a varicocele is diagnosed, there are a variety of surgical procedures to correct the condition. In traditional surgery, the twisted vein is surgically isolated, and sutures (stitches) are used to cut off its blood supply. This, in turn, reduces the temperature of the testicles and helps sperm production to resume.

Among the newest methods is a form of microsurgery pioneered by Dr. Marc Goldstein, professor of urology at the Weill Medical College of Cornell University and director for the Center for Male Reproductive Medicine at New York Cornell–Presbyterian Hospital in New York City.

The procedure, called a varicocelectomy, works much like traditional surgery, to isolate the varicose veins in the testicle and cut off their blood supply. In this instance, however, the surgeon will use a high-powered operating microscope, which, in turn, helps in the preservation of the tiny (one-millimeter) testicular artery, the main blood supply to the testicle itself. This, in turn, lessens the risk of complications, while increasing the success rate of the surgery. Indeed, studies conducted by Dr. Goldstein published in the journal *Fertility and Sterility* have shown

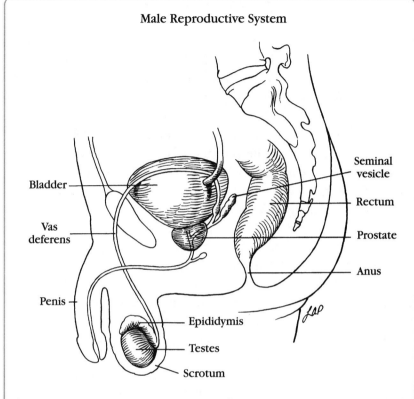

Male Reproductive System

Bladder

Vas
deferens

Penis

Seminal
vesicle

Rectum

Prostate

Anus

Epididymis

Testes

Scrotum

Hot Testicles: One Cause of Infertility

One of the most common causes of male infertility is a condition called varicocele. Here, veins located outside the scrotum become dilated and enlarged, much like a varicose vein on the leg. This reduces the flow of blood to the testicle, which, in turn, causes the temperature inside to rise. When it does, sperm production and motility can suffer.

that even men who had a zero sperm count, or no living sperm, developed living, moving sperm following this procedure.

In a second treatment called a balloon occlusion, tiny implants are used to help stop the flow of blood into the testicles. Should your partner require treatment, his doctor can advise him as to the best method.

The Varicocele Hoax: How to Avoid Unnecessary Surgery

While a varicocele repair can sometimes dramatically improve a man's fertility, in many instances I believe this operation is somewhat *overrecommended*. In fact, unscrupulous doctors routinely recommend varicocele surgery when they diagnose even minor, very tiny varicose veins that have little or no effect on sperm count. For this reason I caution a man not to be persuaded to have this surgery unless there are clear-cut indications that the dilated veins are large enough to cause excess testicle heat. I strongly urge any man who is diagnosed with varicocele as a major contributing factor to infertility to seek a second, or even a third, opinion before proceeding with surgery.

Is Surgery Right for You? How to Decide

If you are having problems deciding whether or not varicocele surgery is right for you, two new diagnostic methods presented at the 1998 World Congress on Infertility can help. Both were designed to measure the effectiveness of a varicocele operation *before* it's performed.

Reporting from Toyama, Japan, researchers from the Department of Urology at Toyama Medical and Pharmaceutical University revealed that Doppler ultrasound—a nonradiation method of tracking blood flow to tissue and organs — can also be used to track the speed at which blood flows into the scrotal veins. As such it can then determine the severity of any varicocele present. Based on that finding, doctors can then determine whether surgery will help your partner.

In studies conducted in the Department of Urology at Rush–Presbyterian–St.Luke's Medical Center in Chicago, a grading system used to mark sperm according to motility appeared to also be able to predict which men will benefit from varicocele surgery. In short, the higher percentage of motile sperm a man has, the greater the chance that the varicocele surgery will be successful. When poor motility exists, the operation rarely helps, and laboratory methods of conception should be explored.

The Testicular Cooler—Does It Work?

In addition to the surgical options for correcting varicocele, a device aptly called a testicle cooler is being used not only for this condition but for any congenital vascular problem that can cause the temperature of a man's testicles to rise too high. Technically called a testicular hypothermia device, it works through the evaporation of water from the surface of the scrotum, reducing its temperature. Resembling a jock strap, it features long thin tubes connected to a fluid reservoir which is attached to a belt worn around the waist. As the water circulates through the tubes, it cools the testicles.

Still somewhat primitive, the water reservoir must be filled every six hours and the device must be worn daily whenever a man is awake and clothed. The unit can, however, be removed for bathing, sleeping, and sex. While most users claim it is fairly comfortable and easy to conceal, it often must be used for prolonged periods of time before positive effects are seen.

When Sperm Can't Leave a Man's Body: Another Cause of Infertility

If the quality of your partner's sperm is good but the overall amount present in each ejaculation is low, or if the size of the ejaculate itself is small, he may have a blockage somewhere in his reproductive tract. As a result, sperm, semen, or both are being stopped before getting to his penis.

Sometimes the blockage is in the vas deferens, the hollow tube that transports sperm from the testicles to the penis, or, more often, in the epididymis, the yards of coiled tubing that sit atop each testicle. When, in fact, either of these scenarios exist, sperm has a problem leaving your partner's body—and that means natural conception is difficult to achieve.

Block Party: The New Diagnostics

Could your partner have a problem with blocked sperm? It's far more common than you think. To help determine if, in fact, this is the case, he can take the following tests:

- **Fluid aspiration:** Here, fluid taken directly from the vas deferens is checked for sperm. If sperm is found, despite not being present in ejaculated semen, then it's likely a blockage exists.
- **The saline test:** A harmless saltwater solution is injected into the vas deferens. If it flows easily inside, then it's likely there is no blockage. If it does not, then the physician can insert an ultrathin catheter into the vas and slowly move it along the inside. Where the catheter meets resistance is usually the site of the blockage.
- **The vasogram:** In the event that either of these tests proves inconclusive, your partner may need a vasogram, a kind of male fertility X-ray. Similar to a hysterosalpingogram used to find blockages in your fallopian tubes, in this test a high-contrast dye is injected into the vas deferens through a small incision in the scrotal sac. Using X-rays to monitor the flow of dye, the specialist can determine where a blockage might lie.

An important warning: Although an extremely effective diagnostic procedure, unless performed by a highly trained, experienced vasogram specialist, this test can harm a man's fertility by damaging the delicate tubal ducts leading to the vas, a problem that must be remedied via immediate emergency surgery. For this reason, this test should only be given in extreme cases.

When the "Well" Is Dry: What to Do

Even if no blockages are found, your partner may still have a problem getting sperm out of his body. The reason could be a simple lack of semen. This is the ejaculatory fluid that acts as the transport vehicle that carries sperm from the vas deferens, where it is made, through the reproductive system and out the penis. This fluid is released from several ducts within a man's reproductive system, including the seminal vesicles, tiny glands located just below the bladder. If these vesicles become blocked, semen will be in short supply.

To check for this problem, your partner's ejaculate will be tested for the presence of fructose or fruit sugar. What can this reveal? Along with semen, the seminal vesicles also release a variety of other biochemicals, including fruit sugar. If fructose is present in the semen, then the vesicles are open and working. If little or no fructose is seen, then it's likely a blockage exists.

Restoring His Sperm Flow: The MESA Solution

In the past, almost any blockage in a man's reproductive system required surgery. Although successful, in terms of opening the blockage, up to 50 percent of the time, only a scant 20 percent of patients were able to regain their fertility. This was particularly true if damage to the epididymis occurred along with the blockage.

Now, however, several far more successful methods of getting sperm out of the body have been developed. One of the most popular is called MESA (short for microsurgical epididymal sperm aspiration). Here, sperm is removed directly from the epididymis. Then, using one of several new forms of laboratory assistance, conception can easily take place.

Although it was once believed that sperm must pass through the epididymis in order to become mature enough for fertilization, new research shows this is only necessary when sperm leaves a man's body on its own. When taken directly from specific areas of the epididymis or testicles, and used for laboratory-assisted conception, the sperm appears to be of high enough quality to bring about fertilization.

PESA: The Nonsurgical Way to Get Sperm Out

Short for "percutaneous epididymis sperm aspiration," PESA works to retrieve sperm from the epididymis without the need for a scrotal inci-

The MESA Procedure: What to Expect

First, your partner will be placed under anesthesia, either general or local. Then, a tiny incision is made into the scrotal sac, the loose area of skin that encloses the testicles. This allows the surgeon to place a thin catheter into the area of the epididymis likely to contain the most sperm. A gentle suction device attached to the catheter helps to gently coax it from the body into the tube. Because, however, it is vital that no blood be allowed to mix with the sperm (this would significantly affect fertility), specially designed microsurgical instruments in conjunction with a specific type of surgical micropuncture are used. This technique not only helps retrieve pure sperm, but also minimizes risk of damage to surrounding tissue. Because sperm residing in the epididymis are so highly concentrated, only a small amount need be aspirated.

To help ensure that the sperm that has been removed is of good quality, it is tested immediately, in much the same way a woman's eggs are tested when they are removed for in vitro fertilization. If the sperm is found to be of poor quality, other perforations are made into different areas of the epididymis and additional samples are aspirated.

sion, something which most men appreciate greatly. However, in order to be considered a candidate for this procedure, your partner must have normal sperm production that is simply blocked by an obstruction in his reproductive tract. You should also know that sperm extracted in this fashion are far less likely to fertilize an egg than those that are extracted using the more complex MESA procedure.

How PESA is performed: Like the MESA procedure, PESA requires your partner to be placed under general or local anesthesia. Then, holding the testicle in a firm but gentle grip, the physician inserts an ultrathin needle into the epididymis tube and begins drawing fluid. That fluid, which comes directly from the center of sperm production, should contain enough motile sperm for a single attempt at laboratory conception. Sometimes, however, it may require several attempts in various areas of the epididymis before enough sperm can be retrieved for

Asking for Directions: Why Sperm Get Lost

In some men, a problem known as "retrograde ejaculation" keeps sperm from ever leaving the body. Most commonly due to nerve damage connected to diabetes, this condition results when the muscle used to close the bladder right before orgasm does not function as it should. As a result, sperm takes a wrong turn and instead of going down the urethra to be ejaculated, some or all of the semen is routed instead into the bladder. If, in fact, a man's urine shows the presence of sperm, this is likely his problem.

Currently, the only treatment specifically for retrograde ejaculation is a series of drugs similar to decongestants, able to induce a restrictive or tightening effect on the opening of the bladder.

Barring that solution, the only other option is to use sperm-harvesting techniques (which you'll learn about in a minute) in conjunction with either insemination or one of the other laboratory-assisted conceptions discussed in Chapters 20 and 21. Although there has been limited success in procedures that attempt to extract sperm directly from the bladder, because they are generally poor quality, pregnancy results are slim—usually only about 10 percent.

conception. If ultimately no sperm can be retrieved—which occurs about 20 percent of the time—then more dramatic procedures, including MESA or a testicle biopsy, must be performed.

The New Testicle Biopsy: The Ultimate Way to Obtain Sperm

In a certain percentage of men, sperm count can be zero. If a physical exam fails to reveal a blockage, the testicles appear small and soft, and blood levels of FSH are high (double the normal reading), a testicle biopsy may be necessary to determine if your partner is capable of making any sperm.

This involves the surgical removal of a small sample of tissue from inside the testicles, which is then examined under a microscope for evidence that sperm is being produced. This is usually done on an outpatient basis, and the surgery itself requires no stitches. Normally, a man can be back at work in just a day or two.

The Biopsy Result: What You Need to Know

If the biopsy sample reveals no sperm, the testicles are assumed to be completely nonfunctioning. There is generally no treatment for this condition. However, it's important to note that a group of Brazilian researchers found that the area of the testicle from which the biopsy was taken can influence whether sperm is found. Indeed, their data show that while one area of the testicle may yield no sperm, taking a biopsy several centimeters away might. Therefore, your partner should always make a request to his doctor that his biopsy yield several samples taken from different areas as well as from both testicles. This is extremely important, since, as you will discover in just a moment, finding even a single sperm means it's possible to biologically father a child.

Zero Sperm Count — and You Can Still Get Pregnant!

In the not-too-distant past, semen that contained no sperm—a condition called azoospermia—was a sign that complete infertility was likely. Although in some instances it could mean a blockage, in which case repair was possible, often it was an indication of severe testicular failure. In essence, few or no sperm was being made. When this was the case, biological fatherhood was impossible.

Today, all that has changed thanks to a procedure known as TESE—short for testicular sperm extraction. Here, doctors use special high-powered microscopes and delicate microsurgical instruments to harvest sperm *directly from the testicle*. In a procedure that is similar to testicle biopsy, retrieving even a single sperm is enough to bring about concep-

Warning: Don't Touch Your Testicles Without This Test

Although both a testicle biopsy and the TESE procedure can help many men father a child, they are considered radical procedures. This is particularly true when other, less invasive treatments may bring about the same result. As such, I always caution my patients' partners to make certain they are tested for LH and FSH before agreeing to these procedures. Why is this so important? When these hormones are low, sperm production can drop dramatically. However, rather than resort to surgery, as you read earlier, often certain fertility medications may be all that's necessary to trigger sperm production and increase fertility—all without an invasive procedure. In fact, these tests are so important, levels of LH and FSH should be taken twice, with the second test thirty days after the first. If levels are borderline or low normal, I recommend treatment with fertility drugs before consenting to a testicle surgery.

tion. This is particularly true when pregnancy is achieved with one of the latest twists on in vitro fertilization, a procedure known as ICSI (intracytoplasmic sperm injection—see Chapter 22).

Indeed, TESE can also be a good choice when a man wishes to father a child after vasectomy—the male "birth control" procedure that creates a blockage in the reproductive system to keep sperm from leaving the body.

Getting Pregnant—No Sperm Necessary!

Can a man who has no sperm at all—even in his testicles—still biologically father a child? Until the late 1990s, the answer was a resounding "no." However, new research has shown that fertilization and ultimately pregnancy are possible even when only a *germ* of a sperm cell is available.

Indeed, one of the newest diagnoses of male infertility involves a problem known as "maturation arrest." Here, a man has all the hormones and other factors necessary to make sperm, but unfortunately he doesn't have what it takes to allow those early sperm cells to grow and mature. As a result, his testicles may be filled with what are called "spermatids" or "round cells"—sperm buds, as you might call them. Containing only the germ of a sperm cell, spermatids are devoid of a tail, meaning they cannot move.

And while spermatids carry only one-half the genetic material of a fully grown sperm, studies show that when combined with an egg (which also contains half of the genetic material needed to make a baby) in a laboratory procedure, fertilization will result.

On the Horizon: Transplanted Sperm Cells!

One of the most dramatic fertility advances of the new century will no doubt be the sperm transplant, a procedure that is already being considered in many fertility centers around the world. Here, precursors to sperm cells will be transplanted into the area of the testicles where sperm are naturally made. Normally, these precursor cells work to generate the production of sperm throughout a man's lifetime. If the transplantation system is perfected, the donated sperm cells should bring about the same result. And that means even some men born without the ability to make sperm will be able to initiate production and eventually become biological fathers.

Love on Ice: How to Freeze Your Fertility Options

Although obtaining sperm via the MESA or TESE procedures certainly makes conception possible, convenience is another story. Indeed, for these laboratory conceptions to be successful, your partner's testicle surgery must be coordinated with the ovulatory/egg retrieval procedures necessary to obtain your eggs. And this means that two surgical teams—one specializing in male fertility, one in female fertility—must be available, simultaneously, at a single facility that is also equipped with two operating rooms. For many centers, this is a difficult reality to achieve.

Now, however, a new option exists. It involves removing your partner's testicular tissue samples up to several months before they are needed and freezing them in liquid nitrogen. On the day of your egg retrieval the tissue is thawed and a single sperm is removed for use in a fertility procedure known as ICSI (see Chapter 22). The first successful pregnancy using this freezing technique was performed at the Reproductive Science Center in Boston, Massachusetts, in 1996. Today, the procedure is available at numerous fertility centers around the nation and is fast proving to be a powerful technique for achieving pregnancy.

Restoring Male Fertility by Reversing a Vasectomy

One of the most important male fertility operations is the reversing of a vasectomy, the male birth control procedure. In the original surgery, a section of the vas deferens closest to the epididymis (the sperm "command central") is cut and the ends sealed with stitches, heat, or clips. So, instead of leaving his body during an ejaculation, sperm is blocked from passage, and it simply dies and disintegrates. The operation to reverse a vasectomy is, in some ways, similar to the procedure used to reverse a voluntary sterilization in a woman's body. It involves opening the area of the vas that was surgically closed and reattaching the cut ends.

If your partner is thinking about reversing his vasectomy he should be aware that the longer he waits, the lower his chances for a successful reversal:

- Men who have had vasectomies ten years or longer have less than a 40 percent chance of conceiving after vasectomy reversal.
- Men who had vasectomies less than ten years have about a 90 percent chance of ejaculating sperm after a vasectomy reversal.

However, it's also important to note that while some doctors recommend bypassing vasectomy reversal and instead opting for MESA or other sperm retrieval techniques, studies published in the journal *Fertility and Sterility* report that, from both a pregnancy standpoint and an economic one, vasectomy reversal is the better of the two options. Indeed, the delivery rate for pregnancies involving vasectomy reversal is

47 percent, compared to just 33 percent when sperm retrieval and assisted reproduction techniques were used for conception. In terms of cost, the total fee for a vasectomy reversal delivery can be up to twenty-five thousand dollars, while the more complex laboratory-assisted pregnancy (which may require several attempts before conception is achieved) could cost as much as seventy-six thousand dollars, or higher.

Before making a decision about this procedure, your partner should also know that in some men the initial vasectomy causes the production of sperm antibodies—which doesn't always reverse itself after the corrective surgery. In fact, up to two-thirds of all men who have vasectomies develop antibodies that can interfere with sperm motility and fertilization after reverse surgery is performed. Although there are some anti-sperm antibody remedies available to help (you can read more about them in Chapter 15), often you may end up having to rely on laboratory-assisted conception to overcome the problem.

Overcoming Impotence: How You Can Still Conceive

One of the most emotionally and physically devastating causes of male infertility is impotence—the inability to develop or maintain an erection. While many people think of this problem as strictly one of sexual gratification, it also represents a serious threat to fertility. In reality, sperm count and motility can be perfect, but unless a man can have an erection he cannot naturally deposit his sperm in his partner's body.

Currently, 10 percent of all male infertility is due to impotence, and there is an increasing number of impotent men in their prime reproductive years—between ages twenty-five and thirty-five. Once thought to be a condition associated only with older men, again, research shows that young men can lose their ability to get an erection as easily as men past age fifty.

In the not-too-distant past it was believed that nearly all causes of impotence were psychological in nature. Today we know that not to be true. While impotence can be due to emotional problems, including depression, anxiety, and fear, in most cases its cause is rooted in a physiological problem—often one that reduces blood flow or nerve stimulation to the penis, such as diabetes or some early forms of heart disease.

The good news is, of course, that even if your partner is totally unable to achieve an erection, he can still father a child. Using one of the new sperm extraction methods described earlier in this chapter, in combination with one of the laboratory-assisted conceptions, fatherhood is possible even for men with injuries that preclude ever being able to have an erection.

However, before you and your partner progress to these advanced methods of fertility treatment, you might want to consider some of the following methods of reversing or improving impotency-related infertility.

How Your Partner Becomes Sexually Aroused

When a man becomes sexually excited, his body's natural reaction is to divert additional blood flow to his penis. There, arteries relax and widen to accommodate that extra blood. As a result, his penis will grow in size, becoming harder and more rigid as more blood continues to flow in. At the same time, veins that normally carry blood out of the penis begin to constrict. *When blood flow into the penis is greater than blood flow out, it maximizes in size, and an erection results.* Under normal circumstances that erection is maintained until just after the point of orgasm or ejaculation. Once this occurs, veins relax and blood flows back out of the penis, which, in turn, relaxes and reduces in size. Any factor along the way that inhibits either blood flow or retention in the penis can result in impotence.

Impotence: The Most Common Causes and the Fastest Cures

- **Cause—environmental factors:** Cocaine, marijuana, caffeine, alcohol, and cigarettes, or even stress can constrict blood supply to the penis necessary for an erection.

   Cure: Discontinuing use of these substances should reverse impotence within a few weeks.

- **Cause—medications:** Drugs used to treat high blood pressure, depression, and anxiety are especially detrimental.

    Cure: Talk to your doctor about substituting a different drug or the safety of discontinuing a medication for a short time. Most often impotence is reversed when drugs are stopped.

- **Cause—increased prolactin levels:** Due to a tumor or other hormonal imbalances, increased prolactin can result in a lowered sex drive and impotence.

    Cure: The medication bromocriptine mesylate (Parlodel) lowers prolactin levels, shrinks tumors, and restores the ability to have an erection about 50 percent of the time.

- **Cause—disease:** Especially harmful are diseases that reduce blood flow to the penis, such as diabetes or hardening of the arteries. In addition, conditions that can damage the nerves leading to the penis, such as stroke, spinal cord injuries, kidney disease, diabetes, or back injuries can also cause impotence.

    Cure: Often proper management of the disease itself can reverse the impotence. When it can't, penile implants and electro ejaculation devices can help (they're both discussed shortly).

- **Cause—leaky veins:** Up to 20 percent of all cases of physiological impotence occur when a leaky vein inside the penis reduces the blood volume necessary to achieve or maintain an erection.

    Cure: Microsurgery. The leaky veins are tied off, keeping blood volume in the penis from dropping.

Viagra: The Ultimate Male Fertility Drug

Because it can help a man regain his ability to have an erection, the somewhat controversial but very promising male drug Viagra (sildenfil citrate) indeed has the potential to function as a fertility medication, particularly when it can help you and your partner forgo costly, invasive procedures, including sperm extraction and in vitro fertilization.

Although for some men the effects of Viagra can seem downright magical, its premise is purely scientific. Quite simply, it works by increasing blood flow to the penis, so that when your partner is sexually aroused, he can more easily obtain and maintain an erection. What Viagra cannot do, however, is cause a man who is not interested in sex to become aroused, nor can it induce sexual desire or in any way act as an aphrodisiac or "love potion." What's more, if no direct genital stimulation takes place, Viagra won't cause an erection. So, for example, if your partner takes the drug and then something occurs that precludes him from having sex, he will not be stimulated into an erection.

From a fertility standpoint, Viagra can help by simply allowing an impotent man to engage in sexual intercourse. It will not, however, increase sperm production, or in any way directly enhance a man's ability to conceive a child. Remember, too, the fact that a man has an orgasm and ejaculates does not mean he is making sperm, or that the sperm he is making is capable of fertilizing an egg. Viagra will also have little effect on a man whose impotence is caused by psychological factors, since its main goal is to correct the physical defects that keep the penis from receiving and maintaining an adequate blood supply.

VIAGRA: THE CONTROVERSY

Although Viagra has, so far, been successfully used by more than a million men for the treatment of some forms of impotence, its success is not without controversy. There can, of course, be temporary side effects, including headache, facial flushes, and, more rarely, upset stomach and visual disturbances. There is also a rare risk of a prolonged erection—a condition that forces the penis to remain painfully erect for an extended period of time. Far more disturbing, however, is the suspected link between Viagra and what has turned out to be an increasing number of deaths in men using this drug. While it's clear that at least some of these men might have died anyway—most had some form of heart disease— Viagra's possible role in these tragedies cannot be ignored.

The latest information yields the idea that this drug may, in fact, be dangerous to some men, particularly those who have a cardiac condition.

More specifically, we know that Viagra should not be used, under any circumstances, by any men who are taking any form of the heart medication nitrate, including the popular nitroglycerin pills often prescribed for angina—a condition wherein blood flow to and from the heart is hampered. The combination of these medications can cause blood pressure to drop dangerously low and that, in turn, can affect the heart, as well as decrease blood flow to the brain. Because there are dozens of medications that fall into the nitrate category, your partner should, of course, always mention every medication he is taking to whatever doctor prescribes his Viagra.

On the horizon: Several new drugs may soon join Viagra as viable treatments for impotence. One of the most promising is a medication known as "apomorphine," which may become widely available in the near future.

Increasing the Safety of Viagra

Make certain your partner always has a complete physical examination before accepting a prescription for Viagra. This should include a cardiac workup as well as testing for diabetes and any back-related problems that could involve spinal nerves. This exam is vital, since some of the conditions that cause impotence—such as undiagnosed heart disease—may increase should Viagra be prescribed.

After a physical exam, your partner should see a urologist, who should also be the person to decide if Viagra is the right treatment. Sometimes, other factors more easily remedied may be responsible for erection problems, and only a urologist is fully qualified to make a complete diagnosis.

Never use "Poppers" when taking Viagra. While this nitrate-based inhaler is often used by men to increase sexual stimulation, when used in conjunction with Viagra the result can be deadly.

Make your partner aware that he should never purchase Viagra from the Internet, or any source, without a prescription from a physician who has personally examined him. Likewise, he should never take a Viagra pill from a friend, or use someone else's prescription.

More Good News: Additional Ways for an Impotent Man to Father a Child

If Viagra is not the drug for you, there are various other ways in which you your partner can deal with his impotence. These can range from simple devices like penile rings and other apparatus used to maintain an erection, to more complex and costly methods such as a penile prosthesis or implant.

Currently two different types of penile implants are available— those that are rigid and those that are inflatable. Both involve a simple installation operation, and both can not only solve the problem of infertility, but also help improve both partners' sexual relations by allowing for lovemaking to resume.

If this is your goal, then the surgeries involved in these potency cures are worth a try. If, however, your goal is simply to achieve conception, it may be ultimately easier for your partner to undergo sperm extraction, and for you to have some form of insemination—a simple and inexpensive laboratory-aided conception fully explained in Chapter 20.

If your partner suffers from a problem called premature ejaculation—an erection is possible but he cannot maintain it long enough to deposit sperm in your vagina—insemination can also be your quickest route to conception.

If Impotence Is a Problem, Don't Wait — Get Help

There is probably not a man alive who at some point in his life will not experience at least one temporary bout with impotence.

However, for some men, it is not a passing incident, but a clinical problem. If your partner goes more than two weeks without being able to achieve an erection (with you, during solo masturbation, or unconsciously while asleep), and if none of the environmental factors linked to this problem is present, then he must see his doctor.

In most cases, treating or eliminating the physical factor will result in a full restoration of potency within only a few weeks. If no physical causes can be found, sex therapy can be successful in overcoming impotence up to 80 percent of the time.

Drugs, Potions, and Other Potency Cures: What Works and What Doesn't

Perhaps the most widespread misconceptions in the world of medicine surround the medications and drugs purported to increase a man's potency. Nearly every week a patient brings to my attention a magazine or mail-order advertisement boasting the ability of various products to stimulate a man's sexual prowess. Some are even billed as fertility drugs, claiming to increase sperm production as well as potency.

Do these products work? Most often they do not. There are, however, a *few* medications that have provided some help for some men.

Papaverine: A chemical derived from the papaya plant, this prescription medication causes blood vessels to dilate throughout the body and can increase blood flow to the penis. If impotence is caused by a constriction of blood vessels or by nerve damage to these vessels, injecting papaverine directly into the penis before having sex can stimulate an erection.

Prostaglandin E 1: This chemical is made naturally in the body and works to stimulate vessel dilation and blood flow to the penis. A supplemental form available by prescription can be injected directly into the penis just before sex.

Yocon (generic name, yohimbe hydrochloride): This prescription drug works by constricting the tiny vessels in the penis, helping to keep blood from escaping. This, in turn, keeps penile blood volume high, which can help men who are able to get an erection but unable to maintain it.

A Final Word

The treatment of male fertility has undoubtedly advanced beyond our wildest dreams—to the point where virtually every man who wants to father a child can do so. Now, more than ever, it's vital for any man who suspects a fertility problem to seek help immediately. If a condition is diagnosed early on, today's treatments can be fast and easy and can bring about conception just a month or two later.

Remember, too, that taking a "couple's" approach to infertility, in which neither partner is considered to "blame" is not only healthier mentally but physically as well. So, do encourage your partner to seek testing, and if necessary treatment. When you work together toward your parenting goals, stress will be minimized—and that can increase fertility for you both.

Chapter Nineteen

Super Ovulation and Other New Ways to a Faster, Easier Conception

Despite all the advances in reproductive treatments, still, the core of female fertility lies in the ability to manufacture and release good eggs. By "good" I mean eggs that begin developing at the start of your cycle, grow to full maturity, release enough estrogen to signal ovulation, and finally, pop from their shell and travel to your fallopian tube so that they may be fertilized.

For many women, this process occurs in a natural, orderly pattern, one that does lead to conception. However, for some, things don't go quite this smoothly. Deficiencies in the hormones needed to stimulate egg growth, development, or release can make conception difficult. If hormone levels drop low enough, complete biochemical infertility can result.

One of the most successful ways to correct these egg-related problems is with fertility drugs, medications that help your body perform the natural, egg-related reproductive activities necessary for conception to occur.

Super Ovulation: A New Way to Use Fertility Drugs

Depending on what your particular problem is, fertility drugs may be the sole basis of your treatment. Indeed, for many women, a few cycles on these powerful medications is all that's necessary to bring about a healthy conception.

However, your doctor may also incorporate fertility drugs into a treatment known as "super ovulation"—an integral and important part of several forms of assisted reproduction, including artificial insemination and in vitro fertilization. In these instances, the medications are used to increase both the amount and quality of the eggs you produce. This can be especially helpful if your partner has a low sperm count, since the healthier your eggs are, the more likely you are to conceive.

The medications most commonly used for super ovulation include human menopausal gonadotropin (such drugs as Pergonal, Humegon, and Repronex) and Metrodin, Fertinex, or newer drugs, such as Follistim or Gonal F, all used in conjunction with a second hormone called human chorionic gonadotropin or hCG (such drugs as Profasi, Pregnyl, and APL).

How Super Ovulation Improves Your Pregnancy

In addition to increasing your egg-making potential, fertility drugs can be a great way to encourage a healthier pregnancy. Studies show these medications may decrease your risk of miscarriage and premature labor and help promote a healthier implantation. How?

   • Fertility drugs help you make more eggs, which in turn means more estrogen. This can help increase the quality of your cervical mucus, which makes it easier for sperm to move through your cervix during intercourse. Estrogen also means a thicker endometrial lining, which makes implantation faster and easier.

   • More eggs also means more corpus luteum, the material found in the shell of your ovulated egg that produces progesterone in the second half of your menstrual cycle. Should you become pregnant, this same hormone will quell uterine cramping and help you avoid miscarriage, as it builds a strong endometrial lining. Again, this promotes a healthy implantation and provides your baby with adequate nourishment right from the start of your pregnancy.

For these reasons I often use fertility drugs to treat any patient whose obstetrical history indicates she is susceptible to either premature labor or pregnancy loss.

Although some couples are concerned that fertility drugs do increase the risk of multiple births by as much as 25 percent, you should know that most often, it is twins.

Understanding Fertility Drugs

There are a variety of medications available to treat a number of fertility-related problems. All, however, work in just one of three ways:

- To encourage egg production or build stronger, healthier eggs, or both
- To stimulate or trigger ovulation—releasing of eggs from ovary and passage into the fallopian tubes so they can be fertilized
- To repair hormonal imbalances that disrupt reproductive functions or to block competing hormones so the reproductive system can function more efficiently

While some drugs may cross categories, or yield more than one benefit (it can help you make healthier eggs, for example, while also correcting an ovulatory problem), every fertility medication you take should be carefully prescribed to treat a specific reproductive problem.

Also remember that it may take a certain amount of experimentation with one or more of these medications, used in varying amounts and combinations, to find the right "fertility prescription" for you. The regimen that helped your best friend get pregnant, for example, might not necessarily be right for you, even if you believe you have similar problems.

The main point: Fertility drugs are medications that help your body do what it does naturally, only better and more efficiently. Generally, they are out of your system by the time conception occurs so they do not interfere with fertilization, and most experts believe they have no residual effects on your baby.

The Most Common Fertility Drugs and How They Work

Medication: Clomiphene Citrate

Brand names: Clomid, Serophene, Lemon-Teva

How it works: By tricking your pituitary gland into believing certain biochemicals are in short supply, it causes your brain to send signals that increase the production of FSH and LH, the hormones which promote egg growth. It also can correct a luteal phase defect (LPD), a problem characterized by a deficiency of the hormone progesterone during the second half of the menstrual cycle. In this way, clomiphene restores the hormonal balance necessary to create a healthy womb where baby can implant and grow.

Method of treatment: Pills or tablets

What you need to know: Used primarily to treat ovarian malfunction, it aids in producing healthy, mature eggs and encourages more regular ovulation in 60 to 80 percent of women, with a 50 percent chance of getting pregnant within six cycles. To check if the drug is working, use an ovulation predictor kit approximately two to three days after you stop taking clomiphene. If you don't get pregnant after several cycles of drug use, you may have other factors contributing to your infertility and should receive additional testing (including an examination of your fallopian tubes to see if they are open). Your partner's fertility should also be tested before you undergo further cycles on this drug.

While taking clomiphene, you should receive regular vaginal sonograms and estradiol blood tests to determine if you are making an adequate number of eggs and to ensure against hyperstimulation, a condition in which too many eggs are made too quickly. This, however, is a rare occurrence when clomiphene alone is used.

Side effects: Minor, temporary effects include hot flashes, blurred vision, nausea, bloating, and headache. This drug has also been associated with an increased risk of ovarian cysts. Additionally, in some women, clomephine may cause cervical mucus to become dry and so sticky it prevents sperm from reaching the egg. To help remedy this problem many of my patients have found that taking daily doses of the cough medicine Robitussin can help. It contains the ingredient guaifenesin which helps thin all mucus secretions and often corrects the problem caused by clomiphene. To promote production of even more mucus your doctor may also prescribe small amounts of estrogen.

Although this medication does slightly increase your chances for a multiple birth, the most common outcome is twins, which results up to 10 percent of the time. One in four hundred women conceive triplets, and quadruplets occur every eight hundred births. This drug is not normally associated with the extraordinary multiple births of five babies or more.

Red flag: There is some evidence to suggest that extended use of clomiphene for longer than twelve consecutive cycles may increase the risk of ovarian cancer, which is discussed more fully later in this chapter.

Medication: Human Menopausal Gonadotropin (Menotropins)

Brand names: Pergonal, Humegon, Repronex

How it works: By supplementing your body with an additional supply of FSH and LH, the hormones that initiate egg production and release. Pergonal is manufactured from the purified urine of postmenopausal women, while Humegon and Repronex are laboratory-created synthetic drugs. This category of fertility medications is used for super ovulation.

Method of treatment: Injection

What you need to know: Used to stimulate egg production, these drugs work only if ovaries are capable of responding to FSH and LH stimulation. They are best used to correct deficiencies in these hormones caused by either inadequate production or delayed timing. Unlike clomiphene, they enhance the production of cervical mucus, which can further help bring sperm and egg together. If you have only one clear fallopian tube, these drugs can also help by encouraging ovulation from both ovaries during every single cycle. This increases pregnancy odds by ensuring that your one functioning tube always receives an egg. Because these medications work only to help you produce eggs, they must be taken in conjunction with hCG—human chorionic gonadotropin (see next category), a drug that helps trigger ovulation.

Side effects: Although they produce no immediate side effects, if not carefully prescribed and monitored, these drugs do increase the risk of "ovarian hyperstimulation" or OHS, a condition wherein you manufacture so many eggs that your ovaries enlarge to painful proportions. This can happen in up to 5 percent of all cycles, and sometimes it cannot be prevented, even by a very experienced fertility expert. In some instances, hyperstimulation may lead to blood clot formation, kidney damage, or abnormal fluid collection in the chest or abdomen, or even affect the health of your ovary. Although it can be serious (in severe cases hospitalization may be required to ensure your overall health), symptoms are transient, and usually last no more than one to two weeks.

Fortunately, there are things that can be done to help reduce your risks: If your eggs are growing too quickly or too large (indicated by sonogram and E2 blood test), your doctor should stop your medication, cancel your cycle, and withhold your injection of hCG, the drug that triggers ovulation.

The chance of multiple births when using these drugs increases by about 20 to 25 percent, with most pregnancies yielding twins. There is also a very slight increase in the risk of a tubal or ectopic pregnancy.

Red flag: Although there are several different brands in this drug category, they often contain specific formulations that are not necessarily interchangeable. For this reason, make sure your pharmacy always fills your doctor's prescription as written. Additionally, some controversy exists concerning the link between these drugs and ovarian cancer. These risks, and the precautions you can take, are discussed more fully later in this chapter.

Medication: Urofollitropin

Brand names: Fertinex, Metrodin

Method of treatment: intramuscular or subcutaneous injection (Fertinex)

How it works: Similar to menotropins (see above), which supply FSH and LH, urofollitropin simply supplies FSH. It works to rebalance the fertility hormone ratio and has a direct stimulating effect on the ovaries, helping to make more eggs. It is, in fact, usually prescribed to stimulate egg development in women who may produce too much LH in proportion to FSH, or for use in helping women over forty get pregnant.

What you need to know: It is often prescribed for women who do not respond to other fertility drugs, particularly Clomid, Pergonal, or a combination regimen. Like menotropins, Metrodin is also extracted from the urine of postmenopausal women, then purified in a lab. Fertinex is made synthetically. Both drugs are used for super ovulation. Since FSH is only responsible for producing eggs and helping them mature, if your supply of LH (the ovulation hormone) is also scarce, you may require treatment with the medication hCG (human chorionic gonadotropin) to help trigger ovulation. This combination is most useful if you suffer with poly cystic ovary disease (PCOD) or if you have not responded to other egg-making drugs. Although Fertinex can be given subcutaneously (an injection under the skin), most physicians have found that the treatment is more successful if the injection is given intramuscularly, thus allowing more of this medication to be absorbed by the body.

Metrodin is currently not being distributed in the United States. However, it is often imported from other areas of the world, where it is still readily used, particularly in patients who do not respond to other forms of urofollitropin.

Side effects: Problems can range from mild to severe, so these drugs should only be prescribed by a fertility expert who is very familiar with how they work. Reported problems include an increased risk of hyper-stimulation, which can progress rapidly over a twenty-four-hour period (see menotropins, above). About 20 percent of patients also experience a harmless but uncomfortable swelling of the ovaries and stomach, with some mild abdominal pain. This usually disappears within several weeks on its own. In addition, there is a small risk of pulmonary or vascular complications, including blood clot formation and pulmonary embolism, most often seen in combination with hyperstimulation. There is also an increased incidence of multiple births.

Red flags: You generally should not use these drugs if you have a very high level of FSH (indicating your ovaries are not functioning), if you suffer from uncontrolled thyroid or adrenal disorders, if you have a pituitary tumor, if you have abnormal bleeding without a cause, or if you have ovarian cysts or enlargement.

Medication: Follitropin Beta; Follitropin Alfa

Brand name: Follistim; Gonal-F

How it works: Acting like natural FSH to stimulate the maturation and development of your egg follicles, this laboratory-created version is similar in action to the medications listed in the category known as human menopausal gonadotropin (see above).

Method of treatment: Daily injections for seven to twelve days

What you need to know: Among the newest fertility drugs, these medications are the first to use a special DNA technology to produce FSH without having to rely on the urine of postmenopausal women. Some believe this may result in a more pure treatment, less likely to cause a negative reaction. It does, however, carry a risk of hyperstimulation and ectopic pregnancy similar to that of other forms of FSH. In order for ovulation to occur, treatment must also be followed with an injection of hCG.

The main difference between the two drugs in this category—Gonal-F and Follistim—is in the way they are administered. Specifically, Follistim requires an intramuscular injection, which uses a larger needle and deeper penetration. Although some women find they are able to give themselves the injection, often it requires a partner. Gonal-F, however, requires only a subcutaneous injection with an ultraslim needle inserted just under the skin. It can be more easily self-administered. Some physicians, however, find that intramuscular injections of Gonal-F are more effective.

Side effects: Although they occurred in less than 1 percent of patients, the following adverse reactions have been reported: ovarian cysts, mild to moderate ovarian enlargement, and body rashes. Other possible problems include an increased risk of vaginal hemorrhage, abdominal pain, and pain at the site of injection. You can reduce the risk of some problems by avoiding strenuous physical activity and vigorous sexual intercourse while taking these medications. Symptoms usually subside shortly after menstruation.

Red flags: If you have a history of recurring miscarriage, you may want to take extra caution when using this drug, since one study has shown there may be a slight increase in the risk of pregnancy loss, as well as ectopic pregnancy. Often you can overcome these risks, however, by following preventative guidelines offered later in this book.

Medication: Human Chorionic Gonadotropins (hCG)

Brand names: Profasi, Pregnyl, APL

How it works: Under normal circumstances, LH is the hormone that triggers ovulation. When, however, due to a variety of circumstances, that hormone is in short supply, doctors usually prescribe hCG. A highly purified version of a substance that is normally secreted by your baby's placenta during pregnancy, hCG is closely related to LH in both structure and form. As such, this drug supplements your natural LH levels and together they work to stimulate the release of your egg (ovulation).

Method of treatment: Injection

What you need to know: This medication is normally given only one time in each cycle, just before ovulation. Your doctor should use frequent ultrasound exams as well as blood tests for estradiol (E2) to determine when your eggs are ready, so that your hCG injection can be properly timed.

Side effects: There is a small risk of headaches, irritability, restlessness, depression, fatigue, and edema.

Red flags: Because there is no way to guarantee against hyperstimulation, if your ovaries are producing too many eggs, or eggs that are overly large, your cycle can be canceled (by withholding your injection of hCG) or your doctor might elect to give you a smaller amount.

Medication: GnRH — Gonadotropin-Releasing Hormone

Brand names: Factrel, Lutrepulse

How it works: Because it stimulates the entire egg production process, this drug is used when your hypothalamus gland does not supply enough natural GnRH to put the process in motion. Working much like the natural hormone, it signals your pituitary gland to produce LH and FSH, which in turn induce egg growth, maturation, and ovulation.

What you need to know: These drugs are usually prescribed only for women who have failed to ovulate when using more common egg-enhancing preparations such as Pergonal, Humegon, Repronex, Fertinex, or even clomiphene. It can also be particularly helpful if you suffer from a luteal phase defect (characterized by low progesterone in the second half of your menstrual cycle), poly cystic ovarian disease (PCOD) or hypogonadotropic hypogonadism. Because GnRH causes indirect rather than direct ovarian stimulation (it works via the pituitary gland and not directly on the ovary), it is often used to help correct difficult ovulatory problems. It carries a very low risk of hyperstimulation, and a high rate of pregnancy success, normally producing ovulation in just three to four weeks.

As helpful as this drug is, it can be difficult to use. Although it is available as an injection, by far the best method is through an infusion pump worn twenty-four hours a day. To deliver the drug to your body, the pump is attached, via a small catheter, to a thin needle implanted under your skin. In this way you can receive a pulsating burst of the drug every sixty to ninety minutes around the clock, which is the way natural GnRH works in your body.

Side effects: Problems include the possibility of pain, redness, swelling, or infection at the injection site, and only a slight risk of hyperstimulation.

Red flags: None

Lupron and Other "Agonizing" Treatments That Help You Conceive

While most patients respond favorably to fertility medications, there is always the possibility that your body will receive too much stimulation, causing hormone levels to rise too high. This can create another type of imbalance that reduces rather than enhances your fertility. To keep this from happening, your doctor may prescribe medications classified as "agonists"—synthetic preparations that shut down your body's natural supply of reproductive hormones, allowing only the controlled amounts supplied by the fertility drugs to circulate through your system. In this way your doctor is more certain of the amount of hormones that are in your body at all times. This can also help ensure more uniform egg production and help to prevent premature ovulation.

The most widely prescribed of these drugs is leuprolide acetate (Lupron) which is given via injection. Other versions include the nasal sprays Naferelin and Synarel, as well as Goserelin and Zoladex, which are under-the-skin implants that remain in place for thirty days. In addition to acting as fertility treatments, these agonist drugs are also used in the treatment of endometriosis and fibroid tumors, which you can read about in Part One of this book.

Temporary side effects include a decrease in calcium, loss of bone mass, hot flashes, decreased sex drive, and vaginal dryness. These effects, however, including loss of bone mass, are reversed once drug use is discontinued.

Bromocriptine: Another Treatment Alternative

A second type of agonist preparation is bromocriptine mesylate (Parlodel). It works to suppress the production of the hormone prolactin. Normally released by your pituitary gland following childbirth to stimulate the production of breast milk, it also disrupts ovulation, which is one reason why most women don't get pregnant while breast-feeding.

In some women, however, an excess of prolactin is present nearly all the time. Known as "hyperprolactemia," this condition can result in a variety of reproductive problems, including inadequate progesterone, irregular ovulation, or total cessation of menstruation, all of which can obviously compromise fertility. Women with hyperprolactemia can often experience a daily leaking of breast milk from the nipples, even when not pregnant or breast-feeding.

Common causes of hyperprolactemia include medications (including certain antidepressant drugs, tranquilizers, blood pressure medications, and antinausea preparations as well as some oral contraceptives), stress, smoking marijuana, a thyroid disorder, or even exercising too much. In some instances, a harmless growth on the pituitary gland may also be responsible, which your doctor can identify with an X-ray. And, up to 30 percent of the time, the cause for hyperprolactemia cannot be found.

In most cases, however, treatment with Parlodel can usually normalize prolactin levels and ovulation. If no other fertility problems exist, this may be the only treatment needed for pregnancy to occur. If, however, conception does not take place, have a second blood test before giving up on this drug. Sometimes you may require a higher dose to gain results.

One note of caution: Be aware that prolactin secretions can be temporarily elevated due to excess sleep, stress, exercise, nipple stimulation, fasting, dieting, and even intercourse. Avoid these activities (particularly fasting) before testing and do all you can to reduce stress levels the day of the test.

Growth Hormone: The New Experimental Fertility Drug

Among the newest fertility drugs now under consideration is a growth hormone simply known as GH. Currently, it is indicated for the long-term treatment of children with a deficiency in growth hormone, or who have growth problems related to a kidney illness. It has also been safely used to replace GH in adults who have this deficiency.

Obviously, because GH has the potential to stimulate growth, it was natural to consider the possible role it could play in stimulating egg development. Indeed, a number of animal studies seem to indicate this may be the case.

Additionally, since men with a GH deficiency seem to have reduced semen quality, this drug may also have a positive effect on male fertility. At least one small study of ten infertile men revealed that GH therapy was able to improve sperm production in half the participants.

Currently, infertility treatment with growth hormone (GH) is considered highly experimental, and there are no specific recommendations for use. In addition, there has been no specific safety evaluations conducted, so it is difficult to ascertain which, if any, patients would benefit from this drug.

However, studies are continuing, and it's entirely possible that in the future, GH deficiency may become a recognizable cause of some types of infertility in both men and women, and that treatment with these medications can help. In addition, there is some speculation that these medications may work to encourage egg production in perimenopausal women. Further, by diagnosing GH deficiencies in children and treating them early on, it's possible this drug may help reduce the risk of some reproductive problems later in life.

Progesterone: The Pregnancy Drug That Helps Your Conception Thrive

For the most part, fertility drugs are medications that help you *get pregnant*. But for many women, the problem is not so much a matter of conceiving, but of getting their pregnancy to survive and thrive.

For this reason, medications that help you sustain your pregnancy can also be considered fertility drugs. Among the most widely prescribed is natural progesterone. Manufactured naturally by your body during the second half of every menstrual period, progesterone helps condition the uterus for a healthy implantation. If no pregnancy occurs, progesterone levels drop, which is actually what triggers the start of your monthly menstrual bleeding. Should pregnancy occur, however, progesterone levels soar and remain elevated. This allows your uterus to begin developing the soft, spongy lining need to maintain a pregnancy.

If, however, your level of progesterone is generally low—something your doctor can determine in the cycles before conception—miscarriage becomes a real threat. What can help: natural progesterone treatments.

Until recently, the most viable forms were either daily intramuscular injections or vaginal suppositories, to be used three times daily. Now, however, there are two additional options.

The first, called Crinone, comes in a relatively new form. It is manufactured as a bioadhesive gel that actually adheres to your vaginal tissue. It is administered twice daily via special applicator. Not only can it be easier to use, its effects are felt directly on the uterus. Additionally, some studies report the gel form of progesterone results in fewer side effects than the injection and is generally available by prescription in most pharmacies. Natural oral progesterone tablets called Prometrium are also now available, which are effective and obviously easier to use.

Although Crinone is indicated as a method of preventing miscarriage in some women, Prometrium is not indicated for use during pregnancy. Generally speaking, however, this warning usually pertains only to a pregnancy that is considered normal and not at risk for miscarriage. In the hands of an experienced fertility expert, all forms of natural progesterone can be used under special circumstances by pregnant women, and they can be helpful.

Finally, some pharmacies are also able to custom-compound natural progesterone into tablet form and provide them, by mail-order, to patients all over the country. For contact information, see the Resources section at the end of this book.

Regardless of how it is administered, side effects of progesterone therapy can include breast pain, headache, breast enlargement, constipation, and nausea, as well as mood swings and depression. You should not use progesterone therapy if you have a known sensitivity to this hormone, or if you suffer from undiagnosed vaginal bleeding or liver dysfunction or disease, or if you have a personal history of breast or uterine cancer. Prometrium should not be used if you have an allergy to peanuts.

For more information on progesterone therapy, please read the chapter on miscarriage earlier in this book.

Are Fertility Drugs Safe? What You Need to Know

Among the most shocking medical headlines of the 1990s were those that questioned the safety of fertility drugs. Specifically, there seemed to be a growing body of evidence to indicate possible links between some of these drugs and breast, uterine, and ovarian cancer. One high-profile case involved the highly respected editor of *Harpers Bazaar,* Liz Tilberis, who developed ovarian cancer following treatments with fertility drugs and succumbed to this disease in 1999. Her outspoken attitude about her personal experience and her valiant efforts to educate women about this disease not only fueled our fears, but helped focus our attention on a subject that clearly needed to be reviewed, particularly since women who suffer with ovarian dysfunction or who never give birth to a child have a naturally higher incidence of ovarian cancer.

Early theories pegged the cancer-drug link to some basic biology we already knew. Specifically, the fewer times a woman ovulated in her life, the lower her chance of developing ovarian cancer. If this was true, said the researchers, then the opposite must be true as well: that increasing egg growth and ovulatory action, as fertility drugs are supposed to do, would naturally increase the risk of ovarian cancer. And some small studies seemed to indicate this could be the case. Other researchers pointed to still another theory: That large eggs, and large numbers of eggs, bursting from the ovaries during each fertility drug cycle might cause ovarian cell damage that eventually leads to malignancy. More recently, new reasearch has shown that the temporary high levels of estrogen caused by some of these drugs may also stimulate breast and uterine tissues to develop abnormal cells.

Although most studies were small and the results considered highly preliminary, they served to launch a number of large international investigations into this issue. Unfortunately, as of the writing of this book, I still cannot give you a definitive answer. Although one of the largest research projects in this area—a study of some fifty-five hundred women conducted by the Australian National Health Medical Research Council—found no evidence linking the use of fertility drugs to ovarian cancer, other smaller studies continue to show there may be cause for concern. And, most recently, a 1999 study in the journal *Lancet* found that women undergoing IVF with fertility drugs had a slight transient increase in the risk of breast and uterine cancer in the year following treatment. But the same study also found infertile women who received no treatment had an increased risk of uterine and ovarian cancer.

And so, all I can offer you at the moment is my personal view of the situation, which I feel is not as bad as some media headlines would have you believe. Indeed, it is my opinion that the only solid information we have to date indicates that when the fertility drug clomiphene citrate is used alone consistently for more than twelve consecutive cycles, the resulting ovarian stimulation may indeed increase the risk of ovarian cancer. However, it's equally important to point out that this is a *highly unusual* protocol. Most women who use these drugs get pregnant much faster and most never require a full twelve cycles of stimulation.

Additionally, there is some strong evidence to show that certain physiological conditions which occur as a result of infertility may in fact be the real underlying cause of this link to ovarian cancer, and not the drugs themselves.

That said, I believe you should always err on the side of caution—and by that I mean, if you have used fertility drugs in any amount, or if you plan to do so, take an aggressive stance in protecting your health. What does this mean?

1. Avoid as many environmental factors linked to cancer as possible. Don't smoke, avoid secondhand smoke, limit alcohol consumption, and when possible, limit or eliminate exposure to pesticides and other harmful chemicals.

2. Take your full complement of vitamins and minerals, particularly high levels of antioxidants, the nutrients which fight against cancer. Grape seed extract and flaxseed oil are two more nutrients that are thought to provide cancer protection.

3. Get regular gynecological exams. If your gynecologist was not your fertility doctor, make certain he or she knows the specific drugs you used, and for how long. Make certain your ovaries are examined manually, by your doctor, at every office visit and be sure that your annual exam always includes a vaginal ultrasound to check the ovaries more carefully for early signs of trouble.

If you follow these three steps, I'm certain you will have little to fear in the way of fertility-related cancer threats.

Fertility Drugs and You: A Commitment to Pregnancy

There is no doubt that fertility drugs can and will increase your ability to get pregnant. However, you, your partner, and your doctor *must* make a joint commitment to your pregnancy.

- Medication must be taken with unfailing accuracy. Timing is often crucial. Since some of the drugs used must be injected, your partner or a good friend can be taught to administer the shot, saving you a trip to the doctor's office and allowing you a more flexible schedule.

- As with all drugs, become familiar with any and all side effects and immediately report any symptoms to your doctor. This is especially important in helping to prevent hyperstimulation syndrome and in alerting your doctor to the need to increase dosages for a faster, easier conception.

- You must make the required trips to your doctor for sonograms and blood tests. Missing even one scheduled session could have disastrous results, or at the very least keep you from getting pregnant.

- For the period during which you are taking fertility drugs you must plan your social and sexual life around your medication regimens. This means weekend trips or vacations must be postponed if they interfere in any way with your checkups. Sex must be timed with your medication in order to make optimum use of its fertility-increasing powers. Remember, however, this will only be for a short time, and I promise the inconvenience will be worth the result.

- You must also consider the possibility of a multiple birth. Although not every couple who uses fertility drugs has more than one baby, the chances increase with the amount of fertility medication you take. Of course, if you have been infertile for a long time, multiples are a great way to *catch up* with your family planning!

Finally, it's important that you not become discouraged if a pregnancy does not result right away. Many different regimens and combinations of fertility drugs are available, and it may take some time to strike the right babymaking "recipe" for you. However, with patience, and the skills of a good specialist, fertility drugs have answered the prayer for motherhood for tens of thousands of women worldwide, and they can help answer your prayers as well.

Chapter Twenty

The New Artificial Insemination:

Nothing Artificial at All

🌿 One of the most exciting advances in reproductive medicine was the development of laboratory techniques to help couples get pregnant. Although new technologies seem to become available almost every year, for many, the first to be developed—known as artificial insemination—remains the most successful.

This relatively simple medical procedure involves placing your partner's sperm (or that of a donor) inside your reproductive tract at the time you are ovulating. The actual creation of your baby then takes place *naturally* inside your fallopian tubes, just as it would if you and your partner made love. In fact, the only thing *artificial* about insemination is that it facilitates the process of getting the sperm to your egg. Everything else about your conception follows the natural course.

Can Artificial Insemination Help You?

Originally developed as an effective means of conceiving if your partner was not able to ejaculate or have an erection, a number of key advances in the process have made artificial insemination a viable solution for millions of couples with a vast array of reproductive problems, including:

- Marginal to low sperm counts
- Poor sperm motility

- Sperm antibodies (in you or your mate)
- Seminal fluid deficiencies
- Hostile cervical mucus
- Vaginal, cervical, or uterine abnormalities

In addition, I have personally used artificial insemination to successfully treat a great number of couples with unexplained infertility, where a pregnancy cannot occur but no physiological reason can be found. Researchers theorize that minor defects in *both* partners' reproductive systems (too slight to be measured by any test) may come together to create a barrier to conception that insemination seems to overcome.

Not All Inseminations Are Alike: How to Tell What's Right for You!

Depending on the type of physiological problem that is causing your infertility, different kinds of insemination processes are used. Each places the sperm in a slightly different area of your reproductive tract, and each solves a distinct type of fertility problem.

For most couples, however, one of the following three basic procedures is used:

- **Vaginal insemination:** The first type of insemination developed, this involves placing sperm inside your vagina, which then must swim, on its own, to your fallopian tube. This method works best when your partner's sperm is good, but he cannot maintain an erection or ejaculate during intercourse, or when you have unexplained infertility.

- **Intracervical insemination:** This process places sperm a little higher into your reproductive tract, at the mouth of your womb, which is located at the top of your cervix. It is often used when infertility is caused by deficiencies in your cervical mucus, by vaginal abnormalities, or when your partner has a low to low-normal sperm count or poor sperm motility.

- **Intrauterine insemination (IUI)**: This method bypasses the vagina and cervix completely and places sperm directly into your uterus, very close to the opening of your fallopian tube. This method allows sperm to bypass certain problems, including insufficient or hostile mucus and antisperm antibodies, as well as endometriosis, irregular ovulation, low sperm count, and poor sperm motility.

Looking for Love: Another Insemination Option

For the most part, fertility experts believe that all fertilization takes place in the fallopian tubes. As you read earlier, the fimbriated or "fingerlike" ends of the tube "catch" your egg as it is ovulated and gently guide it inside. There it meets with sperm and conception occurs.

However, another theory holds that fertilization may also occur outside the tube, in an area at the back of the uterus called the cul de sac, or "Pouch of Douglas." Here it is thought that sperm may swim from the vagina through the uterus, *down* the fallopian tubes *out the other side.* There it meets the egg in the cul de sac, where conception actually occurs. Then, only after the egg is fertilized do the fallopian "fingers" come into play, sweeping your embryo back into the tube for incubation and passage to your uterus.

This theory became the basis for still another form of insemination, known as IPI—intraperotoneal insemination. In terms of complexity, it is viewed as halfway between IUI and in vitro fertilization. Here's how it works:

1. First, your doctor will use ultrasound to check on your egg production. When ovulation is imminent, you will undergo a procedure called *transvaginal follicle puncture.* Here, an ultrathin catheter needle is inserted through your vagina and into your ovary, where it siphons out your ripened eggs and surrounding follicular fluid. Although the procedure is brief, your doctor can relieve any discomfort you may feel by giving you an injection of a pain medication such as Demerol before starting.

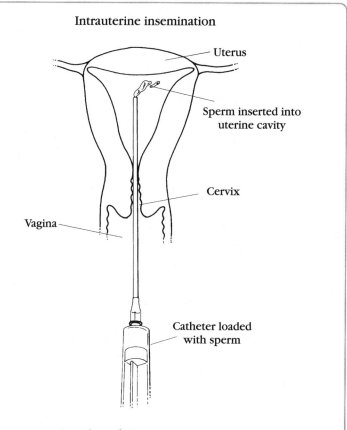

Intrauterine insemination

Uterus

Sperm inserted into
uterine cavity

Cervix

Vagina

Catheter loaded
with sperm

Artificial Insemination

One of the most popular forms of artificial insemination is called IUI—
intrauterine insemination. In this procedure, your partner's sperm is
placed directly into your uterus, very close to the opening of a fallopian
tube. This is thought to give sperm a good "running start" and increase
the chance that it will reach your egg. Best used for sperm that has poor
motility, or when your mucus is considered insufficient to help carry
sperm through your reproductive system.

Illustration courtesy of the American Society of Reproductive Medicine

2. When the catheter containing your eggs and fluid is withdrawn from your ovary, it is then immediately released into the cul de sac "Pouch of Douglas" area of your uterus.

3. With the needle still in place, your partner's sperm is loaded into the catheter and released into this same area of your uterus, as close to your egg as possible. This eliminates the need for sperm to travel through your reproductive system, which can be particularly helpful if there are any obstructions along the way or problems with your cervical mucus.

The entire procedure should take about five minutes. If all goes well, your egg and your partner's sperm will combine in this cul de sac area in much the same way they do in the small glass dishes used to form an embryo during in vitro fertilization. But unlike IVF, which requires that the embryo be implanted into your uterus, in IPI, your fallopian tubes do all the work, gently guiding your embryo inside where it can incubate. Within a few days it begins traveling to your uterus for implantation.

The projected success rate for IPI: Providing fertility drugs are used and at least one fallopian tube is open, 20 percent of couples who try this procedure get pregnant within three cycles. If you do not succeed within three tries, you should consider other forms of assisted reproduction.

Getting Pregnant FAST: The Newest Insemination

Among the most advanced forms of artificial insemination is FAST—fallopian sperm transfer system. This means that your partner's sperm is placed directly into each of your fallopian tubes, the site where most natural conceptions take place. Since you should be ovulating at the time of your insemination, your doctor will strive to place the sperm as close to your egg as possible, thus making fertilization faster and easier. How effective is FAST? Small but significant studies published in the journal *Fertility and Sterility* have shown that when combined with fertility drugs to stimulate egg production, FAST achieves a 40 percent pregnancy rate per cycle, as compared with 20 percent for standard IUI (intrauterine insemination).

Researchers theorize it's because FAST can remove small obstacles from your tubes that might otherwise keep sperm from reaching your egg. What also increases fertilization: location, location, location! Unlike other forms of insemination, in which some sperm is always lost en route to the egg, in FAST, the full volume of available sperm is deposited right next to the egg, so you get the full benefit of everything your partner has to offer.

Also important: FAST costs about one-third as much as standard in vitro fertilization and in many instances can offer similar pregnancy rates. For this reason many fertility experts now suggest trying FAST before advancing to more complex and costly fertility treatments.

On the downside, FAST may increase the risk of multiple births, and there is some concern that it may also increase the risk of ectopic pregnancy and increased production of antisperm antibodies. A discussion with your fertility expert should help you determine where your personal risk factors lie, and how much this procedure may or may not help you.

How Your Body Helps Your Partner's Sperm

When you conceive via sexual intercourse, it is cervical mucus that helps transport sperm to your uterus and tubes. It also helps separate sperm from its semen, which is necessary because once outside a man's body semen becomes highly toxic to sperm, causing it to die within a few hours.

Additionally, while semen is considered a harmless fluid in the vagina, once it travels through your cervix and into your uterus, it can cause cramping so violent, pregnancy would be impossible. Semen also contains bacteria and other debris that can hamper fertilization, as well as dead sperm (which can affect healthy sperm) and white blood cells, which can also be toxic to your conception. And, too, it is only when sperm is separated from semen that it gains the power to swim through your fallopian tube and reach your egg. So, it's easy to see why the filtering actions of your cervical mucus is so important.

But there is also another vital step your mucus performs. In a process called "capitization," it helps sperm release a group of enzymes located in the head. Why is this important? It is these enzymes that give sperm the power to biochemically "drill" through the tough outer layer of your egg's shell, which is the only way it can get inside so fertilization can occur.

When either a vaginal or cervical insemination is performed, sperm does make some of this important contact with mucus. In IUI (intrauterine insemination) or FAST, however, cervical mucus is totally bypassed, meaning the important capitization process won't occur.

To the rescue: A sophisticated laboratory process called "sperm washing," a procedure that simulates some of the cleaning and capitization actions naturally performed by your cervical mucus and, in the process, optimizes sperm performance and fertilization success.

How Sperm Washing Is Done

1. The ejaculated sperm is placed in a container and left to liquefy at room temperature for about a half-hour.

2. Next the ejaculate is floated on top of a harmless chemical called Isolate, which has a kind of "scrubbing bubbles" property that isolates the most active sperm. The entire solution is placed into a centrifuge, a machine that rapidly spins the contents. The chemical reaction caused by the bubbles and the spinning motion allows the most motile sperm (the best swimmers) to fall to the bottom of the container, where they can be collected.

3. This concentration of the fastest sperm is then removed and mixed with a culture medium—a type of fluid that will further encourage the capitization process.

4. Once again, the mixture is placed into a centrifuge and respun. This fully separates the sperm from the unwanted seminal fluid.

5. After about ten minutes, the sperm form a small, concentrated pellet that falls to the bottom of the container. Often, steps 3 and 4 are repeated to ensure purity.

Unless your partner's count is exceptionally low, his sperm is now ready to be inseminated.

A *Caution Your Doctor Must Not Ignore*

Until very recently, the solution used to "float" the sperm (step 2) was a chemical called Percoll. However, new studies have shown that Percoll appears to have a toxic effect on animal embryos, thus reducing the chance for a healthy conception. While no effect on human embryos has been shown, Percoll was voluntarily recalled by the manufacturer. The newer, much safer version—called Isolate—is what should be used to wash your partner's sperm.

Sperm Helpers: The Latest News

Even though a sperm can appear healthy and normal, it doesn't always have the ability to fertilize an egg. Various deficiencies, including a lack of the proper enzymes in the head of the sperm, can make penetrating your egg difficult, or even impossible, even with the washing process.

Fortunately, science is here to help. One of the newest procedures involves incubating (or soaking) your partner's washed sperm in a combination of two chemicals: pentoxifylline (a natural enzyme present in seminal fluid) and deoxyribonuclease (another natural seminal enzyme that is also present in a woman's reproductive tract). Together they work to increase a sperm's ability to penetrate an egg. (An older method, which is still used occasionally, involves incubating sperm in the anti-clot medication heparin just before insemination.)

Because the sperm of some men simply takes longer to complete the enzymatic action, it is sometimes left alone to incubate for up to twenty-four hours before insemination.

Getting Your Body Ready for Insemination: What to Do

In addition to what can be done to enhance sperm performance, there are things that you can do to increase the success of your insemination. First and foremost: Make certain your procedure is performed at the time when you are ovulating. I cannot emphasize this enough.

Why? When you conceive on your own, your natural cervical mucus helps sperm remain alive in your reproductive tract for up to seventy-two hours, maybe even 120 hours. That means you can have intercourse up to three to five days before ovulation, and still have a chance of achieving a pregnancy.

Yet most forms of insemination bypass your cervical mucus, which means that sperm cannot survive for any significant amount of time in your body. In order for your insemination to be successful, your partner's sperm must be deposited at the same time your egg has ovulated. If, in fact, ovulation does not occur within hours of receiving sperm, it's highly unlikely that a pregnancy will occur.

To help make sure that your insemination is properly timed, use your BBT and cervical mucus to chart your ovulation time frame, beginning a month or two before your insemination is to take place.

However, to be certain your timing is right, you should also use the ovulation predictor methods described in Part Two of this book (such as the CUE II or ovulation predictor kits), beginning about a month or two before the cycle in which you plan to be inseminated.

When you believe ovulation is imminent, your doctor will perform a vaginal ultrasound. If your egg follicle has collapsed, it means you have already ovulated and you should be inseminated immediately. If your follicle is about to rupture, ovulation is likely to occur within twenty-four to forty-eight hours, in which case you should also be inseminated right away, followed by a second procedure in twenty-four hours to ensure

Ovulation Helpers: The Medications You Might Need

As research into reproductive endocrinology advanced, scientists began noting that women who required fertility drugs to make eggs actually had more successful inseminations than those who relied solely on their own eggs. Theorizing that the drugs could make even healthy eggs stronger and easier to fertilize, many doctors began routinely prescribing these medications for all women undergoing insemination.

Now, a new study of 930 couples shows that not only can fertility drugs enhance the conception rate of inseminations, when used properly, for some couples this one-two punch may take the place of more sophisticated fertility treatments that cost far more.

The research, published in 1999 in the *New England Journal of Medicine,* found that the women in the study who underwent super ovulation (using fertility medications to develop several eggs in a single cycle) and were then artificially inseminated were twice as likely to get pregnant as those who underwent only one form of treatment—either fertility drugs or insemination. The combination regimen also yielded a pregnancy rate three times that of women who used no fertility treatments of any kind.

If you decide to enhance your insemination with fertility medications, don't worry about tracking your ovulation or monitoring your LH surges. Instead, your doctor will use frequent ultrasound exams to track egg development. When the test shows you are ready to ovulate, you will receive the egg-releasing medication, which should be followed by your first insemination within thirty-six to forty hours. Within twenty-four to forty-eight hours after that your second insemination should take place. (You can read more about fertility medications in Chapter 19.)

success. In fact, I strongly advocate the use of two consecutive inseminations under all circumstances, since a second procedure will raise the likelihood that sperm is deposited at the right time.

The Insemination Process: What to Expect

On the scheduled day of your procedure, your partner will be asked to supply a sample of fresh sperm. This will be needed about one to two hours before the actual insemination is set to begin. The sperm can be obtained via masturbation into a sterile container provided by the lab, or via sexual intercourse into a specially prepared condom (we'll tell you how in a minute).

1. As soon as your partner's sperm has been washed, it will be aspirated into a long, thin catheter with a syringe at its end.

2. You will then be asked to lie on an examining table and your feet will be placed in stirrups. A speculum will be gently inserted into your vagina to hold it open during the procedure. Because insemination is relatively painless (it feels about the same as a Pap smear), it is not likely you will need any type of anesthesia.

3. Next, your doctor will insert the catheter into your vagina (vaginal insemination) or into your cervix (cervical insemination) or uterus (intrauterine insemination), or into your fallopian tube (FAST procedure). Once this is in place he or she will slowly depress the syringe and release the sperm into your reproductive tract.

4. To help lock the insemination into place, a small plastic-covered fertility sponge is inserted into your vagina, directly in front of your cervix. It remains in your body for about six hours, after which time you can remove it, using an attached string similar to a tampon.

In an alternative method, a small plastic cap is placed over your cervix before the insemination. The sperm is then injected through a small opening in the cap, which snaps shut the moment the catheter is withdrawn. This prevents any chance of spillage and ensures that all the inseminated sperm remain inside your body. You remove the cap in six hours yourself.

Natural Sex: Still the Best Route for Sperm

When it comes to supplying the sperm for your insemination, many fertility centers will routinely instruct your partner to masturbate, either at home or in a private room at the clinic, which is often equipped with magazines, soft lighting, even adult videos—the way samples are provided to sperm banks.

However, research continues to show that natural sex may be the most beneficial for sperm. Why? First, the more intense level of stimulation offered by sexual intercourse may allow more sperm to pass into the vas deferens, and ultimately that means more sperm available for fertilization. Intercourse also usually leads to a more intense orgasm, which, some researchers report, allows more of the young, newly matured sperm lying near the epididymis to come forward and leave the body, which may also increase the likelihood of conception.

Studies conducted at the Andrology Institute in Lexington, Kentucky, for example, have shown that sperm counts in semen samples obtained during natural intercourse were 324 percent higher than those obtained in the lab. In some cases, the increase was significant enough to push men with a low sperm count into the normal range. In addition, motility was up by 16 percent, along with a 20 percent increase in normal-shaped sperm, particularly in those men who had produced only abnormal sperm in the lab.

Intercourse and Insemination: How They Can Work Together

To use the benefits of intercourse for insemination, your doctor can provide a sterile container and a specially prepared sterile condom, free of spermicide. It is worn while you make love and serves to collect the ejaculate. The condom is then carefully removed from your partner, placed back into the sterile container, and brought to the lab. Here, the embryologist empties it into a test tube and begins the washing process.

If sperm is collected at home, it must be kept warm during the transport. The best temperature is body temperature, and many women find that carrying the container in their bra, between their breasts, is the optimal way to preserve sperm quality. If you live farther than an hour away from your fertility center, the embryologist can show your partner how to empty sperm from the condom into a container filled with a special medium to preserve it for several hours.

Should Your Partner Be Present During Your Insemination?

If your partner wants to be there, I recommend it! Sharing the insemination experience can help you bond, not only to each other but to your baby as well. But because, some men find the idea of insemination very disturbing (especially if donor sperm is needed), it may be easier for him not to be present during the process. If this *is* how your partner feels, don't be alarmed: The reaction is normal. Do, however, discuss how he feels about being present well before your day of insemination. This can help you avoid any excess stress immediately before the procedure.

Increasing Your Insemination Success: What to Do

In much the same way that lying still after sex can help keep sperm inside you, so too does minimizing movement after insemination. Although some doctors disagree, I believe that remaining on the examining table with your buttocks raised slightly upward for about twenty minutes following your procedure will help encourage conception. In addition, I believe you should also spend at least a few hours in bed as soon as you return home. I have used both these techniques to encourage successful conceptions, particularly in those couples whose previous inseminations were not successful.

Donor Sperm: Improving Your Conception Odds

Even with all the new sperm-enhancing technologies, problems can still persist. In essence, some men simply cannot produce enough high-quality sperm to make an insemination work. When this is the case, donor sperm may be the answer to your fertility crisis.

Choosing a Sperm Donor: What You Need to Know

For many couples, a donor is selected from a sperm bank—a laboratory that collects, tests, and processes samples from otherwise anonymous donors. If this gives you an uneasy feeling, you are not alone. Many couples have this same concern, and some women have a particularly difficult time thinking about creating a child with a man they will never know. For others, however, it is considered highly acceptable and easy to do.

Regardless of where your feelings fall, if a sperm bank is an option you are considering, there are some important things you should know.

Banking on Success

In 1988 the American Society for Reproductive Medicine published guidelines recommending that laboratories no longer provide fresh sperm from anonymous donors. In addition to insisting they be regularly screened for sexually transmitted diseases, including HIV, the new recommendation also suggested all donor sperm be frozen (called cryopreserved semen) and stored for three months before being offered for insemination, thus allowing for retesting for HIV infection.

In 1990, that quarantine period was extended to 180 days, with an additional recommendation not only to retest the sperm before releasing it for insemination, but also to retest the donor. Although there are no federal laws regulating the operation of sperm banks, the use of frozen sperm as opposed to fresh has been endorsed by not only the American Society for Reproductive Medicine, but also the Centers for Disease Control and the Food and Drug Administration.

So, as long as your sperm bank adheres to this policy, you can feel fairly confident that the sperm you will be receiving is safe. Indeed, since these new recommendations have been issued, the National Centers for Disease Control have not received a single report of HIV transmission via sperm bank donation.

Protecting the Family Jewels

For the most part, sperm banks routinely rely on a patient's medical and family history to determine which, if any, genetic tests are required before declaring the sperm healthy enough for donor insemination. But does this data really offer a true picture of what your child's future medical history might be? At least one group of researchers believe it may not.

Indeed, studies conducted at the Genetics and IVF Institute in Fairfax, Virginia, revealed a number of serious genetic-related diseases, including several types of cancer, may be silently passed from one generation to the next and activated when certain environmental or biological conditions come into play.

As such, your donor may have no obvious signs that more in-depth genetic testing is necessary in order to fully ensure your child's future health. The answer, say the experts, lies in the need for greater, more detailed genetic screening for all sperm donors, particularly for these otherwise "silent" disorders. In the meantime, you can talk to your sperm bank about the level of testing it *does* use to screen donors, and when possible, request that thorough testing be done, particularly for any of the same genetic flaws that may be present in your family history. This step can help protect not only your child, but your child's children as well.

In addition, the American Association of Tissue Banks (AATB) hopes to further ensure insemination standards by providing an additional set of guidelines for the collection, storage, and tracking of donor sperm and offering a special accreditation to those sperm banks that meet the requirements.

To be accredited a sperm bank must open its doors to on-site inspections for compliance with all of AATB's regulations, including not only quality control and donor selection criteria but also patient histories, safety of operation, even recordkeeping. If the sperm bank is accepted by AATB, the accreditation holds for just three short years, after which time the entire inspection and application process must be repeated. To check whether your sperm bank is accredited with AATB, write them at the American Association of Tissue Banks, 1350 Beverly Rd., Suite 220A, McLean, VA, 22011, or call them at 703-827-9585.

Making the Final Choice

While most sperm banks do their best to adhere to rigid health guidelines, when it comes to other specifics—including how much information they will provide about your donor—there can be a wide margin of difference from bank to bank.

The information they provide can be as limited as routine physical characteristics and basic health history, or as in-depth as personality and character portraits that include IQ, education, occupation, hobbies, talents, family and ethnic background, religion, and marital status. It's entirely up to you to decide how much you want or need to know about your donor.

Additionally, some sperm banks have regulations regarding how much information they will release about the donor to your child once he or she turns eighteen years of age. Currently, at least one California laboratory confirms that on request, it will release the name, driver's license, Social Security number, and last known address of the donor/father. Soon, more sperm banks may follow suit, so if this is an important aspect of your decision-making policy, be certain to get the bank's protocols concerning this issue in writing before deciding to use their sperm.

Finally, you should also talk to your sperm bank concerning the number of times a man may be a donor. Although the industry standard recommendation is to father no more than five children in a single state, and no more than five additional children out of state, these are only guidelines. And since there is currently no federal registry of sperm donors in the United States, there is no way of tracking or enforcing any type of limitations on sperm donation. If this is important to you, again, get the policy in writing.

Friend or Foe: When the Donor Is Someone You Know

If, regardless of the safety standards, you still don't feel comfortable using anonymous donor sperm, you may want to consider a friend or relative. This is also an option if you insist on fresh rather than frozen sperm, since the only time the freezing guidelines are waived is when the donor is a personal friend or non–blood relative of the mother (such as a brother-in-law or the husband's cousin), or in some instances a very distant cousin of the mother herself.

As with anonymous sperm, however, you should also be concerned with the general and the reproductive health of any donor you choose.

Unfortunately, this isn't always as easy to verify as you might think. Some surprising studies have shown that sometimes those who are closest to us may not be as forthcoming about their lives as we would like to believe, particularly in regard to sexual behavior. This is why many fertility experts still encourage adhering to the freezing/testing standards, even if the donor is a friend.

Fresh Versus Frozen: Which Is Best?

If you're thinking that, much like fruits and vegetables, fresh sperm is always better than frozen, this is not necessarily the case. Although it may take a bit longer to get pregnant using frozen sperm (between eight and twelve cycles, as compared to five to seven cycles for fresh sperm), the overall conception rate is pretty much the same. There is, however, one precaution worth noting: A retrospective study conducted at Queens University in Kingston, Ontario, Canada, revealed women who conceived via IUI (intrauterine insemination) using donor sperm were significantly more likely to experience preeclampsia (a dangerous form of high blood pressure occurring during pregnancy) than women who used their partner's sperm. Researchers theorize the reason may have to do with the fact that your body has no "biological familiarity" with the donor sperm, as it has with that of your partner. As such, your body may actually "reject" the donor's sperm, with a kind of immunological response that ultimately causes the preeclampsia. This theory is further supported by studies that show the risk of preeclampsia is greater among couples who get pregnant after long-term use of condoms, as well as those who conceive after a short-term sexual relationships—both situations are indicative of a lack of biological familiarity.

Consider Your Partner and Your Child

Additionally, you might also want to think about the psychological impact of choosing a donor who is already a part of your life. Questions to consider include whether you plan on telling your child how he or she was conceived, if you would reveal the identity of the biological father, and perhaps most important, whether your donor will go along with your plans, regardless of what you decide.

Also important to consider: How your partner will feel about having your sperm donor remain an active part of your lives. Discussing all these issues before making a donor choice can help keep many problems from occurring in your new family life.

Single Mothers and Donor Sperm: A Pregnancy Option

While the majority of women who conceive via insemination do so to overcome specific fertility problems, the procedure also opens the door for another pregnancy option: single motherhood.

If your doctor refuses to inseminate you because you are single, seek another physician. Your candidacy for insemination should be based solely on your ability to conceive, deliver, and care for a healthy baby. Do not allow any physician or fertility center to judge your right to be a mother.

A Final Word About Insemination

No longer looked upon as a treatment strictly for male inadequacy, artificial insemination is viewed by today's couples as a joint effort to create a perfect and healthy baby, regardless of which partner is the focus of that treatment.

Remember too that artificial insemination is not artificial at all. Your conception and your pregnancy is natural, and your baby will be as normal as any other.

Chapter Twenty-One

The A.R.T. of Conception:

The New In Vitro Fertilization and How It Can Help You Conceive

In 1978 an Englishwoman named Lucy Brown gave birth to a baby who forever changed the way we look at conception. The reason? Lucy's child, a daughter she named Louise, was the world's first "test-tube" baby—the only child ever conceived via what was then a revolutionary procedure developed by doctors Robert Edward and Patrick Steptoe. It was called in vitro fertilization (IVF) and Louise's birth was one of the most outstanding medical accomplishments of the century—one that revolutionized reproductive medicine for all time.

Perhaps most important: Lucy Brown and her blond, blue-eyed baby, Louise (now a healthy, grown woman), became the symbol of hope for millions of infertile couples for generations to come. I hope you will view them as your new symbol of hope as well as we begin your personal journey of exploration through not only the newest forms of IVF, but also some of the most advanced and exciting new ways science has developed to help you get pregnant.

The A.R.T. of Conception

Although there are now a plethora of new and exciting fertility enhancing treatments available, all are categorized under a single umbrella heading of A.R.T.—short for assisted reproductive technologies. While each procedure is slightly different (and you'll read more about each of them in the chapters that follow), all stem from that basic IVF process first developed in 1978.

And while it is more than two decades old, impressive advances in nearly all phases of today's IVF have allowed it to remain a major player in the high-stakes game of scientific conception. With improvements in both the success rate and the ease with which IVF can now be performed, it is often the first procedure of choice when a couple cannot conceive.

How In Vitro Fertilization Works

As complex as IVF can seem, the concept behind it is really quite simple. It allows for fertilization to take place outside your body, in a carefully controlled laboratory environment developed to encourage conception. By extracting your eggs and your partner's sperm and placing them together in a glass dish, science helps nature take its natural course—and fertilization usually occurs.

Viewing the laboratory dish as a kind of "glass fallopian tube," the sperm penetrates your egg and the conceptus begins to divide, much the same way it would if conception took place in your body. When the resulting embryo reaches a certain size, it is transferred into your uterus, where it implants and begins to grow. The remainder of your pregnancy progresses naturally, as if conception *had* occurred via sexual intercourse.

Can IVF Help You?

One of the chief advantages of IVF is that it allows conception without the fallopian tubes. Normally, your tubes are the passageway through which your eggs travel and eventually meet sperm. It is also where the initial uniting of sperm and egg take place. So, if tubes were damaged, pregnancy was nearly impossible. The IVF procedure, however, bypasses the tubes, making pregnancy not only possible but highly successful. So, if you do have tubal damage, you are a prime candidate for IVF.

Research has shown IVF can also help you overcome a variety of reproductive problems, including:

- Male factor infertility
- Unexplained infertility
- Cervical or uterine damage, especially that caused by exposure to DES
- Antisperm antibodies
- Annovulation (lack of ovulation)
- Advancing maternal age

While it may not be the first line of defense for all these problems, when other treatments, including insemination, fail to help, IVF often succeeds.

Preparing Your Body for IVF

The more eggs a woman has available for fertilization, and the healthier those eggs are, the more likely she is to get pregnant. Thus, the use of fertility medications designed to encourage egg growth are a part of the IVF process. The concept is called "super ovulation" (see Chapter 19), and most women undergoing IVF are treated with at least one cycle of these drugs.

There are, in fact, a variety of medications and dosing regimens available to be used during the IVF procedure, and each doctor or clinic has particular favorites.

However, in my experience, most women can develop the most eggs of the highest quality by using the following regimen:

- Lupron injections administered approximately a week before menstruation and followed with a lower dose after bleeding begins
- Follicle-stimulating drugs, such as Follistim or Gonal-F, administered from the beginning of the cycle (continued until two days before egg retrieval), often in combination with some amount of the fertility drugs Humegon, Pergonal, or Repronex

In certain instances—if your egg production remains poor—the fertility medication Clomid may be added to the next cycle.

You will also need at least one medication designed to mature the eggs and trigger ovulation, usually hCG (human chorionic gonadotropin), which works like the natural hormone LH to help ready eggs for release.

In addition, because the dosages needed to make multiple eggs is generally higher than what is needed to simply induce the development of a single healthy egg, both you and your doctor must be extremely vigilant about preventing hyperstimulation—the condition involving overproduction of eggs that is fully explained in Chapter 19. If, in fact, hyperstimulation seems inevitable, all fertility medication must be stopped and your IVF cycle canceled. You will, however, be free to try again right after the start of your next menstrual cycle.

Assuming, however, that no hyperstimulation problems occur, between the twelfth and fourteenth days, your eggs will be mature and ready for retrieval. Instead of allowing your eggs to pass from your ovary on their own, however, they will be aspirated and removed by your doctor.

Your Egg Retrieval: Some Special Advice

When IVF was first developed, the primary methods of retrieving eggs were either via a sonogram-guided needle inserted into the abdomen or laparoscopy, minor surgery that involved making a small incision through your navel. And in some instances, these methods are still used, particularly if your ovaries are located high in the pelvic cavity or if your eggs are difficult to locate. Sometimes, if a woman has had previous surgery, such as a myomectomy to remove fibroid tumors, her ovaries may have been repositioned in such a way as to demand egg retrieval be done in this manner.

For most women undergoing IVF today, however, eggs are retrieved via a transvaginal, ultrasonic guided needle aspiration (see illustration, page 463). Here your doctor will gently insert the long, thin ultrasound wand into your vagina and lightly press it against your ovaries. Visualizing the entire inside of your ovary (displayed on a computer screen) he

Baby Aspirin and IVF

To help ensure not only your egg-making potential but also your IVF pregnancy, talk to your doctor about taking low doses of aspirin (baby aspirin is a good choice) in the weeks before your procedure. New studies show that IVF patients who took 100 mg of aspirin daily along with egg-stimulating drugs produced twice as many eggs and were 50 percent more likely to get pregnant than those women who took no aspirin. Researchers aren't certain why. Earlier studies have shown baby aspirin may reduce the risk of miscarriage by helping to prevent blood clots in the vessels that transport nutrients from the mother's body to the developing baby.

or she will insert a thin, double-barreled needle into each separate follicle—one barrel used to provide a liquid that flushes the follicles, the second used to aspirate the fluid that contains your eggs.

That fluid is then deposited in a sterile container that is quickly passed to the embryologist—the IVF team member who is an egg specialist. He or she examines the fluid and isolates and then "grades" each egg for growth and maturity status. (Under a microscope, fully matured eggs resemble a sunburst or a newly blossoming flower!) While normally only the ripe eggs ready for fertilization are considered for combination with sperm, sometimes otherwise healthy but immature eggs are given a second chance to grow by being placed in a special culturing solution for twelve to twenty-four hours to enhance maturation. This can be particularly helpful if your egg harvest is less than plentiful.

The entire egg retrieval process normally takes between twenty and forty minutes, although occasionally, if eggs are difficult to locate, it can require up to sixty minutes. Because the procedure causes some discomfort, your doctor will likely give you a light, fast-acting anesthetic, or at the very least, a pain medication in combination with a drug to calm and relax you. Afterward, you spend one to two hours in the recovery room, and then you are free to return home and resume most of your normal activities.

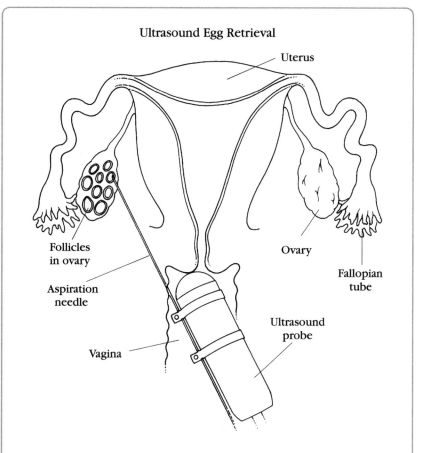

Ultrasound Egg Retrieval

Uterus

Follicles in ovary

Ovary

Aspiration needle

Fallopian tube

Vagina

Ultrasound probe

The Ultrasound Egg Retrieval

In order to retrieve eggs from inside your ovary, your doctor will often use an ultrasound probe. Here, a thin needle is attached to the traditional ultrasound vaginal wand. The images from the wand are relayed onto a computer screen, which your doctor then uses to guide the needle to your ovary, puncture the follicle, and gently suck out the eggs one at a time.

Illustration courtesy of the American Society of Reproductive Medicine

Timing Is Everything

Even though, technically, aspirating your follicles means you will not be ovulating the eggs that develop within your ovary, still, you will need to take an ovulation drug (human chorionic gonadotropin—hCG) to mature your eggs just before removal.

The reason? The normal ovulation process includes a very vital step called "meiosis." This is a natural reduction of chromosomes within the egg that is necessary for fertilization to take place. The ovulation drugs help your eggs go through this vital process so that when they are aspirated and retrieved they will be healthy and ready to be fertilized.

Additionally, in order for your IVF fertilization to succeed, your eggs must be aspirated approximately thirty-four to thirty-six hours after you take your egg-maturing medication (hCG). The actual IVF fertilization (the combining of your partner's sperm with your egg in a Petrie dish) then takes place in a laboratory, usually within several hours, according to egg and sperm quality.

I cannot emphasize enough the important role that the exquisite timing of these steps, particularly the injection of the egg-maturing drug hCG, plays in the success of your IVF treatment.

Preparing Your Partner for IVF

On the day of your egg retrieval, your partner usually gives his sperm sample. As in artificial insemination, he can do this by masturbating at home or at the fertility center or doctor's office. Sperm can also be collected via sexual intercourse, at home, using a specially prepared sterile condom (see Chapter 20).

Because your partner's sperm will not be traveling through your cervical mucus as it would if you conceived naturally, as in insemination, sperm washing becomes necessary.

Your doctor may also put sperm through a second procedure called the "swim up." Here, the already washed sperm is placed into a test tube containing a special culture medium, and then into an incubator set at body temperature, for up to two hours. During this time, the healthiest, most motile sperm swim up to the top of the container—hence the name.

Although a successful IVF pregnancy has been achieved with sperm counts as low as one million per milliliter, the more healthy sperm available, the greater the chances for conception.

Making Your Baby: The Next Step

Having chosen the best and highest-quality eggs from those retrieved, the embryologist places them into an incubator, where they remain for several hours. This helps simulate the natural climate in which your ovulated eggs would reside if they were waiting inside your fallopian tube for sperm to arrive.

After the incubation period, the following steps take place:

1. If sperm count is high, the eggs are individually placed in shallow glass dishes and a portion of sperm is added to each one. The ratio ranges from fifty thousand to 1 million sperm per egg.

2. If sperm count is low, the eggs are placed together in one dish and all the sperm is added to a single container, or the embryologist might prefer to perform a second procedure known as ICSI (intracytoplasmic sperm injection), which you will read more about in the next chapter.

3. After sperm and egg are combined, they are placed in an incubator where the fertilization process occurs. It is estimated that 80 percent of all mature eggs become fertilized during IVF. If more than one sperm penetrates an egg (a situation called polyspermy), an abnormal embryo results, which would not survive. Since your doctor can easily diagnose this problem, these embryos are not transferred into your uterus.

4. Within twenty-four hours after fertilization, your egg becomes a two-celled embryo. Within forty-eight hours four cells result, and within sixty hours eight cells. In the past, we often transferred the embryos into the uterus in about forty-eight hours, and under certain conditions it might be necessary to do this today as well. However, for most women,

Sperm Penetrating Egg During Fertilization

Sperm head

Tail

Sperm

Zona pellucida

Polar body

Cytoplasm

Egg membrane

Granulosa cells

Sperm Penetrates Egg and Fertilization Occurs

After intercourse occurs, many sperm begin swimming furiously toward the fallopian tube, where they anticipate finding an egg. Special enzymes in the head of the sperm help in penetrating the zona pellucida, the egg's hard outer shell. Although many sperm try to get in, normally only one succeeds. And as soon as it does, the other sperm automatically stop trying. During in vitro fertilization, essentially the same thing occurs, only this time it all happens in a shallow Petrie dish: Sperm are placed right next to the egg, and the process of gaining entry begins. When the sperm reaches the nucleus or center of the egg, they fuse together, and conception is said to occur.

Love, Italian Style!

Traditionally, the initial fertilization step—the combining of sperm and egg in an incubator—took place over a twelve- to eighteen-hour period. Indeed, research seemed to indicate that it would take this long for sperm and egg to commingle and for conception to occur. Now, however, a group of Italian researchers have given a new meaning to the words "chemical attraction." Their research shows it may, in fact, take only moments for sperm and egg to connect, and that the less time they spend in the incubator after fertilization, the more likely a pregnancy will occur. The reason, say the scientists, is that when they are left to incubate for long periods, waste products are produced that ultimately affect the embryo. And while the long and short incubation periods appear to yield about the same fertilization rates, the short incubations seem to produce a healthier embryo, one that is more likely to implant and grow. This, in turn, translates into a higher pregnancy rate overall. If after several IVF attempts you are not pregnant, and no reason can be found, you might want to mention this new Italian-style conception to your doctor.

the embryos will be allowed to mature a full seventy-two hours before the transfer takes place. In some instances, embryo transfer may be done five days after retrieval, in a procedure known as blastocyst transfer, which is explained more fully later in this chapter.

When Science Plays Mother Hen: Assisted Hatching

When you conceive naturally, your newly fertilized egg remains inside your fallopian tube for about six days. As it slowly travels the length of the tube it continues to divide but still remains cloistered within the zona pellucida, the hard outer covering or "shell" of your original egg. As it approaches your uterus—usually on the sixth day—a kind of "hatching" action takes place. The hardened shell begins to thin, thus making it eas-

For Your Eggs Only

A brand-new technique for helping eggs hatch involves the eximer laser—the same equipment used for radial keratotomy, the operation that corrects nearsightedness. Pioneered at Hadassah University Hospital in Jerusalem, the laser is used to drill a small hole in the shell of the egg, producing an opening with a specific size that has been shown to encourage the hatching process.

Unlike chemicals, which can damage the egg, and other lasers, which may produce a harmful charring effect, the eximer reportedly yields a cleaner hole with little or no risk to the embryo. So far, a baby girl and a baby boy have been delivered to two separate mothers as a result of the laser-assisted hatching. In both cases the women had undergone seven or more unsuccessful IVF attempts before conceiving with this new method.

ier for the embryo to attach to the lining of your uterus and start to implant, something that usually begins on the seventh day after conception.

When, however, your baby has been created outside your body—in a laboratory Petrie dish—this "hatching" process may not occur as completely as it should. And that can make implantation difficult or impossible. It may also be the reason past IVF attempts have failed to produce a pregnancy. Indeed, some researchers believe that when an IVF pregnancy fails to thrive—particularly in women under age thirty-six—the main reason is that the shell does not thin enough for a strong and healthy implantation.

The good news is that science can become your "mother hen" via a procedure known as "assisted hatching" (AH). Here, either a minute amount of dissolving fluid (similar to digestive acids) or ultrathin microsurgical instruments are used to manually thin the shell of your egg before implantation.

While this has been shown to increase pregnancy success, there is a slight risk of damage to your embryo. This is why it's vitally important that your fertility team have experience in the egg-hatching procedure and know how to avoid such problems. In addition, there is some discussion about whether assisted hatching is helpful for women over age thirty-six (see Chapter 24), so be sure to discuss all aspects of this procedure with your doctor.

Giving Your Baby Back to You: The Embryo Transfer

In the very last stage of your IVF procedure, your doctor places your fertilized egg (the embryo) in your body.

Initially, you will be asked to drink water to fill your bladder, then you will lie on your back with your legs in the traditional stirrup position. Your doctor will then perform an abdominal sonogram to locate your uterus and help find the best area to deposit your fertilized embryos.

The actual transfer is then done via a thin plastic tube that is inserted into your vagina and gently eased up through your cervix and into your uterus (see illustration, page 470). A thin catheter containing all the embryos is then inserted into the tube. A syringe attached to the outside of the catheter is gently depressed, then, using the sonogram as a guide, your embryos are gently injected through the tube and into the proper place inside your uterus. I cannot emphasize enough the need for this procedure to be done slowly and gently. Indeed, if injected with full force, they can rush from the catheter and hit your uterine wall at speeds up to six hundred miles per hour—a situation not conducive to implantation. The goal, rather, is to gently nudge the embryos into your uterus so they stick to the surface and begin to implant and start to grow.

Confirming Your Pregnancy: A Cause for Celebration!

While the excitement surrounding your IVF may indeed cause you to "feel" pregnant as soon as your embryos are transferred, it actually takes

In Vitro Fertilization

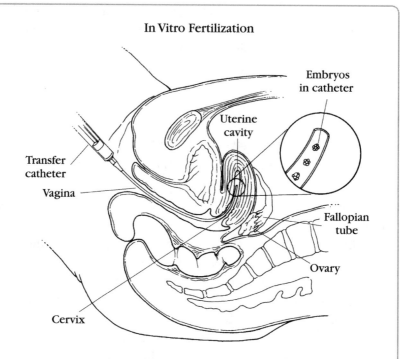

Embryos
in catheter

Uterine
cavity

Transfer
catheter

Vagina

Fallopian
tube

Ovary

Cervix

In Vitro Fertilization: The Embryo Transfer Procedure

After your partner's sperm has fertilized your egg, the resulting embryos are loaded into a slim, flexible catheter attached to a syringe. The catheter is gently threaded through your vagina, up into your cervix, and to your uterus. Once in the proper place, the syringe is lightly depressed, releasing the embryos, where, one hopes, they will adhere to the uterine lining and begin to grow.

about two weeks before a pregnancy can be confirmed. Many of my patients have confided that this waiting period is the most difficult phase of their IVF. It is during this time that most fertility experts begin to truly appreciate the fact that for all our scientific advances, the success of our efforts is still governed by Mother Nature. I know this is the way my in vitro team and I feel after every IVF procedure.

At the end of the two-week wait, however, you will be given your first pregnancy test. If the result is positive, one to two weeks later you will be given a blood test (quantitative hCG), followed by a sonogram to identify how many babies you are carrying (the average IVF pregnancy is twins) and to confirm the strength of your babies' heartbeats—usually seen four weeks after embryo transfer. Your pregnancy should then continue in a "normal" manner, as if you had conceived naturally.

Improving Your Pregnancy Rate: The Newest Technologies

One of the most exciting improvements on basic IVF came in late 1998, when a group of scientists found a new way to extend the life of an embryo outside the body. Normally, a fertilized egg could survive no more than two or three days before it had to be transferred back into the uterus. Because this was up to three days sooner than if fertilization took place naturally inside the fallopian tube, often the IVF embryos had not reached optimum maturity (called the "blastocyst" stage) when the transfer took place. And that naturally decreased the chance for implantation.

The only way to compensate was to transfer numerous embryos, which, of course, naturally increased the risk of multiple birth.

Now, however, there is a new alternative. The development of a new type of amino acid–based culture fluid is allowing embryos to survive in the laboratory longer than ever before—up to five days, or until they reach that important "blastocyst" stage. And that means your doctor can transfer an older, more mature embryo to your uterus, thus increasing your chance for a successful IVF pregnancy. Ultimately, this means fewer embryos are needed to ensure a pregnancy, so your chance for a multiple birth is decreased.

In addition, research shows that by using this new method, the overall IVF pregnancy rate can be as high as 60 percent. For example, studies conducted at Monas University in Australia, one center that pioneered the "blastocyst transfer," found the new procedure enabled women to get pregnant even after ten or more previous IVF procedures had failed.

How Many Embryos Does It Take to Make a Baby?

Sound like a trick question? It is—sort of. Of course, regardless of how conception occurs, a single embryo is all that's needed to develop a baby. However, because not every embryo that is transferred into your uterus will implant and grow, to increase the chance of pregnancy, multiple embryos must be transferred during each IVF attempt. But is more necessarily always better?

Another "trick" question. The answer: Yes, but only to a point.

First, the more embryos transplanted, the greater your chance for a multiple birth. In fact, the only reason fertility treatments are associated with such a high degree of multiples is that it's necessary to transfer more than one embryo in order to help ensure that conception does occur. However, depending on how many babies result from the transfer, their health, as well as the health of the mother, may be compromised, particularly if she is not under the care of an obstetrician who specializes in high-risk, multiple births.

So, how many embryos should your doctor transfer with each IVF attempt? Currently, the November 1999 guidelines set by the American Society of Reproductive Medicine are as follows:

- For women with optimum prognosis for conception—usually those under age thirty-five—two good quality embryos
- For women with above-average chance of conception—three embryos
- For women with average chance of conceiving—usually aged thirty-five to forty—four embryos
- For women with a low chance of conceiving—aged forty or over, or with multiple failed cycles—five embryos

A number of studies, including a 1998 report published in the *New England Journal of Medicine,* reveal that transferring four embryos into your uterus may not increase your chances for conception over what they would be if you received only two embryos—thereby eliminating the risk of conceiving three, four, or more babies.

If past IVF attempts were unsuccessful, or you feel strongly about limiting the number of babies you conceive, talk to your fertility expert about whether this new technique could help you. However, I must caution you that waiting for the blastocyst stage to develop is not always advisable for all women, particularly those over age forty. The reason: Sometimes several embryos will die in the process, because they are simply not strong enough to survive the five-day wait in the laboratory. Since women over forty may have a limited supply of eggs, they cannot risk losing even a single embryo before implantation.

The Natural Cycle: An (Almost) Drug-Free IVF

There is no question that, from a patient standpoint, one of the most complex parts of an IVF procedure involves super ovulation—the use of fertility drugs to increase egg production. Not only can the drugs be expensive, sometimes costing thousands of dollars per cycle, but in some women they can cause a number of unwanted side effects that can make the entire conception process more uncomfortable than it has to be.

And while fertility drugs do increase the chance for a successful IVF—the more healthy eggs you have, the more likely it is for fertilization to take place—still, doctors have been working long and hard to find ways to eliminate or reduce the use of these medications without sacrificing pregnancy success rates. Now, it appears, that time may soon come.

A new method of performing the egg retrieval process of basic IVF appears to eliminate the need for at least two types of fertility preparations: egg-stimulating medications and ovulation-induction drugs. The technique, developed by fertility expert Dr. Jeffrey Russel and colleagues at the Reproductive Endocrine and Fertility Center of Delaware, is called "immature oocyte retrieval." Essentially, it involves the use of transvaginal ultra techniques to locate and remove unstimulated, still immature egg follicles, then allowing them to mature outside the body, in laboratory dishes, until they are ready for conception.

The key to making it all work, experts say, is proper timing—

removing your follicles and allowing them to mature within the same time frame that your uterus is building the spongy nest ready for implantation. So far, the process goes something like this:

1. On day two or three of your menstrual cycle, a transvaginal ultrasound helps determine your number of follicles available for retrieval.

2. A second ultrasound—performed anytime between days five, six, and seven, helps assess uterine lining. At this time you will also receive small doses of estrogen, equal to that which your body would normally produce if your eggs were allowed to develop on their own. This will help the lining of your uterus develop.

3. Depending on the length of your cycle, your egg follicles—from five to fifteen in number—will be retrieved somewhere between days seven and fourteen.

4. After retrieval, your follicles will be transferred to the in vitro lab, where they will be left to mature for thirty-six to forty-eight hours. As maturity is reached, and the follicles become eggs, they will be combined with your partner's sperm.

5. Once your embryos have formed, they will be transferred into your uterus using the same techniques as the basic IVF process.

Although a drug-free IVF procedure may yield a slightly lower rate of conception than when fertility medications are used, there are some advantages as well. First, eliminating the drugs can cut the overall cost of a procedure by 50 percent or more, which for some couples is a very important consideration. Additionally, a drug-free IVF means you can escape not only the unpleasant side effects that can occur while you are taking certain fertility drugs, but also the negative consequences that some believe may result years after these medications have been used.

However, I must caution you that this technique is still considered experimental, so success rates have not been verified. And while I believe that, ultimately, this procedure will be an acceptable option, it may not be right for every woman undergoing IVF, particularly those over age thirty-eight.

Will Your IVF Be Successful? How to Tell Before You Try!

Whether or not fertility drugs are used, there is no question that IVF is both costly and time-consuming. This is particularly true when more than one procedure must take place before a pregnancy results.

For this reason, I believe it's always best to know as early as possible if, in fact, your IVF has a significant chance of succeeding. Fortunately, science is here to help. As reproductive technologies continue to develop, so too have a number of tests that can help us narrow down the number of couples who may need to move past standard IVF to more sophisticated fertility treatments. What follows is some of the more successful diagnostics that can help you and your partner, together with your doctor, determine which fertility procedure is right for you.

The Tests That Can Help

Clomiphene challenge test: As you previously read, FSH (follicle-stimulating hormone) helps eggs develop and grow. When this test begins, your doctor will measure your level of FSH on day three of your cycle. You will then receive 100 mg of the fertility drug clomiphene citrate on days five through nine of your cycle. On day ten, your blood will again be measured for FSH. By comparing levels from day three to levels on day ten, your doctor can determine, to some degree, your fertility status. If hormones levels are abnormally high on day three *and* day ten, conception using any method may be exceptionally difficult. Pregnancy is not impossible, but you are considered to be at very high risk for infertility—meaning both you and your doctor must take every possible precaution to ensure your procedures are successful. Giving up smoking, for example, may help, since smokers tend to have abnormally high FSH levels at an early age. Conversely, when FSH levels register low on days three and ten, the likelihood of pregnancy is great. Likely, an IVF attempt will be successful.

The reason the test is thought to be a good predictor of fertility is that egg quality generally declines just before FSH begins to rise. If levels are already high, then it's likely egg quality is such that fertilization may be extremely difficult.

While different laboratories can yield different and confusing FSH test results, generally speaking, as levels begin to exceed 20–25 IU/L (international units per liter), pregnancy rates begin to diminish. As rates climb above 25 IU/L, chances for conception continue to diminish.

The estrogen test: Along the same lines as the clomiphene challenge test comes the estradiol day three reading. Here, high levels of this form of estrogen on day three of a menstrual cycle generally mean a perimenopausal condition exists, so a pregnancy may be difficult to achieve. The estrogen level that seems to indicate the breaking point is 80 pg/mL (picograms per milliliter).

Color Doppler and pregnancy success: This special type of ultrasound exam tracks blood flow patterns—and according to researchers at McGill University in Montreal, Canada, this can help determine if you have the ability to get pregnant. Indeed, according to their research, certain blood flow patterns within the uterus are associated with higher rates of pregnancy, while others are indicative of problems conceiving. What's really important here, however, is that blood flow patterns can improve within a day or two. So should your test indicate problems in this area, your ovulation injection can be withheld for twenty-four to forty-eight hours, thus giving your uterus more time to prepare. And this, in turn, may help improve your pregnancy odds.

Additional studies are also looking at the possibility that small doses of nitroglycerin—the same drug used to stimulate the heart—may stimulate the beneficial blood flow pattern to the uterus.

In addition, the Canadian researchers believe that by observing Doppler blood patterns to the ovaries, it's possible to determine the optimal amount of fertility drugs necessary to stimulate ovulation.

The new fertility ultrasound: Putting a slightly different spin on the uterine blood flow test, Chicago radiologist Dr. Michael Applebaum has developed a way to predict embryo death before implantation takes place. Using a new type of ultrasound procedure, the test evaluates blood flow to the lining of the uterus, which must reach a certain level in order to keep embryos alive. If that flow is inadequate, the embryo will not survive. By having this information before implantation, doctors can help patients avoid an unsuccessful IVF and freeze and preserve the embryos for transplant during another cycle, when uterine blood flow patterns improve.

Ovarian response testing: If your ovaries respond to egg-making medications, then your IVF is likely to be successful, regardless of your age. According to a large-scale study conducted in the Netherlands and reported in the journal *Fertility and Sterility,* women who developed three or more follicles using egg-stimulating medications were far more likely to conceive than those who developed fewer follicles, particularly when the size was also small. While the number of available eggs and the rate of successful implantation does appear to decrease as a woman ages, the pregnancy rate does not significantly drop after age forty in those women who respond well to the egg-stimulation medications.

Using ultrasound exams to test ovary response after the first failed IVF attempt may help determine whether more aggressive treatment is needed for subsequent tries at pregnancy.

Ensuring the Health of Your IVF Baby

Among the most heartbreaking of all IVF experiences is when the child you worked so hard to conceive is born with genetic abnormalities— sometimes so severe the baby cannot survive. While the risk of birth defects in IVF babies is no higher than in children who are conceived naturally, still, the efforts involved in pregnancy can be so great that the problem can hit with even greater impact and sorrow.

Fortunately, a new system of preimplantation genetic diagnosis (PGD) may help spare parents this tragedy. Essentially it is used to identify the presence of certain genetic abnormalities in an embryo long before implantation takes place. Indeed, three days after fertilization is confirmed, it's possible to remove one or two cells from an eight- or ten-celled embryo without disturbing further development.

Then, by performing certain genetic tests on those two cells, doctors can rule out the diagnosis of some serious genetic abnormalities. So far, they are able to identify embryos that are affected by cystic fibrosis (CF), Tay-Sachs disease, Lesch Nyham syndrome, Duchenne muscular dystrophy, a-l-antitrypsin deficiency, Fragile X syndrome, Charcot-Marie-Tooth disease, Down's syndrome, hemophilia A, retinitis pigmentosa, and Turner's syndrome.

Most recently, Dr. Kangpu Xu of the Weill Medical College of Cornell University in New York City became the first researcher to successfully use PGD to help a couple who were both carriers of sickle cell anemia to give birth to a child who is disease-free. Reporting in the *Journal of the American Medical Association,* Dr. Xu writes that out of the seven embryos that were conceived in the laboratory, PGD indicated that four were normal, two were carriers, and diagnosis on one was not possible. Three of the normal embryos were then implanted in the mother's uterus, and thirty-nine weeks later she gave birth to healthy twins.

Unfortunately, PGD is very expensive, and currently most insurance companies do not cover the costs. Thus, today it is often limited to couples of which one or both parents are at very high risk for transmitting certain genetic abnormalities.

In the future, however, PGD may become the standard way of increasing the success of all IVF pregnancies, since it can selectively filter out those embryos that may be genetically too weak to survive.

In what is still considered a highly experimental version of this new technology, doctors flush a naturally conceived embryo from a woman's uterus and test it. If it proves healthy, standard IVF transfer techniques are used to place it back in the patient's body. If the method proves worthy, doctors may one day be able to dramatically reduce the number of babies born with genetic abnormalities long before any significant fetal development begins.

Improving the Odds of Your IVF: What You Can Do

Although much of your IVF success is predetermined by the quantity and quality of your eggs and your partner's sperm, there are also a number of things that you can do to help improve your odds for a successful IVF pregnancy.

Pay Strict Attention to Prenatal Nutrition

As mentioned in Part Two of this book, I am a strong believer in the power of vitamin supplements and prenatal nutrition to help all women get pregnant, particularly those undergoing laboratory procedures. I advise that you begin taking one to two prenatal vitamins daily (including extra folic acid) before you plan to conceive and follow a balanced diet with adequate caloric intake during this prenatal time as well. (The fertility diet featured earlier in this book is a good place to start.)

Talk to Your Doctor About Progesterone Supplements

Taking natural progesterone supplements, beginning just after your embryo transfer, and continuing for several weeks into your pregnancy can also be a big help. How? Studies show it may increase the health of your uterine lining and offer your baby proper nourishment right from the very start of your pregnancy.

You should also ask your doctor about the possibility of taking 333 mg of the antibiotic erythromycin twice daily for several days after your egg retrieval. Studies show it may help minimize the threat of infection that could later interfere with your implantation.

Get Adequate Bed Rest

Following the final step of your IVF procedure, when your embryos are transferred into your uterus, you should remain in bed in the recovery room for at least two hours. Upon returning home, you should go right to bed and remain there for up to seventy-two hours. While some IVF programs advocate resuming normal activities after just two or three hours, I believe that this extra rest, in a nonstressful environment, gives your conception an extra measure of security. This is especially vital if you have miscarried in the past.

Do Not Smoke — and Avoid Secondhand Smoke

Important studies from Sheba Medical Center in Tel Hashomer, Israel, have revealed that regular, daily cigarette smoking in almost any amount can adversely affect the success of IVF. The reason: Smoking decreases estrogen levels, which is important to follicular development. Additionally, nicotine in the bloodstream at the time when your eggs are developing can adversely affect the zona pellucida, the hard outside covering of your egg.

If you are contemplating IVF, give up smoking and, if possible, have your body free and clear of all traces of tobacco for at least three months before your procedure.

Limit Exercise

Because heavy exercise decreases blood flow to the uterus, which in turn can affect your pregnancy, it is vital that you limit this type of activity for at least the first three months of your IVF pregnancy. In addition, limit all exercise, even light workouts, for the first three weeks following your embryo transfer, extending that to eight weeks if you are prone to early miscarriage. While you don't have to lie in bed, it's important that your body is not physically overstressed or overheated during the first few important weeks of your IVF pregnancy.

A Final Word

According to the latest analysis, the success of laboratory-assisted conceptions is greater than perhaps anyone ever thought it could be: In the United States alone, nearly 25,000 babies have been conceived and delivered through 1997 as a result of advanced fertility techniques. Indeed, sooner or later, almost all couples who walk the road that technology has paved will realize their parenting dreams.

For some, that walk will be short and sweet, with pregnancy occurring on the first try.

For others, however, having a baby will be a longer, more arduous task. Indeed, as good as our technology is, it cannot perform miracles—and more important, it doesn't always yield a pregnancy on the first try. For many couples, two or even three IVF procedures are needed before a successful pregnancy occurs.

I know this can be difficult for many of you reading this book—particularly since these procedures are generally costly, and many states still refuse to force insurance companies to cover women for these treatments. I hope that will change in the near future, as the insurance industry comes to recognize that infertility is, indeed, a true medical disability.

In the meantime, however, remember that studies show your chances of IVF success do not diminish with each subsequent try. Each time you attempt an IVF procedure you have a fresh chance at becoming pregnant. And don't forget that the younger you are, the more successful your IVF can be—so don't wait too long before you seek treatment!

Chapter Twenty-Two

The GIFT of Life—and Other New Technologies

❧ Among the most fascinating advances in reproductive medicine are new treatments that combine both nature *and* science in a way that offers patients the advantages of both. Not surprisingly, these same techniques are rapidly proving to be the most successful in terms of achieving pregnancy.

In this chapter you will learn about three such groundbreaking treatments. The first procedure is called GIFT—gamete intra–fallopian tube transfer. And for the tens of thousands of infertile couples it has already helped conceive, it truly is a *gift of life*.

What Is the GIFT Procedure—and What Makes It Special?

In the most basic sense, getting pregnant with GIFT involves removing mature eggs from your ovaries and placing them, together with your partner's sperm, into your fallopian tube—in the precise place where fertilization is most likely to occur. While it draws on some of the same technology used in standard IVF, there is one important difference. Rather than combining sperm and egg in a laboratory, the GIFT fertilization is *all natural*—occurring inside your body.

This may be one reason why GIFT is so successful—in many instances far more likely to result in pregnancy that the basic IVF. According to the French scientist Dr. Yves Menezo (who invented the fluid in which all sperm and egg are pretreated in the laboratory), nutrients secreted inside the fallopian tube may play an important role in the fertilization process. Specifically, they can help nourish your baby from the start, leading to a healthier embryo—one far more likely to implant and grow.

But that's not the only reason GIFT can be more successful. When fertilization occurs inside your body, it allows your embryo to take the natural route to implantation—in just the precise amount of time (about five to six days) necessary to ensure your uterus is ready to accept implantation. This can be harder to duplicate with basic IVF, since the embryo-transfer (putting your fertilized egg back in your uterus) must often take place sooner than nature had in mind. And that can result in either an insufficiently prepared uterine lining or a weak or young embryo, not yet ready to implant. In either case, the chance for a successful pregnancy diminishes.

With GIFT, however, everything takes place on a "natural" timetable, and the rate of pregnancy success goes up.

How much more successful is GIFT than basic IVF? That depends on whom you ask. In the past, GIFT was believed to be more than twice as likely to result in pregnancy. Over the years, however, improvements in various aspects of basic IVF have helped increase the pregnancy rates of that procedure, so today, the gap is not as wide. In fact, some researchers contend that rates are so similar one procedure has no advantage over the other.

I, however, continue to believe that GIFT is far more successful, and the overall fertility statistics culled from reproductive centers around the nation indicate this is the case. Indeed, although many couples choose GIFT because the conception is considered natural, it can also be a way to achieve pregnancy when basic IVF has failed. I, personally, have seen GIFT help many patients who came to me after numerous IVFs failed to produce a pregnancy.

Can the GIFT Procedure Work for You?

The three main factors that determine whether GIFT will work for you are your ability to make good eggs, that you have at least one disease-free fallopian tube, and that your partner has healthy sperm.

If this *is* the case, GIFT can be the solution for many infertility problems, including:

- Unexplained infertility
- Male-factor infertility
- Endometriosis
- Cervical factor infertility
- Damaged fimbria (the fingerlike ends of your tubes)
- Lack of ovulation
- Antisperm antibodies
- Juxtaposed tube and ovary (one good tube, one good ovary on opposite sides of the body)

How the GIFT Procedure Helps You Get Pregnant

Like basic IVF, GIFT usually begins with the super ovulation fertility drug regimen featured in the previous chapter, followed by the same egg-monitoring steps. Your partner's sperm will also be pretreated with the washing and swim-up techniques featured in Chapters 20 and 21.

In addition, once your eggs are ripe and ready for fertilization, as in IVF, they must be retrieved. Once this takes place, however, the similarities between GIFT and IVF end.

The GIFT Conception

While eggs harvested for IVF are shuttled off to a Petrie dish to be combined with sperm and allowed to fertilize, in GIFT, eggs are outside your body just long enough for the embryologist to determine that they are healthy. If so, they will be placed on top of a droplet of sperm and loaded into an ultrathin catheter ready to be placed into your body. Using the same incision made to harvest your eggs, the tiny catheter is inserted into your pelvic cavity and guided into your fallopian tubes. The syringe is gently depressed, releasing both sperm and egg at the location where they would normally meet if sexual intercourse had taken place.

The GIFT Procedure

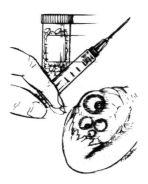

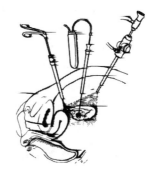

Step one: Fertility drugs, which can include both oral medications and injections, are used to help increase the production of healthier, more plentiful eggs, and ready the eggs for retrieval. (slide A)

Step two: Using an ultrasound vaginal probe, the eggs are located; then laparoscopic surgery is often performed to help the surgeon retrieve the eggs.

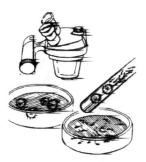

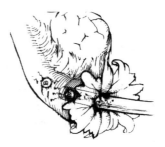

Step three: The retrieved eggs are mixed with sperm and placed into a culture medium for a short time.

Step four: The sperm/egg mixture is loaded into a catheter and then gently injected into the fallopian tube.

Illustration courtesy of the American Society for Reproductive Medicine

If you were able to make a sufficient number of eggs—from twelve to sixteen—the same procedure is then performed on your other fallopian tube, thus further increasing your chance for pregnancy. On average, between six and eight eggs should be placed into each tube to maximize the chance for fertilization.

Once the eggs and sperm are deposited, the catheter is gently removed, and one small stitch closes your abdominal incision. The entire procedure lasts from sixty to ninety minutes. The sperm and egg usually fertilize within hours, and this conception is considered *totally natural*.

Increasing Your Pregnancy Success Odds: The IVF/GIFT

In some women, even the most potent fertility medications will yield only a few eggs—just enough for a GIFT procedure in a single tube. For some, however, egg production is abundant, with far more follicles becoming ripe than what can be used in a single GIFT attempt. In fact, although the number of eggs put back into the body is often determined by a woman's age (the older she is, the more eggs are placed in the tube to increase the success rate of fertilization), generally, no more than eight or ten eggs are normally placed in a single tube.

When there are extra healthy eggs available, often doctors will combine them with the partner's sperm, in a laboratory dish, to see if fertilization can take place. This can then be used as a barometer to predict the success of your GIFT pregnancy. Sometimes, these testing embryos can be frozen to be used in a future IVF transfer. Sometimes they are immediately transferred into your uterus during the same cycle as your GIFT procedure. This is usually done within two to three days of your GIFT surgery, using the standard IVF embryo transfer technique (see Chapter 21).

Since it does not require any incision or anesthesia, this transfer is safe to perform, even if your GIFT conception has already occurred. Known as the combined IVF/GIFT, this extra step may help seal your pregnancy success. Be aware, however, that taking this step will also further increase your chances for a multiple pregnancy, which I personally believe is a great idea if you are planning to have more than one child.

A GIFT Precaution

The type of anesthesia used during the GIFT procedure could affect your pregnancy. That's the result of new studies conducted by the University of Iowa College of Medicine. Here it was learned that the anesthesia known as propofol/nitrous oxide was associated with a far lower rate of laboratory pregnancy success when compared with the drug isoflurane/nitrous oxide. Be certain you check with your doctor, and more important, your anesthesiologist about which drug will be used during your procedure, and when possible, insist on isoflurane.

Your Post-GIFT Recovery: What to Expect

As with basic IVF, the same posttransfer precautions apply after GIFT. These include a few hours of rest in the recovery room, followed by bed rest for at least seventy-two hours at home. Although postoperative pain is minimal, you may experience pressure under your diaphragm or shoulders as a result of gas in your abdomen. You may also feel some slight soreness in your abdomen, due to the incision. If necessary talk to your doctor about a pain-relieving medication, such as Tylenol, which may help.

To further increase your chances for a healthy implantation, ask your doctor about treatment with natural progesterone injections, tablets, or gel, alone or in combination with the hormone hCG.

Natural Pregnancy After GIFT

One of the most exciting benefits of the GIFT procedure was something neither doctors nor researchers had anticipated: For some women a *natural* pregnancy follows the delivery of a GIFT baby! A growing number of patients continue to report they have conceived spontaneously while making love several months after their postpregnancy menstrual cycles returned.

Why does this occur? Researchers theorize *some* of the initial obstacles to fertility may be overcome by the GIFT pregnancy: Hormones are rebalanced and, through the stretching of certain organs, the ravages of scar tissue may be eliminated and vital passageways reopened.

More Conception Options: The ZIFT Pregnancy

While researchers learned early on that getting sperm to fertilize an egg was relatively easy, successfully implanting the resulting embryo and getting it to survive and thrive was quite another story.

Part of the problem was solved by the GIFT procedure. Allowing sperm and egg to remain in the fallopian tube until the uterus was ready seemed to increase pregnancy odds. Still, GIFT is not without its drawbacks—specifically, if a pregnancy fails to occur, there is no way of checking if fertilization had taken place. And that means there is also no way of knowing what went wrong or how to fix it.

To the rescue: ZIFT—zygote intrafallopian tube transfer, a fertility treatment that combines most of the benefits of GIFT and IVF to offer you still another pregnancy alternative.

Here's how ZIFT works:

1. It begins with all the same follicle-stimulating drugs and egg retrieval steps, and all the sperm-washing techniques used for both GIFT and IVF.

2. After the eggs are retrieved, they go through the same culturing process as IVF, then combine with sperm in the same type of laboratory dish, allowing conception to take place.

3. Then, once the eggs are fertilized, the resulting zygote—the first stage of a fertilized embryo—is transferred back into your body. Unlike IVF, in which doctors wait until that embryo would start to develop before placing it in your body, in ZIFT, the transfer takes place within two days, and sometimes just hours after fertilization occurs. Additionally, unlike IVF, which places the embryo inside your uterus, the ZIFT trans-

fer is made to your fallopian tube, in much the same manner as the GIFT procedure.

4. Once inside your tube, the embryo remains for several days, absorbing the natural nutrients from your body and growing stronger. In the meantime, your uterus gets the message that an egg is on the way and continues building a strong and healthy lining.

5. As your embryo develops naturally, inside your tube, it begins moving closer to your uterus. By day six—the optimum time for implantation—it very naturally moves into your uterus, where, one hopes, it engages in a strong and healthy attachment, one that allows it to survive and thrive.

You're Halfway There!

Like GIFT, your ZIFT pregnancy has nearly all of nature's advantages—including development inside your fallopian tube and the option of waiting until your uterus is fully ready to accept implantation before trying to implant.

But like IVF, ZIFT gives your pregnancy an important "running start" by letting you know before the transfer takes place that your egg has been fertilized. You are, in a sense, "halfway there."

For this reason, ZIFT often becomes the procedure of choice for those couples who want to maximize advantages that the new technologies offer.

What Can Go Wrong: The Statistics You Must Consider

As with natural conception, not every pregnancy goes as planned. You should be aware that the risk of ectopic pregnancy—a conception somewhere outside the uterus—is increased when certain reproductive technologies are used, particularly GIFT and ZIFT. Although the actual risk is quite small, less than 5 percent, still, this is two to four times greater than what occurs via natural conception.

IVF, GIFT, and ZIFT pregnancies also may increase your risk of delivering a preterm baby, or one that has a low birth weight. This is particularly true if you are pregnant with multiples, which tend to arrive earlier and be smaller than singletons. To help offset these risks, be certain to follow both the fertility diet plan laid out in Part Two of this book and the vitamin and mineral plan. By getting enough calories and ensuring your nutrient intake, you can give your baby the best possible chance to grow healthy and strong. In addition, don't smoke, and avoid even secondhand smoke, both of which could weaken your implantation and lead to preterm delivery problems.

Indeed, a few simple precautions, beginning just before or right after you conceive, can go a long way in helping to ensure that your IVF procedures yield a normal, healthy, and problem-free pregnancy for you and your baby.

ICSI: The New "Couple's IVF"

Although a couple's fertility problems could be limited to factors in either the man's or the woman's body, in my experience, more often than not they are the result of factors in both partners' reproductive systems. Sometimes, a slight defect or problem in a woman's body, or a man's, might go completely unnoticed until they pair with a partner who also has a slight problem. Then, their two small defects come together to make conception impossible, and infertility becomes an issue.

That's one reason I'm so excited about a brand-new fertility procedure called ICSI—intracytoplasmic sperm injection. Because it does involve significant manipulation of sperm, many doctors consider it to be a treatment for male infertility. But since it does involve treatment for both partners, I prefer to view it as the *Couple's IVF*—a fertility procedure that often works to help the reproductive systems of both partners to function better and more efficiently. ICSI not only works when a man has sperm-related problem, but it can also help if his partner is not producing enough eggs, or she is over age forty, making natural fertilization more difficult.

Is ICSI Right for You? How to Tell

As exciting as ICSI is, however, it's not right for everyone. Indeed,whenever a new and exciting fertility breakthrough comes along, the tendency is for every infertile couple to leap at the chance to try it. And doctors too can sometimes be guilty of being overzealous about a new procedure, particularly when they sincerely want to help a couple get pregnant. As a result, inappropriate procedures are sometimes performed, resulting in a waste not only of money but also time, a commodity that is particularly precious when your biological clock is running down.

According to Dr. Gianpiero D. Palermo, professor of embryology at Weill-Cornell College of Medicine and one of the physicians who helped discover and develop ICSI in Belgium—as well as the first to introduce it to the United States—you and your partner should consider this procedure only when the following infertility factors are present:

In your partner:

- Severely compromised sperm, with concentrations of less than 500,000 progressively motile spermatozoa in a single ejaculate, with the frequency of normal sperm less than 3 percent
- Antisperm antibodies bound to spermatozoa
- Inability to fertilize an egg in previous standard IVF attempts

In you:

- antisperm antibodies
- mild endometriosis
- tubal factor infertility
- unexplained infertility

In addition, you and your partner might be considered candidates for ICSI if several attempts at standard IVF have failed, particularly if fertilization did not take place.

How ICSI Works: What You and Your Partner Need to Know

In the most basic sense, the main goal of this procedure is to deposit your partner's sperm directly into your egg. In doing so, it eliminates several steps that your partner's sperm alone may not be able to accomplish, including swimming to your egg, then releasing the enzymes necessary to penetrate the shell. It also means that as long as a single sperm is alive, a pregnancy can occur.

For the most part, your ICSI procedure will begin in the same way as any standard IVF. You will most likely receive a cycle of fertility medications to help you make an abundance of healthy eggs. Those eggs will be retrieved vaginally, as explained in the previous chapter.

Your partner will obviously need to supply sperm, and in many instances it can be retrieved via the same techniques described earlier in this book.

In order to isolate the sperm from semen and its components, such as white blood cells, the sperm-washing techniques explained in Chapter 20 are also employed.

It is also important to note, however, that when underlying problems lead to extremely low sperm count, or even no sperm at all, the new harvesting technologies detailed in Chapter 18 can also be used in conjunction with the ICSI procedure.

Although the beginning stages of ICSI proceed as in any standard IVF, once sperm and egg are ready to be combined for fertilization, a dramatic turn of events occurs, with both sperm and egg receiving special treatment.

Preparing Your Eggs for ICSI

Remember I told you earlier that ICSI involves depositing sperm directly into the egg? In order to do that accurately, your fertility team must be able to handle each egg with uncanny deftness. To make this possible, your eggs must be "washed" using a special, nontoxic acidic solution. This works to loosen a gel-like coating and sticky layer of cells known as the cumulus corona. Normally, they help your newly ovulated egg stick to the fibriated ends of the fallopian tube and be swept inside. Now, however, the coating simply gets in the way of the micromanipulation necessary to place your partner's sperm inside. Removing these cells also helps in accessing the true quality of your egg, making certain it is perfect for fertilization.

Once the coating is loose, the eggs are passed back and forth through tiny glass straws, which helps free them of the excess cells, and they are rinsed again of all residue.

Preparing Your Partner's Sperm

Once your eggs are ready, they can be combined with your partner's sperm. The good news here: Even a single sperm with just the slightest hint of motility is enough to bring about an ICSI pregnancy.

No matter how slowly the sperm moves, however, it is still going faster than the human hand can move. It's also slippery to the touch, and the two elements combined can make catching the sperm seem a little like fishing with your bare hands. To help the process along, the sperm is slowed by combining it with a drop of a solution known as PVP—polyvinylpyrrolidone—the same substance that has been safely used for many years as a plasma extender in patients who could not immediately receive a transfusion. By slowing the sperm to a kind of "crawl," the solution makes it easier to pick them up, and the stickiness of PVP also slows the injection into the egg, so a much more gentle approach can be taken.

Sperm Bashing: How It Helps the ICSI Conception

During natural conception, your partner's sperm fuses with the membrane inside your egg, causing a chemical reaction that immobilizes the tail. Indeed, while a rapidly moving tail is what helps sperm swim their way through your reproductive tract and get to your egg, once inside, that same tail movement would harm the nucleus and prevent conception from occurring.

When, however, sperm is injected into the egg, as it is in the ICSI procedure, tail movement doesn't stop. If left to its own devices, the sperm would continue to swim happily inside the egg and eventually destroy it. For this reason, the sperm tail must be "paralyzed" before it is allowed to enter. This is done by using a tiny glass tube to pin the sperm to the bottom of the dish and pinch the tail. This is no easy feat—particularly since a sperm tail is no more than one-fifteen-thousandth of a inch in diameter!

Once the tail is crushed, however, your partner's sperm is ready to be injected inside your egg.

The ICSI Conception—Step by Step

1. Sperm and egg meet: One of the most complex aspects of ICSI fertilization is getting the egg in the exact position before injecting the sperm. The reason: Unless sperm enter at a precise point, the nucleus of the egg will be damaged and no pregnancy will occur. Using a powerful microscope, the embryologist will first secure the egg with a tiny suction tube, and then align it with a kind of "clock" formation. When the egg is in position, an ultrathin glass tube will be used to pick up the sperm, gently puncture the egg membrane, and ultimately deposit that sperm inside (see illustration).

2. The incubator honeymoon: To help encourage fertilization, the newly combined egg and sperm—still in the laboratory dish—are placed in an incubator, where the early stages of embryo formation begin.

3. Room service: Approximately twelve to eighteen hours later, the eggs are checked for defects—a critical step that must be performed with the utmost care. This is because not all eggs that receive sperm will fertilize—and not all will go on to develop as perfectly as nature intended. This is true not only in ICSI, but in all forms of IVF, and in natural fertilization through intercourse as well. If an egg is not fertilized, however, it is not wasted, as it can be used again for a second ICSI procedure.

4. Checkout: Not all the eggs your doctor retrieves are able to be fertilized. Of those that are, approximately 60 to 80 percent will, after fertilization with sperm, develop into two- and four-cell embryos—the very earliest stage of growth. So, if your procedure began by harvesting fifteen of your eggs, ultimately, only three to six may progress to the embryo stage.

Further, only the two-day-old embryos that have four equal-sized cells (called blastomeres), and a nucleus that is clearly visualized, are the most likely to develop into a healthy pregnancy.

5. Special delivery: the embryo transfer: Normally, the healthy embryos are transferred back into your body within seventy-two hours, or in certain circumstances within one to two days. Your pregnancy can then be verified, usually within about twelve days—and it should progress in a normal fashion.

ICSI: Your Pregnancy Odds

For the most part, ICSI is the answer for almost any type of male fertility problem. Although it can't promise that every infertile man will become a father, it does level the playing field so that his chances are equal to that of men who have no fertility problems.

Indeed, the only element limiting the success of ICSI is egg quality—usually the result of a woman's advancing age. Indeed, the older the egg the more likely there will be problems getting pregnant no matter which method of conception is used.

To help calculate your potential success with ICSI, here are some statistics that can help.

AGE OF WOMAN	PREGNANCY RATE (PER ICSI TRY)	MISCARRIAGE RATE
Under 30	50%	Under 5%
30 to 36	35%	15 to 20%
36 to 40	Under 35%	30% or more
40 and over	5 to 10%	50% or more

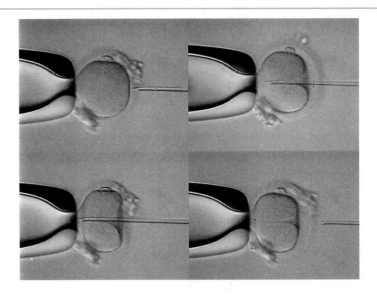

ICSI: Placing the Sperm Inside the Egg

The key function of the ICSI procedure is to place a single sperm directly inside an egg, thus clearing the way for fertilization to occur unhampered by any outside factors. In order to do this, the embryologist looks through a powerful microscope and secures the egg with a tiny suction tube (top left). Then, a thin glass tube picks up the sperm and gently punctures the egg membrane (top right), pushes deep inside the egg (bottom left), and releases the sperm. The tube is then gently removed from the egg (bottom right), and the edge automatically seals itself shut.

Improving Your Pregnancy Odds:
The ICSI-GIFT of Life

As you read earlier in this chapter, some research indicates that the GIFT procedure results in what may be the highest rate of success among all the new reproductive technologies. Therefore, my colleagues and I began thinking about the possibility of a combination procedure, one that would blend the pregnancy success rates of GIFT with the extra advantages for male fertility found in ICSI.

The result: Our team was among the first in the United States to develop and perform ICSI-GIFT. It begins with the same egg-stimulation medications used in the regular GIFT procedure, taken at the start of your cycle. When your eggs are mature (in roughly thirteen or fourteen days), you will be placed under light anesthesia, your eggs will be retrieved through the vagina, then passed to the embryologist, who locates them in the fluid. They are then passed to a second embryologist, who begins performing the ICSI procedure, placing the sperm inside the eggs. Ideally, by the time your doctor finishes the retrieval process, the embryologists will have completed the ICSI procedure on at least four or five embryos. And here is where our procedure takes another really important twist.

Rather than placing the ICSI egg/sperm combination into an incubator, you will be immediately sedated with a slightly more potent anesthetic, and your doctor will quickly perform a laparoscopy, during which the ICSI eggs will be transferred directly into your fallopian tubes.

After this, the completion of the fertilization process will take place in the most natural way possible, inside your body. Your resulting embryo then travels to your uterus, where it undergoes implantation at the precise time it would if you had conceived naturally via intercourse.

I'm happy to report that several months ago I delivered our first ICSI-GIFT baby—a healthy robust boy. Since that time we have gone on to perform this procedure many times, with good success. In fact, some patients who previously failed to get pregnant using other IVF techniques were able to conceive via ICSI-GIFT.

The Benefits of ICSI-GIFT

Because ICSI places the sperm inside the egg before being placed in the fallopian tube, fertilization is more likely to occur than with the regular GIFT procedure, which relies on sperm and egg combining in the tube. Indeed, once ICSI is added to the mix, the only real requirement for conception is a healthy egg and at least one healthy fallopian tube.

And while we do have the opportunity to better ensure conception using the ZIFT procedure (mainly because an already fertilized embryo is placed inside the fallopian tube), doing so requires two surgeries—

one to retrieve your eggs, the second to probe your fallopian tube and put the embryo inside. In ICSI-GIFT, only one procedure and one anesthesia is necessary, since everything is done at the same time.

ICSI-GIFT also has the added advantage of limiting the amount of time the egg and sperm are out of their natural environment, and that may also increase pregnancy success. In addition, ICSI-GIFT does not use incubators, or force sperm and egg to spend extensive time in a laboratory dish or endure unnecessary exposure to outside media, such as cultures or chemicals. I believe that all these small differences can come together to help make a healthier embryo and a stronger, healthier implantation. Ultimately, this may increase pregnancy rates, particularly in older women, as embryos appear to survive more readily in their bodies than in a laboratory.

Is ICSI Safe? What You Need to Know

From almost the very beginnings of the ICSI procedure, researchers began questioning its safety, particularly in regard to potential birth defects. One reason is that the nature of the procedure itself does away with one of the most important steps in human reproduction—natural selection. Here, a woman's egg chooses which sperm is allowed in, and it does so based on which one is the healthiest and the strongest. The end result is usually a healthy pregnancy.

In ICSI, however, natural selection is replaced by scientific choice. And although fertility experts do their best to choose the sperm they believe are healthiest, often it comes down to a matter of the best of the worst. Indeed, couples who use ICSI often do so because sperm *is* somehow inadequate, which could represent more than just a fertility problem. Many believe poor-quality sperm are also genetically defective—a situation that can seriously affect the health of the baby.

Conversely, other experts maintain that appearances aren't everything, even in sperm! That it looks or acts deformed does not mean the DNA is not normal.

And there are studies that illustrate both points of view:

- In one recent report published in the journal *Lancet,* eighty-nine Australian babies born via the ICSI procedure demonstrated a shocking increase in developmental delay during the first year of life, when compared to babies born via other IVF procedures or through natural pregnancy.

- In a second study, also published in *Lancet,* two years of research on some two hundred ICSI babies two years of age found absolutely *no difference* in mental development when compared to babies born using standard IVF.

So the debate over the safety of ICSI continues.

What should you believe? I would venture to guess that nearly all experts, myself included, do not take the threat of any illness or disease lightly. The possibility that any fertility procedure may cause subtle, complex, or even far-reaching changes in the genetic basis of the next generation, or even the generation after that, is indeed a fear and a threat we cannot afford to ignore.

That said, I also want to personally reassure you that, in my opinion, ICSI is generally a safe and effective treatment that you should consider. Indeed, studies on more than one thousand ICSI babies have shown that this treatment represents no major threats to your baby.

To be fair, however, I must tell you that there is one genetic flaw that does appear to result from the ICSI procedure: Male babies conceived in this manner are at risk for the same genetic infertility problems as their fathers. The reason: Sperm appear to carry the genetic code for the very defect linked to infertility, whether it be low sperm count, motility problems, enzyme-related difficulties, or even the shape of the sperm itself. Whatever the problem is specifically, it can be passed on. This, however, is not much different from any genetic trait that a parent may pass to a child, such as short or long legs, or thin or wavy hair.

Ensuring Your ICSI Baby: How Your Doctor Can Help

It is my personal belief that you can go into your ICSI procedure, or any form of IVF, with full confidence that you will conceive and deliver a healthy baby, one that is more likely than not to be normal.

If, however, you still have concerns over safety issues, here are a few suggestions on how to reduce the risks:

1. By selecting the very best and most normal sperm your partner has to offer, your doctor can minimize the threat of a problem know as DNA breakage—a situation wherein some of the genetic material inside the sperm may become disturbed or disrupted.

2. Ask your doctor to screen your partner's sperm for abnormal levels of "oxidized DNA products," present in semen and urine. If levels test abnormally high, indicating a higher-than-average risk of transmitting defective DNA to your baby, you should consider genetic counseling before going ahead with your ICSI procedure.

3. Genetic screening before ICSI should be considered for carriers of sperm-related disorders such as cystic fibrosis (CF), a chronic respiratory disease. This should be a prime consideration if your partner is missing the part of his reproductive system known as the vas deferens, which can occur as a result of the CF gene.

4. Talk to your doctor about the possibility of embryo biopsy—a method of testing your conception for chromosomal defects. Although not perfect, some of these tests can be quite good at identifying the risk of specific diseases such as hemophilia or CF. Once an embryo has been biopsied and deemed healthy, it can still be successfully transferred and result in a healthy pregnancy. Analysis may also tell whether your embryo is male or female, which can also affect the risk of transferring certain sex-related genetic abnormalities. Be aware, however, that this is extremely expensive and generally not covered by most insurances.

5. If you would consider terminating a pregnancy when a severe birth defect is found, then be certain to talk to your doctor about testing your baby via amniocentesis and chorionic villus sampling as early in your pregnancy as possible.

A Final Thought

If you can come away from this chapter with only one thought, let it be that you should never give up on your parenting dreams, no matter how remote they seem to be. This is extremely important to remember as you go forward with your fertility plans, since no matter what treatment you choose, it will likely require numerous tries before you get pregnant. And I don't want you to give up hope.

At the same time, I want you to also keep in mind that you shouldn't waste too much effort on any given procedure, or even on any one doctor or clinic. Sometimes even small changes can make a huge difference to the success of your treatment.

The main point to remember: Hold that positive attitude, give yourself room to fail, and promise yourself you will succeed.

Chapter Twenty-Three

The Science of Motherhood:

Donor Eggs, Frozen Embryos, and
More New Ways to Have a Baby

For most women the process of ovulation—making and releasing eggs—more or less continues on a regular basis from puberty until the middle thirties. In fact, the only time the cycle should be interrupted is if a pregnancy should occur.

After age thirty-five, however, the process slows down just a bit. You are still making and releasing eggs, just not quite as regularly. That's one of the reasons why it can take so much longer for older women to get pregnant.

As you enter your forties, things slow down even more, with ovulation occurring far less frequently—three or four times a year, or sometimes less. Although getting pregnant naturally is not impossible (I'm sure you know of several women with "change-of-life" babies), it is usually more difficult.

But something else also happens as a woman ages: Her eggs are not quite as healthy or strong as they were when she was younger. Not only does this affect the rate at which pregnancy occurs ("old" eggs are harder to fertilize), but even if she does conceive, the risk of both birth defects and miscarriage increases, even when technologies such as IVF are used.

In fact, while your uterus may be in the perfect condition to carry a child, and your body strong enough to handle labor and delivery, if your eggs are weak, or in short supply, having a baby is going to be a challenge.

Indeed, regardless of your age, if you cannot make healthy eggs—

something which can also affect younger women—you must turn to technology for help.

Stopping Your Biological Clock: What You Can Do

For many women, the answer to their egg-making dilemma can be found in fertility drugs. As you read earlier in this book, these are medications that stimulate your body's own egg-making potential.

For some women, however, a bit more help is necessary, in the form of donor eggs. Here, the precious "seeds of life" are taken from a donor's body and mixed with your partner's sperm in a laboratory, and the resulting embryo is placed inside *your* body, where it will be nourished by you. Providing you are in otherwise good health, donor eggs can extend your childbearing potential by a considerable margin. In fact, you may have already read about several women who have used donor eggs to give birth in their sixties! While I certainly don't recommend you wait this long to get pregnant, it's clear that when donor eggs are used, your biological clock can stop time for quite a number of years.

Your Donor Pregnancy: The First Step

The very first donor egg pregnancy actually took place quite a number of years ago—in 1984, in Australia. Although first developed to help young women with ovarian failure, since then, the technology has expanded so that a woman of virtually any age can take advantage of what science has to offer. In addition, the process of extracting eggs is now much simpler and easier to endure, so more women are encouraged to become donors, thus increasing the available supply of eggs.

If you are considering using donor eggs, your first step is, of course, to find a suitable donor. For many women, a close friend or relative turns out to be the best choice. If, in fact, a close relative is chosen, such as a sister, then your embryo may ultimately contain at least some of the same genetic material that would be in your own egg, particularly in terms of physical characteristics. However, that your egg donor is related is not a guarantee that your baby will be any closer to you, physically or in any other way. By way of example, let me remind you of the many sisters and brothers you have known who were not anything alike, either in physical appearance or in personality.

If, however, choosing a friend or relative would make your egg-donation process harder, you are not alone. Many couples choose to keep their donor activities exceedingly private, so that no one, not even their families, knows how their pregnancy was achieved. If, for any reason, you would feel more comfortable with a donor you do not already know, then you do have a variety of options from which to choose.

Selecting a Donor

In many instances, your fertility doctor will have access to egg donors—women who are willing to give up their eggs to those couples who cannot conceive on their own. In other instances, your doctor can connect you to a "surrogate agency"—a professional, medical organization that matches egg donors with women who want to get pregnant. While the American Fertility Society and others frown on the concept of "selling" eggs, they do agree that the donor should be compensated for the risks involved and the time it takes to complete the donation process, usually a sum between one thousand and three thousand dollars. Most surrogate agencies also charge a fee for screening donors, a sum that ranges from as low as one thousand dollars to as high as six thousand dollars or more.

Secrets, Anonymity, and You

In the not-so-distant past, egg donation was a completely anonymous experience. The donor had no idea who was getting her eggs, and the recipients had no personal identifying information about their donor. And, in fact, even today, most donor databases remove all identifying information from their files.

Donor Screening: What You Need to Know

Much like sperm banks, agencies representing egg donors can vary greatly in the amount of information they provide about donors. In some instances they will offer only basic characteristics of the donor, such as hair and eye color, ethnic background, and general health data. In other instances you may find an entire dossier of information including IQ, hobbies, religion, education—even food preferences. In many instances this can help in choosing a donor who is most like you. Although there is no guarantee that the egg she delivers will also have these same characteristics, the odds are in your favor.

In order to become a donor, a woman must undergo specific medical testing, including a Pap smear, cervical exam, and numerous blood tests. In some instances you may also request that she undergo genetic testing, particularly if your partner is considered at risk for any diseases. Sometimes you may also be able to request that your donor undergo drug testing.

However, many egg-donation agencies now operate with a new kind of "open door" policy that offers both donors and recipients the opportunity to make their identity known to each other. In some instances, they even meet before a selection is made, and some become quite close friends during the donation and subsequent pregnancy. You may also choose to simply speak to your donor by phone, or communicate only by mail, and never meet face-to-face. For the most part, the choice is up to you and your partner, in conjunction with the agency supplying your egg donor.

Because certain legal issues are involved in egg donation, lawyers will also likely be a part of the process. In this respect, binding documents will be drawn between you, your partner, and your donor with respect to legal ownership of any children conceived with the donor egg (your baby will legally be yours from the moment of implantation), as well as the future use of any embryos that are conceived using your

Consider This: Factors That Influence Donor Choice

Although there are a variety of new services available to help you locate and choose an egg donor, this is a new area of expertise, one that currently requires no license and no degree. Therefore, there are no legal parameters to determine what an agency should or should not do in the process of matching donors to recipients. Indeed, you are pretty much on your own in terms of finding out what you need to know. To help reduce the risk of problems I suggest you rely heavily on either your own fertility specialist or a related medical academic center to recommend an egg-donation program. Many times medical centers with fertility programs will also have an egg-donation program in place. Other times they may work with specific outside agencies that can be trusted.

To further ensure that you will be treated fairly, you should also consider these factors when choosing a donation program.

- Length of time the program has been in business, and the success rate
- Fee structure, including whether you have to pay up front or can pay in installments. Also, discuss any refund policy, particularly if you change your mind about a donor for any reason.
- What lengths will the broker go to to fulfill your donor requirements—and any additional fees for extra services
- Does the donor have a separate fee—and will you also have to cover her medical and other expenses, such as the cost of fertility drugs and egg retrieval? If this is the case, who will itemize those expenses?
- The health screening policy for donors, including tests for sexually transmitted diseases such as chlamydia, gonorrhea, and HIV, and who pays for what
- Anonymity policy
- Recordkeeping—particularly on anonymous donors—including the number of times they have donated eggs. Does the donor have an exclusive contract with the agency, and if not, who is keeping track of her egg donations?

donor's eggs but not implanted into your uterus during your initial fertility procedure. Most often the donor may have legal representation on her own, and the donor center will have a legal representative who can counsel you. However, you may want to retain your own attorney to make certain you fully understand the legal obligations of everyone concerned.

Getting Pregnant: The Donor Egg Process

Once you have made a decision concerning the woman who will supply your donor eggs, the next step is to plan the pregnancy itself. The method used to conceive your baby will be IVF—in vitro fertilization—or the ZIFT procedure. Because both are generally more successful when more than one embryo is implanted, it's necessary to fertilize more than one egg. As such, your donor will usually receive treatment with fertility drugs to help ensure she makes multiple eggs. At the same time, you will be treated with estrogen and other hormones to ensure that your uterus begins building the spongy "nest" necessary to sustain your baby throughout a pregnancy.

While it was once necessary for the menstrual cycles of both donor and recipient to be carefully coordinated—her eggs had to be ready to ovulate at the precise time your uterus was ready to accept an embryo—this is no longer necessary, thanks to an innovation called cryopreservation, or embryo freezing. The process works this way: When your donor's eggs are mature, they are surgically retrieved (see Chapter 21), and then mixed with your partner's sperm in a laboratory dish to form an embryo. If your cycle has been synchronized with that of your donor, those embryos will be transferred into your body within three days. If, however, your cycles are not synchronized, the embryos are instead medically frozen and stored until your body is hormonally ready to sustain a pregnancy. When this occurs, the embryos are thawed, cultured in a laboratory to ensure healthy growth, and then transferred into your body.

Although frozen embryos are an important alternative (freezing also means your donor may be able to forgo fertility drugs and participate in a natural cycle), there is a downside—most notably, that about 20 to 30

Ensuring Your Donor Implantation

To help ensure that your uterus is receptive to the donor eggs, talk to your doctor about a regimen of low-dose aspirin to be taken along with hormones in preparation for pregnancy. Studies show that while the aspirin won't increase the thickness of your uterine lining, it does appear to increase the rate of embryo implantation, thus making it more likely for a pregnancy to occur. You should also receive antibiotics such as tetracycline to reduce the risk of infection, which could interfere with the success rate. In addition, you should always receive progesterone supplementation to ensure that your uterine lining remains healthy and able to supply good nutrition to your baby.

percent do not survive the process. You should note, however, that the earlier the stage of development in which an embryo is frozen, the greater the chance for survival. Additionally, loss of embryos should not be a problem if your donor supplies multiple eggs, since more than one embryo is usually created.

In addition to freezing embryos in conjunction with donor eggs, many couples undergoing IVF with their own eggs also make use of this technology, particularly when a single cycle yields more eggs and more embryos than are needed for a successful IVF. If the extra embryos are frozen, a subsequent IVF can be performed without the need for another round of fertility drugs.

Bonding to Your Donor Baby

Many women confide to me that they are reluctant to use the donor-egg technology because they are afraid there will be no emotional or physiological bond to the baby they carry and deliver. I, however, am always happy to reassure them that this is almost never the case.

Why?

First off, you will be carrying a baby that is very much the product of your partner's genes, something that will automatically bring the two of you closer together and will bring you closer to your baby as well.

Perhaps more important, it is your body, your blood, your life that is sustaining this child and allowing him or her to come into the world: This child, in fact, belongs more to you than to anybody.

Egg Freezing: The Newest Technology

Although cryopreservation—freezing human tissue—has been in use on sperm since the 1940s, and on embryos since the mid-1980s, it wasn't until the late 1990s that advances in freezing technology allowed eggs to be frozen as well. A pair of twin boys were recently born to a Georgia mother who received embryos made from eggs that had been retrieved from a donor and frozen for twenty-five months. Unfortunately, however, to date, frozen eggs have yielded only a few such successful births. Why? In most instances, the freezing process damages the egg and prevents fertilization. This, however, is likely to change in the near future.

The very latest research—award-winning studies conducted at the Institute for Reproductive Medicine and Science of St. Barnabas Hospital in Livingston, New Jersey—found a new way to freeze both embryos and eggs that may revolutionize the process. Their technique involves a simple change in the culture medium used in the freezing process. More specifically, if the sodium is removed from the solution and replaced with a natural substance known as choline, survival, fertilization, and development of frozen eggs improves dramatically.

Meanwhile, research conducted at the Florida Institute of Reproductive Medicine in Jacksonville found that simply removing some of the water in the freezing solution, increasing the level of sucrose, and then using a super-rapid cooling system increases the success of egg freezing.

As advances in this area continue, it is possible that in the future, all young women will have the opportunity to bank their own eggs beginning as young as age eighteen or twenty—a time when potency is high and reproductive health is excellent. Then, they would be free to conceive twenty or even thirty years later, using their own healthy eggs. The freezing process could also help women who are forced to undergo chemotherapy for cancer. By removing and preserving their eggs before treatment, they can be free to conceive with healthy eggs at a later time. Additionally, studies conducted at Robert Wood Johnson Medical School in Camden, New Jersey, have shown that frozen eggs are far less likely to result in ectopic pregnancy than fresh eggs, so this may be an alternative for women at higher risk for this problem as well.

It is, however, important to note that several studies have shown that while frozen eggs are more likely to result in pregnancy in women over forty years of age, for those under age thirty-five, fresh eggs still yield the higher pregnancy rate.

Good Eggs — No Pregnancy: What to Do

The Cytoplasm Transfer

For most women, it is the quality of their eggs that determines how successful any assisted reproductive technology will be. However, as in all things in life, there are exceptions to every rule. You may be one of a small but significant group of women who manufacture perfect follicles and yield many eggs—and yet every embryo conceived fails to develop.

For many years this seemingly contradictory situation puzzled scientists. The answer, however, came when we discovered an important new role of cytoplasm, the gel-like fluid that lines the shell of each egg.

What we learned: When a defect in the cytoplasm exists, even the most perfect fertilized egg does not have the biochemical power necessary to properly divide and multiply into a normal embryo.

The end result: Good eggs, but no pregnancy.

For a long time, it was believed that when a cytoplasmic defect existed, a woman's only option was donor eggs. Then, like a light going on in the middle of the night, another treatment option was illuminated: Why not simply replace the cytoplasm with that of a donor, leaving the egg intact?

Unlike donor eggs, which preclude any biological link between birth mother and baby, donor cytoplasm would allow the chromosomal material inside the mother's own egg to form the basis of the embryo. The donor material—the cytoplasm—acts only as a helper.

Thus, the theory behind the IVF procedure known as cytoplasm transfer (CT) was born. Here's how it's done:

1. Your eggs are retrieved using the procedure described in Chapter 21.
2. Your donor's eggs are also retrieved, and then, using a slender needle, up to 5 percent of the cytoplasm is extracted, leaving the nucleus of her egg untouched.
3. Using a variation of the ICSI procedure, the donor cytoplasm and your partner's sperm are loaded into an ultrafine catheter and injected directly into the egg that was taken from your ovary. After a period of incubation and fertilization, the resulting embryo is transferred into your uterus, where it implants and grows.

The first child born using this procedure was a beautiful baby girl name Emma, who arrived in April 1997, thanks to the work of Dr. Richard Scott and his team at the St. Barnabas Medical Center in Livingston, New Jersey. During the sixteenth week of pregnancy, and later at Emma's birth, the doctors used DNA fingerprinting to test her chromosomal cells. In both instances, tests confirmed her chromosomal characteristics were those of her birth mother and father. Little Emma had, in fact, no biological traces whatsoever of the donor who provided the cytoplasm transfer material.

More Pregnancy Options: The Future of Egg Technology

Among the most exciting new fertility options are those that work to further expand the pregnancy potential of women with less-than-satisfactory eggs. Herein are a few of the more advanced techniques, some of which may become widely available soon.

- **The "designer" egg:** In this procedure, the nucleus of the intended mother's egg is removed and placed inside the "shell" of a younger woman's egg, which is then fertilized using an injection of the father's sperm. The end result is an embryo that is stronger and healthier than if only the mother's original egg was used on its own. So far, studies show that embryos developed from this process suffer no particular genetic consequences. If research continues to show good results, it could become an important new option for older women trying to conceive.

- **Using baby eggs to make a baby:** As I told you earlier, every woman is born with all of the "follicles" she will need to make and ovulate mature eggs in her adult life. Well, this is the premise upon which a somewhat controversial new egg-enhancing technology was developed. In this procedure, follicles are harvested from the ovaries of fetuses that, for whatever reason, were not born. Once the seeds are removed, they are matured in a laboratory and later used as donor eggs. A second variation involves removing the entire ovary from a fetus and transplanting it into a woman whose own ovaries are not functioning. Although this technology may hold the answer for many women, any procedures involving a fetus holds center stage in ethical debates. While it has the support of many scientists and researchers, just as many are critical of this procedure and openly oppose it, as do many government-sponsored commissions. I too believe this new technology raises more ethical questions than it answers biological needs. However, I also know that science marches forward—and at some point this procedure will likely become a fertility reality.

- **The embryo transplant:** Still one more fertility possibility involves using your partner's sperm to artificially inseminate an egg donor. Once conception occurs and a pregnancy is verified, the embryo is gently flushed from the donor's body and placed inside your uterus. This technique is most advantageous for women who are infertile due to complete, irreversible ovarian failure, or when conception in their own bodies would risk transmitting a serious genetic disorder. The key to the success of this treatment is synchronization of the menstrual cycles of both donor and recipient. It is vital that your body be ready to receive your donor's embryo exactly five days after it has been conceived. If more than five days pass, the embryo is so firmly attached to your donor's uterus that it will not survive attempts to remove it.

- **Ovarian transplant:** In the not so distant past, freezing an embryo was considered a technological marvel. Today, not only is this possible but a brand-new technology is also allowing women to freeze ovarian tissue to be transplanted back into their bodies at a later time.

Indeed, the world's first human ovarian tissue transplant took place in February 1999 by Dr. Kutluk Oktay, director of reproductive endocrinology and infertility in the Department of Obstetrics and Gynecology at New York Methodist Hospital and a professor at Cornell University. The patient was a thirty-year-old ballerina, who one year earlier underwent surgery for a medical problem that included removal of her ovaries. Rather than tossing the tissue away, doctors froze it in a procedure known as cryopreservation.

Because her ovaries were removed, the surgery threw the then twenty-nine-year-old into instant menopause. She did not get a menstrual cycle, and by all accounts, production of reproductive hormones stopped. Just one year later, however, her biology turned around again.

After assessing the frozen ovarian tissue, Oktay and his team found that, while half the cells were damaged, a good 50 percent remained healthy. So, after thawing the tissue, he isolated the healthy sections, then began sewing, attaching approximately eighty separate pieces of the ovary into two separate strings. Then, using laparoscopic surgery, a type of pocket was created in the patient's pelvic wall, and the two strings of the healthy tissue were stitched into place.

Much as a skin graft placed in a bed of vascular activity eventually begins to grow, so too did the ovarian tissue thrive.

Three months later, the ballerina received treatment with a variety of fertility medications for approximately eleven days, after which time an ultrasound exam revealed an egg had developed in one of the grafts. As the follicle grew, it produced hormones in amounts similar to that of a normal ovary.

Before long, the woman ovulated the new egg, and experienced a normal menstrual cycle! Doctors are hopeful that one day a pregnancy may also be possible—and I share their enthusiasm and hope. Certainly, as long as the woman's body does not reject the transplant, and she continues to make eggs on even a semi-regular basis, there is no reason not to believe that, with the help of fertility procedures, a pregnancy will one day occur.

Although technically the procedure did allow a woman to return from a menopausal state and regain her reproductive potential, experts say it may not help women over thirty-five, since the freezing process itself destroys some of the ovary's egg-making potential. And since women over thirty-five generally produce fewer and less healthy eggs, doctors fear there would be too little healthy tissue to work with.

However, younger women, particularly cancer patients who must undergo chemotherapy, can benefit greatly from the new procedure by having their ovarian tissue removed prior to treatment, and then transplanted back after they are cancer-free. Indeed, in anticipation of this procedure, which has been successful in animals for quite some time, thousands of cancer patients around the world have been freezing and banking their ovarian tissue, with hopes of one day resuming their childbearing potential.

And, while it's not here yet, I can only assume that at some point women will also be able to use this new technology to freeze ovarian tissue while young and most fertile, and then undergo the transplant later in life, when they want to resume their baby-making potential.

The New Surrogacy: Another Way to Have a Baby

If you are like most women, your introduction to the term "surrogate mother" may have been from sensationalist headlines surrounding several cases—most notably, the "Baby M" file. Here, the woman who contracted to have another woman's baby decided to keep the child. Unfortunately, the publicity generated from this one case—including a television movie—helped cast the entire surrogacy issue in a negative light.

In reality, however, surrogacy can be a wonderful alternative for any couple who cannot become parents naturally. It can also help those who have been failed by even the most advanced reproductive technologies.

While most folks think of surrogacy in only one context—one woman having another woman's child—there are actually three different types of surrogate relationships:

- **Traditional surrogacy with artificial insemination:** In this instance, your surrogate agrees to undergo conception via artificial insemination with sperm from your partner. The surrogate carries the baby to term, and after the birth, relinquishes all rights to the child. You will then participate in a stepparent adoption process to establish your rights as the child's legal mother.

- **Gestational surrogacy:** Here, you and your partner participate in the first steps of IVF, each contributing egg and sperm, which are combined in the laboratory to form an embryo. Rather than being transferred into your uterus, however, the embryo is instead handed over to a "surrogate uterus"—a woman who agrees to carry your child, and to give birth. Normally, this is done if you can make eggs, but either you have no uterus (the result of a genetic defect or a hysterectomy) or your health is otherwise such that you could not undergo gestation, labor, and delivery. In this instance, you and your partner are also the biological parents, and your surrogate is considered a "host" uterus. Often, a mother or sister volunteers to carry a child for a woman who cannot do so on her own.

- **Donor egg/gestational surrogacy:** In this unique situation, three women are involved—the one who donates the egg, the one who carries the embryo and delivers the baby, and finally the intended mother who eventually adopts the child. Here, a donor egg (often anonymous) is fertilized with your partner's sperm, and the resulting embryo is transferred into the second woman, known as the "gestational carrier." After giving birth, she relinquishes all rights to the child, who you will then adopt.

As is the case with finding an egg donor, finding a surrogate willing to participate in any of these scenarios can be difficult. And since the risk of emotional attachment to the child can be great in surrogacy, I strongly suggest you use a professional surrogacy service, as well as retaining legal advice, when pursuing any of these options. While you may be tempted to rely on the help of family or friends, in this instance you should not do so unless some psychological counseling is involved, for both you and your surrogate. Definitely speak to your doctor about all possibilities and ask for his or her help in making your surrogate decision.

If, in fact, you do decide on a family member or friend, be certain to have the entire agreement drawn up legally, with representatives for both sides. While it may seem unnecessary, particularly if your surrogate is a close relative, in the long run it will benefit everyone involved, including your baby, to have each person's role in the birthing process, as well as future obligations, clearly outlined and defined.

Motherhood: A Final Thought

As a fertility expert I am often asked by my patients, as well as by members of the press, whether all these new technologies somehow diminish the concept of "true" motherhood—and more important, how these seemingly "unnatural" forms of conception are likely to affect the children they bring into the world.

Well, speaking from a strictly scientific point of view, I am happy to report that, for the most part, children conceived via most forms of laboratory conception are as healthy as those conceived naturally. In many instances, they can be far healthier than those who were conceived naturally by parents who had borderline fertility problems.

But perhaps more important, I am even happier to report that couples who conceive with the new technologies have every bit the natural "parenting" instincts and feelings they would have if conception had occurred naturally. From an emotional standpoint, the impact of feeling a child growing inside you is a wondrous and all-encompassing experience, regardless of who provided the egg.

Moreover, the overwhelming feeling of joy and the natural nurturing instincts that come when your new baby is placed into your arms for the very first time are both universal and automatic—whether that baby came from your body or from that of another woman. After helping to introduce thousands of couples to their precious new role as parents, I can tell you with confidence that at the precise moment you glance down at that tiny, loving face and feel those ten tiny fingers wrap around your hand, the bond of motherhood cannot be denied. You are this child's mother—and no less a loving parent than if your conception had been totally natural.

Chapter Twenty-Four

The Midlife Pregnancy:

What You Need to Know

Among the most outstanding advances not only in reproductive health but in medicine in general are the tests and treatments that have dramatically extended our life expectancy. Indeed, on nearly all fronts, researchers and scientists have made enormous strides in helping us live not only longer but healthier lives.

It makes sense, then, that we should also turn our attention to an expansion of our reproductive years, particularly with regard to women. Although men have always had the ability to retain their fertility somewhat throughout their entire lives, women had no such luxury. A woman's biological clock begins to tick the moment she's born and is preset for a certain predetermined number of cycles. And for many decades there was little, if anything, medicine could do to reprogram a woman's fertility timetable.

Not so anymore.

While there are certainly still some limitations, both physically and emotionally, the good news is that for most women, the childbearing years can now extend far beyond what we could have imagined even just a decade ago.

In fact, as long as your overall health is good, it's not only possible but probable that you can have a baby up to and even past your mid-forties. For some of you, a baby may be possible even after menopause has already started!

Now I'm not saying that it's going to be easy—far from it. Indeed, the older a woman gets, the harder it becomes not only to get pregnant, but to have a healthy baby. And we'll tell you more about why in a moment. However, if you are one of a growing number of women past the age of forty who are committed to having a child, there is important new information that can help make your parenting dreams come true.

Before you fully understand what *can* be done, it's important to know a little something about how your reproductive system ages.

A Woman's Body: The Baby-Making Changes

One of the most profound physiological differences between men and women is the longevity of their reproductive systems. While both you and your partner began your reproductive lives around the same time—puberty—if all goes well your partner will continue to manufacture the hormones necessary to initiate sperm production throughout his lifetime. And while the quality of that sperm may decline somewhat as he ages, for the most part, a man can still conceive a healthy child well into his eighties and nineties.

For you, however, quite a different timetable prevails. As you have already learned, each woman is born with a predetermined egg-making potential. That is, not only are your ovaries programmed to turn out just so many eggs, but there is also a time limit on production. At puberty your body begins regularly making the hormones necessary to stimulate egg growth and release. But unlike your partner's, your hormone production will only last a set number of years. Although the exact timetable is different for every woman, once production stops, your chance of getting pregnant naturally is lost.

But that's not all that happens. As you age, the quality of your eggs also decreases, with significant changes occurring with each decade. This means that as you age, not only is your egg harder to fertilize, but it could be more difficult for you to have a healthy baby. While no one is certain why this happens, leading theories suggest that as part of the aging process, communication within the cells of your ovary breaks down. That means the older you are, the less likely it is that your follicles will receive the appropriate biochemical signals necessary to grow healthy and strong.

If all this sounds discouraging, please don't despair. Although the younger you are when you attempt pregnancy, the less likely you are to encounter fertility problems, this is not a hard-and-fast rule. Indeed, I have had many patients past the age of forty get pregnant and deliver beautiful, healthy children, sometimes with nothing more than a change in diet necessary to encourage their natural fertility.

Additionally, today there are a plethora of fertility treatments developed specifically to cater to the reproductive needs of women over forty. Indeed, as this chapter continues to unfold, I hope to offer you the most encouraging news available today to help make motherhood a reality for you.

However, I still must add just a few words of caution: If you are at least forty years old and want to get pregnant, see a fertility specialist right away. In fact, before you read any more of this book, sit down and make an appointment. Right now. The reason? Once a woman passes age forty, *every single day* makes a big difference in terms of the success rate of fertility treatments. So the sooner you seek treatment, the more likely it is for your pregnancy to become a reality.

You're Only as Old as Your Eggs!

Have you ever spent a few moments looking back on family pictures, or even glancing through your high-school or college yearbook? For most women, that trip down memory lane frequently elicits the same response: "I can't believe how much better we look today!" Indeed, whether you are comparing yourself at age forty-two to how your mother or grandmother looked at that age or simply holding up the mirror of time and gazing at your own reflection, it's likely you will see a better picture today than what was present in the past.

While part of that reaction is due to a psychological phenomenon that influences how we see the past, in many ways there is also a stoic truth to the saying, "We're not getting older, we're getting better." Changes in everything from skin care to cosmetics, hair styling, and body shaping, to the clothes we wear and activities we participate in all go a long way in blurring the lines of biological change from one decade to the next. I have even found this to be strikingly true in my own medical practice.

Whereas thirty years ago it was relatively easy for me to identify a patient's age by simply looking at her, today a glance around my waiting room no longer automatically reveals which new patients are here for obstetrical care, and which ones are seeking menopause treatment!

The truth is that when it comes to reproductive medicine, there can be a big difference between a woman's chronological and her biological age. Even more important, women of the same chronological age may not be of the same biological age, particularly in regard to reproduction. I have some patients who, at age forty-five, are still producing significant amounts of FSH and LH necessary to stimulate egg production and growth, while others of the same age have already completed their menopause. And while a woman's reproductive life is often linked to family history (if, for example, your mother had an early menopause, then you probably will too), nothing is cast in stone. That's one reason age alone cannot act as the sole barometer of your fertility potential.

What does matter? A factor doctors call your "ovarian reserve." In essence, this means not only the number of egg follicles left in your ovary (the seeds that can mature into eggs), but also the ability of those follicles to respond to stimulating medications—essentially, egg-making fertility drugs.

Together, these two factors form your reproductive biological age, and regardless of your chronological age, they are the main barometer of your ability to get pregnant.

In a few moments I'll tell you more about how your ovarian reserve can be determined, and how to judge your true reproductive age. But right now it's also important that you understand something about how the rest of your body ages—and how that can also affect your pregnancy goals.

Preserving Your Good Health

When your doctor tells you to eat more fiber, increase your calcium intake, exercise regularly, limit alcohol consumption, and stop smoking, he or she is not just helping you protect your heart and bones and reduce your risk of cancer. On some level your doctor is also helping you preserve your fertility. How can this be?

First, the most obvious answer: If your overall health is good, your body is much more likely to "go with the flow" of pregnancy. If truth be told, a forty-five-year-old woman with strong bones, good muscle tone, and general good health is more likely to have a problem-free pregnancy and an easier labor and delivery experience than a twenty-five-year-old couch potato who smokes, consumes a lot of alcohol, and eats nothing but junk food.

Equally important, however, is that when your overall health is good, your reproductive hormones are more likely to function at peak capacity, and your egg-making potential can soar. Likewise, studies show that when even serious health problems are diagnosed and treated before pregnancy, conception is more likely to occur.

For this reason, once you are age forty or beyond, your "fertility exam" should begin not with your reproductive specialist but with your internist. As I mentioned earlier, it's imperative that you seek the help of a fertility doctor as early as possible. But at the same time you should also make it a point to check in with your internist, and tell him or her that you are planning to get pregnant. Not only can he or she reassure you that your body is primed and ready to accept the challenges of labor and delivery, but often your doctor can pinpoint one or two undetected health problems that, once corrected, could make getting pregnant faster and easier.

Your Fertility Exam: What You Need and Why

For the most part, the fertility portion of your prepregnancy exam should include all of the key factors covered in Chapter 16, particularly an evaluation of your fallopian tubes, your cervical mucus, and the condition of your uterus. Depending on what these tests show, you might also benefit from an endometrial biopsy on day twenty-one of your cycle, as well as a prolactin-level test. Your partner must have a semen analysis, and

Over Forty: The Medical Checkup You Must Have

If you are over age forty and considering getting pregnant, your internist will use your personal as well as your family history to determine which tests you need before getting pregnant. There are, however, also some essential protocols that are considered important not only to your fertility but also to the health of your pregnancy.

What do you need?

- Baseline electrocardiogram
- Baseline mammogram
- Chest X-ray
- Glucose tolerance test (for blood sugar)
- Fasting cholesterol and blood lipoprotein
- Blood chemistry panel (SMA 12/60)
- Thyrotropin (sensitive thyroid-stimulating hormone)
- Antinuclear antibody, lupus anticoagulant, anticardiolipin antibody
- Complete blood count with platelet

It's also a good idea to see your gynecologist for a basic pelvic-health exam, including a sonogram and a Pap smear, as well as tests for any STDs to which you may have been exposed.

his doctor might also consider a hamster penetration assay and an anti-sperm antibody test. All these procedures are fully explained in Chapters 17 and 18.

Most important for you, however, are tests to determine your ovarian reserve—the ability of your ovaries to respond to fertility medications. I can't emphasize enough the importance of having these tests right from the start. When treating younger women, fertility specialists often go slowly, spacing tests out and performing certain diagnostic procedures only after several attempts at conception have been tried. For the woman over forty, any time lag can be highly detrimental to her pregnancy goals.

What tests do you specifically need?

- **Baseline FSH**: Measuring blood levels of follicle-stimulating hormone, this test reveals your ability to make eggs. Because it is often elevated just before egg-making potential ends, this test can provide a good barometer of the "age" of your ovaries.

- **Baseline estradiol**: This test measures the amount of estrogen in your bloodstream. Since estrogen is made by your ovaries, testing levels can help indicate how well your ovaries are functioning.

- **FSH—day three**: If you are still having a menstrual cycle, elevations of FSH on day three of your cycle mean pregnancy will be difficult to achieve without adequate stimulation from fertility drugs.

- **Pelvic ultrasound**: Although FSH is a good barometer of your egg-making potential, readings are not conclusive. For this reason it's also important that your doctor back up the findings with an ultrasound exam to confirm follicle growth inside your ovary.

The New Hormone That Predicts Fertility

One of the ways in which your egg follicles are nourished is through certain cells inside the ovary itself. Called the *granulosa cells,* they act as a kind of communication system helping to direct egg production and growth. A direct product of these cells is a hormone known as "inhibin B." If testing shows levels are low, it could mean that cells inside your ovary can no longer produce the signals necessary to stimulate egg follicles to grow.

As valuable as this screening may one day be, right now there are no laboratory standards regarding normal inhibin B levels. Therefore, it can be difficult to pinpoint when they are low, particularly when a borderline problem exists.

Until this test is perfected, it should only be used to draw one segment of your fertility portrait and never viewed as conclusive evidence of your ability to get pregnant.

The Fertility Test You Don't Need After Age Forty

If you are under age forty, one of the most telling fertility tests can be the clomiphene challenge described in Chapter 21. Because, however, the test involves tying up at least one menstrual cycle, during which no attempts at conception can be made, this diagnostic is not a good idea for older women.

The reason? The older you are, the more valuable each and every cycle is. It's probably not a good idea to waste one on testing, particularly when the test may not necessarily yield accurate results.

Getting Pregnant: The Quickest Route to Success

Although getting pregnant after age forty can present a unique set of challenges, in many ways, infertility can be more easily treated in older women than in younger ones. Why? If you are thirty and can't get pregnant, chances are you may have a more serious problem—one that could require complex treatment. When, however, you are forty-two and are having trouble conceiving, chances are your problems result from the natural aging process. This, in turn, often means that only slight medical manipulations are necessary to help you conceive. This can be particularly true if you have already had one or more successful pregnancies earlier in your life.

The first and often the most successful treatment for pregnancy after age forty is intrauterine insemination (IUI) paired with fertility drugs—usually a combination of Clomid and hMG. You will find a full explanation of this procedure in Chapter 20.

However, I must caution you again about the time constraints on your fertility. As such, you should pursue no more than three cycles of IUI, particularly if you take a rest between each one. In fact, if your doctor suggests resting between cycles—meaning you will go off fertility drugs—you should continue to use your BBT and other ovulation prediction methods and then have natural intercourse during your window of ovulation opportunity. Occasionally, I have had patients who could not get pregnant during their IUI cycles, but did go on to conceive in the natural cycles that follow. You should always take every opportunity to get pregnant, no matter how small your chances for conception.

In addition, if you are taking the fertility drug Clomid, you must insist that your doctor pay special attention to your cervical mucus, routinely monitoring it throughout your drug regimen. Why? Regardless of the age of the patient, Clomid has a tendency to reduce cervical mucus. When you are over forty, the quantity of your mucus has already decreased—meaning Clomid is likely to affect your cervical environment even more. Although IUI bypasses cervical mucus by placing sperm directly into your uterus, attempting pregnancy during your natural cycles, or via cervical insemination, requires that mucus production be adequate to help transport sperm. Therefore, it's probably a good idea to monitor mucus production. Should levels drop dramatically, other fertility medications, such as estrogen, can help.

IVF After Forty: What You Need to Know

There is no question that IVF—in vitro fertilization—is one of the most important tools in the fertility workshop. However, if you are over forty, this may not automatically be the right treatment for you. Studies show that while IVF can increase the pregnancy odds in younger women—with a "motherhood" rate of more than 13 percent—in older women, the chances of coming away with a successful pregnancy drop dramatically, to just a bit over 3 percent.

Fortunately, by making certain modifications in your IVF treatment cycle, your doctor can significantly improve those odds. What can help? The keys to your IVF success include:

- A high dose of the hormone progesterone during the second half of your menstrual cycle—after your eggs have been retrieved but before the embryos are transferred back into your body. This helps to ensure that you build a strong and healthy uterine lining able to sustain your pregnancy.
- Careful monitoring of your uterine lining. When ultrasound scans show it has remained too thin, your IVF cycle should be canceled, and your embryos frozen, to be used in subsequent tries.

To Hatch or Not to Hatch

As you read in an earlier chapter, a procedure called "assisted hatching" can often improve the success of an IVF cycle. This procedure, which manipulates the outside casing of your embryo before it is transferred into your body, can make implantation easier and more successful.

However, not everyone agrees it is equally useful to women of all ages. While some studies show it does offer benefits to any woman undergoing IVF, more recent evidence has begun to mount showing that women over thirty-six are not helped by this procedure.

My advice to you: The one thing we do know for certain is that assisted hatching in no way harms your embryo or decreases your chance for conception. At worst, it may not help you. At best, it could make a significant difference. If you happen to be one of the older women who falls into the subgroup for which this procedure works, then it can give your baby-making potential a real boost. Rather than wasting a lot of time and energy trying to figure out if assisted hatching can help you, I say why not give it a try? Since it can't hurt your pregnancy odds, and can only help, why not take every advantage you can to obtain your parenting dreams?

In addition, it's important to the success of your IVF that you have at least three healthy embryos available for implantation. In fact, studies show that if you respond well to the fertility medications and have at least three good embryos available for transfer, the chance for a successful IVF is much greater—with a pregnancy rate of nearly 27 percent, which is considered very, very good.

What can increase your odds even further is a new procedure known as embryo defragmentation. How does this work? After your egg is fertilized by your partner's sperm, it begins to divide—from one cell to two, two cells to four, and finally, four to eight cells. During that cell division, your embryo can become fragmented—that is, tiny bits of cytoplasm can come loose. This generally indicates some problem within the structure of the cell wall of the embryo.

As a woman ages, her risk of fragmentation increases, and the higher the rate of fragmentation, the lower the rate of implantation.

However, if those fragments are removed (a relatively simple procedure) before transferring the embryo into your body, implantation rates go right back up to normal.

The GIFT for Women Over Forty

Although there is clearly a group of older women who can benefit from an enhanced IVF treatment cycle, there is also much evidence to show that three of the newer "cousins" of this procedure may work even better. I'm speaking of GIFT (which places sperm and egg together into your fallopian tube), ICSI-GIFT (which places sperm directly into your egg before being placed in your fallopian tubes), and ZIFT (which places your fertilized embryo into your tube). Any of the three (which you can read more about in Chapter 22) may actually be the most beneficial treatment for getting pregnant after age forty, with studies to show each can boost pregnancy rates by a significant margin in this age group.

In one study of some 150 menstrual cycles in women seeking to get pregnant, researchers at the University of California found that while the pregnancy rate was just 5 percent for standard IVF, it jumped dramatically to 29 percent with GIFT. Even more impressive was the pregnancy rate for ZIFT—a startling 45 percent!

While the exact reasons for the difference in these rates remain unclear, I believe the success has much to do with the subtle differences that arise when conception is allowed to take place in the fallopian tubes, where it occurs naturally. While this probably doesn't do much to affect the conception of the embryo itself, I believe it offers hormonal as well as other benefits that help prepare the uterus for implantation. Ultimately, this will help improve the implantation rate, which is the true barometer of the success of an assisted pregnancy. In fact, while it may seem as if fertilization is the most difficult step to achieve, it's actually the easiest. When left alone—even in a laboratory dish—sperm and egg can't seem to stay away from each other! Indeed, the hardest part about achieving a successful pregnancy is in achieving a healthy implantation—and GIFT, ICSI-GIFT, and ZIFT appear to work best in this regard.

Increasing Your Pregnancy Odds Even More

While I believe every woman, regardless of her age, should give herself every opportunity to get pregnant with the minimal amount of laboratory assistance, once you pass age forty, time is of the essence. For this reason, if pregnancy is not forthcoming after two or three cycles of treatment (either IVF, GIFT, or ZIFT), you should consider donor eggs. This is particularly true if you were able to conceive, but your pregnancy did not survive.

As you read in the previous chapters, there are various ways in which you can make use of donor technology, and most important, it may be the fastest, easiest way for you to conceive.

Studies show that when donor eggs are used in conjunction with any of the laboratory-assisted technologies, pregnancy rates improve dramatically. In one study of some some forty cycles in women over age forty, donor eggs boosted the success of IVF from 5 to 29 percent. The rates for GIFT (67 percent) and ZIFT (57 percent) soared even higher!

The best news: When donor eggs were used, the rate of pregnancy loss was cut by more than 50 percent!

Are Donor Eggs Right for You?

It can be a difficult decision, I know. If you are like most of my patients, your inclination is to keep on trying on your own as long as possible. While I do encourage this, I also know that, like many of my patients, you may need a gentle nudge before you start seriously considering donor eggs—encouragement that I am offering you now.

Indeed, your parenting dreams can only become a reality if you yourself are realistic about your reproductive health. So, if, after six months of treatment—including IUI, IVF, GIFT, ICSI-GIFT, or ZIFT—you do not get pregnant, or cannot sustain a pregnancy, I strongly urge you to consider donor eggs. This is particularly true if your levels of FSH register at twenty or above.

Although it may be difficult for you to accept the idea that you and your baby will not be genetically linked, once you are pregnant, I promise that all feelings of natural motherhood will kick in—and you *will* feel like your baby's mother.

Also remember that you may be a candidate for cytoplasmic transfer—the newest form of donor technology, which allows you to maintain a genetic connection to your baby (see Chapter 23).

Protecting Your Pregnancy: What Older Women Need to Know

Regardless of which new technologies help you *get* pregnant, you may soon discover that *staying* pregnant is the tough part. Indeed, maintaining your gestation and guarding against miscarriage often turns out to be an older mother's greatest challenge. Unfortunately, research does show a dramatic rise in pregnancy loss, particularly at the seven-week stage, in women over thirty-five. Unless precautions are taken, by age thirty-eight your chance of pregnancy loss can be as high as 25 percent.

These risks can be magnified even further if your partner is over fifty years old. In fact, while a man certainly retains his fertility throughout most or all of his life, the quality of his sperm can suffer with age. And that, in turn, can play a role not only in conception, but also in the growth and development of a healthy baby. In the chapter on miscarriage you will find many important tips on how to decrease your risk of loss right from the start of your pregnancy.

In addition, however, it's vital not only that you participate in prenatal counseling, but that you get more than adequate prenatal care. You must also take steps to ensure your pregnancy by following strict prenatal dietary recommendations, taking prenatal vitamins, and avoiding smoking, alcohol, and caffeine, both before and especially after you conceive. The reason? All risks associated with pregnancy, including such maternal health problems as gestational diabetes, high blood pressure, bleeding and ruptured membranes, and even fetal or maternal death, increase with a mother's advancing age. While it's important to note that some of these risks, such as fetal death, are small (about 992 out of every

1,000 pregnancies turn out just fine), nonetheless, risks do continue to increase with age. In the event that a problem does occur during your pregnancy, bring your symptoms to your doctor's attention at the very earliest stage, so you can minimize complications and keep your pregnancy on track.

Preventing Birth Defects: What You Can Do

While science has definitely come a very long way in helping to extend a woman's reproductive potential and her childbearing years, our advances were not without a price. The older a woman is when she conceives, the more likely her child is to develop a number of birth defects. In addition, if either mother or father carries the genetic markers for any inherited diseases, risks for these problems can increase with age as well.

Fortunately, there are a variety of diagnostics able to help. Blood tests, including the AFP triple pregnancy screen, as well as amniocentesis (which tests your baby's embryotic fluid), can help rule out many problems at the very earliest stage of pregnancy, including Down's syndrome, a form of mental retardation the risk of which increases as a result of advancing age in either the mother or the father.

In addition, another brand-new technology called preimplantation genetic diagnosis (PGD) tests the embryos formed in the first stage of IVF for a variety of genetic diseases, all before they are transferred back into your uterus.

By identifying which embryos are genetically the healthiest and transferring only those to your body, your doctor can help reduce the risk of birth defects considerably. And the healthier the embryo is, the less risk there is of miscarriage, so in many women, PGD can also work to protect their pregnancy from loss.

Although not all genetic diseases can be identified in an embryo, the list of those that can be—including Down's syndrome—is growing rapidly. In time, it should be possible to confirm or deny the risk for any disease for which we have gene identification. There are, however, some important precautions associated with PGD, so do read Chapter 21 for more information on this procedure.

Finally, never forget the power of good nutrition, particularly vitamins such as folic acid, to help guard your baby against birth defects. Do
be certain to follow the dietary and nutritional guidelines found in Part
Two of this book.

The Older New Mom: Some Final Advice

Getting pregnant—at any age—is a thrill. It is even more rewarding
when you have suffered the pains of infertility and have tried very hard,
for a long time, to make your motherhood dreams come true. As hopeful as I am that your pregnancy will turn out fine, I must leave you with
a few words of caution.

By all means, maintain a positive attitude! At the same time, however, never lose sight of the fact that pregnancy in the older woman is
special, and needs special care. Once your conception is verified by your
fertility doctor, seek the care of a high-risk prenatal specialist, and be certain to follow his or her advice to the "letter." If you should encounter
problems during your pregnancy, seek your doctor's advice right away.

You can also help yourself and your baby by remaining as stress-free
during your pregnancy as possible. Although it is almost second nature
for a mother-to-be to worry, reassure yourself as often as possible that
everything is going to turn out all right. If fear and worry begin to consume your thoughts, confide your feelings to your doctor. In most instances your obstetrician will be able to assure you that everything is
progressing just fine.

Finally, be certain to make your partner a part of your pregnancy,
and whenever possible, include him in your doctor visits and other pregnancy-related activities. Remember, not only are you an older mom—in
most instances he will also be an older dad. If it is the first child for both
of you, then life adjustments will be fast and furious once baby arrives.
If you help him "feel" the presence of your baby in your lives right from
the start of your pregnancy, you will both gain much from your childbearing experience.

I also want to leave those of you struggling to get pregnant after forty—or at any age—with this thought: Several years ago a patient came to me for gynecological treatment. A bright and energetic college professor in her early forties, she was experiencing what she thought was perimenopausal PMS. After having seen me on many television shows, she sought my help in overcoming her symptoms. When she arrived at my office I noticed that, in addition to whatever PMS symptoms she was experiencing, she was also very stressed and seemed somewhat depressed. During our preexamination talk I found out why. For more than seven years she had been trying, unsuccessfully, to get pregnant. After five different doctors told her to give up hope, she finally conceded, and, she told me, abandoned her parenting dreams.

After examining her, and seeing that she had no serious gynecological or reproductive problems, I bypassed the usual hormonal treatments for PMS and instead asked her to follow a high-potency vitamin-mineral plan and a special diet, both similar to the plans featured earlier in this book. I also encouraged her to continue enjoying sexual relations with her mate. While I didn't want to get her hopes up about the prospect of pregnancy, I had a strong feeling that motherhood might still be possible for this woman. I told her to come back and see me in six months—and certainly to call if her PMS symptoms got any worse.

It was not quite five months after our visit that my receptionist buzzed me to tell me this patient was on the line and insisted on seeing me as soon as possible. I told her to come in that afternoon.

When she arrived I could see in her eyes she was angry and upset. Once inside my private office, she really let me have it! "I followed your diet and vitamin plan," she said, "and the only thing it did was throw me into menopause! I haven't had a period for over two months!"

Perhaps you've already guessed the end to this story—it was a happy one indeed. My angry college professor wasn't in menopause—she was pregnant! After seven years and five fertility doctors, she had conceived naturally, on her own, with nothing more than a change in diet. Later that same year, at age forty-four, she delivered a healthy, beautiful baby girl. She was, in fact, so happy, she agreed to appear on several talk shows with me—programs that we hoped would give new optimism to all women struggling to conceive.

Although a simple change in diet worked for this patient—and it may work for you as well—some women may need more than just good nutrition to get pregnant. However, always remember that motherhood can be just around the next bend—so don't give up hope. I'm quite certain there is a treatment that can help you realize your motherhood dream. At the same time, however, be aggressive about obtaining your goals. Don't let a doctor discourage you from getting pregnant solely on the basis of your age, and don't let even the top fertility doctors in your town waste your time by trying the same procedure over and over.

Take charge of your life and your pregnancy goals, and never let age stand in your way.

Your Personal Pregnancy Planner: A Six-Month Guide to a Safe and Healthy Conception

Planning Your Pregnancy
Step-by-Step

In addition to following the suggestions your doctor offers during your pre-conception exam, there are also things *you* can do on your own to get your body ready to have a baby. Indeed, whether you are just beginning to plan for a pregnancy, and believe you will conceive naturally, or you have failed to get pregnant and have decided on a laboratory-aided conception, your Personal Pregnancy Planner can help. Based on the latest medical research and many hours of conversation with my patients, this six-month program is designed to lay the foundation for a healthy pregnancy.

To illustrate how it works I've chosen July as the target date for conception. The months in which you take these steps will depend, of course, on the conception target date that you and your partner select. To chart the correct months in your own pregnancy timetable, simply count back six months before your target date (exclude your conception month from that count).

Also, don't be concerned if you can't complete the steps in the time allotted. Remember, it is only a guide to help point you toward a faster, healthier conception.

Countdown Calender of Events
(Target Date for Conception: July)

January: Pre-Conception Month Six

Goal: To be free of as many potentially toxic substances as possible by the time you conceive

Strategy: Reduce your intake of alcohol and caffeine and begin total elimination of tobacco, recreational drugs, diet pills, sugar, artificial sweeteners, and diet sodas.

Helplines: If you are seriously addicted to any of these substances, especially if you are dependent on one or more, consider getting professional help in overcoming your habit before setting a final target conception date.

February: Pre-Conception Month Five

Goal: To achieve the best weight for a healthy conception

Strategy: Use the chart in Chapter 9 to establish your ideal pre-conception weight, and come as close to that as possible within the next three months. If you need to lose weight, avoid crash diets, diet pills, any form of fasting or starvation, and liquid diets. If you need to gain weight, add calories in the form of complex carbohydrates and protein rather than fats. Also avoid commercial weight-gain products.

Helplines: Because dieting often causes tricky shifts in hormonal activity, some of which can affect your fertility, pre-conception weight loss or gain must be sensible and slow. In addition, because even those slow changes in body fat can have some effect on reproductive biochemistry, your system needs time to stabilize after any significant weight change before you attempt conception. Unless drastic losses or gains are required, you should be able to achieve your goals within three months and then use the eight to ten weeks that follow to stabilize before conceiving.

March: Pre-Conception Month Four

Goal: To overcome nutritional deficiencies that could affect your fertility or the health of your baby

Strategy: Follow the Fertility Diet 2000 featured in Part Two and remember to take one to two prenatal vitamins starting daily now. In addition, add supplements of vitamin C, folic acid, and zinc if you smoke, drink alcohol, or take birth control pills. Also important:

- Avoid junk food, preservatives, processed foods, sugar, artificial sweeteners, caffeine
- Eat fresh fruits, vegetables, nondairy or low-fat dairy sources of calcium, and fiber, and drink lots of water

April: Pre-Conception Month Three

Goal: To avoid fertility- or pregnancy-related complications that arise from medication or birth control pills

Strategy:

- Discontinue taking birth control pills and substitute a barrier form of contraception for a period of at least three months before attempting conception.
- Limit the use of unnecessary medication, both prescription and over-the-counter drugs, including cold remedies, pain relievers, sinus medications, cough medicines, diet pills, diuretics, tranquilizers, and antibiotics.

Helplines: Should your doctor prescribe any medications during the pre-conception period, make certain that he or she is aware of your target date and ask whether the drugs in question could have adverse reproductive effects. If possible, wait at least thirty (and better sixty) days after discontinuing medication before attempting conception.

Once you stop taking them, all traces of birth control pills are normally out of your body in several weeks. However, each woman's metabolism is unique, so residues can sometimes remain longer than the average.

The risk of birth defects is slightly higher for babies accidentally conceived while birth control pills are being used, so it's wise to remain pill-free for as long as possible before conception.

May: Pre-Conception Month Two

Goals: To ensure that all previously diagnosed medical problems are under control; to ensure that no fertility-robbing conditions have developed since your last exam; to establish your ovulation pattern

Strategy:

- See your doctor for follow-up pre-conception counseling exam. This is extremely important if you are currently using an IUD for birth control.
- Begin establishing your BBT chart and your cervical mucus patterns as described in Chapter 13.

Helplines: Although your first prepregnancy checkup should have included all the tests and diagnostic procedures needed before pregnancy, this second visit, six to eight weeks before your target conception date, is important as well, especially if you have been using birth control pills or if you use an IUD. Your second exam should include the following:

- A review of your medical records and follow-up exam for any previously diagnosed problems
- Removal of the IUD, followed by a repeat test for chlamydia and a prescription for 250 mg of tetracycline antibiotic, taken four times a day for seven days. This will help reduce the risk of infection that can sometimes follow the removal of an IUD
- A pelvic exam to ensure that no fertility-related abnormalities have developed since your previous checkup, including fibroid tumors, ovarian cysts, endometerial lesions, or adhesions

June: Pre-Conception Month One

Goal: To achieve maximum fertility potential
Strategy:

- Restrict alcohol consumption
- Avoid all recreational drugs
- Stop dieting
- Keep exercise to a minimum
- Avoid stress
- Avoid caffeine

Helplines: Although it's vital that you clear your body of all potentially toxic substances before attempting conception, it's also important that changes in your life be gradual and not abrupt. Any sharp decline in activity or sudden alteration in body chemistry (even for the better) can throw your reproductive system into a frenzy and actually keep you from conceiving, sometimes for a year or longer. For best results, cut down negative factors gradually, giving your body time to adjust before you try to conceive.

July: Your Target Conception Month

Goal: To get pregnant! If you have followed the six-month prepregnancy program and all the advice of your physician, you should be ready for a fast, easy, and healthy conception. However, it's important to keep your "target" date flexible. Even the healthiest couples don't always conceive when they want to, so remain relaxed and confident even if a pregnancy does not occur right away.
Remember:

- It can take up to a year to get pregnant, even if you and your partner are in perfect health.
- The success rate for pregnancy in healthy, normal couples is only 14 percent, with just three pregnancies possible for every twenty-five acts of intercourse during your most fertile time.

The main thing to remember: One of the best ways to get pregnant is to be relaxed and feel good about yourself and about the idea of becoming a parent. Use the Personal Pregnancy Planner as a guide, but don't get bogged down with routines and schedules, especially in love-making. Keep your sex life spontaneous and fun!

The Forty-Eight-Hour Conception Boost: Surefire Ways to Increase Your Fertility Right Before You Conceive!

Things You Should Avoid

- Pantyhose
- Artificial sweeteners
- Excessive sugar
- Cola beverages, especially diet sodas
- Coffee, tea, chocolate
- Hot tubs, hot showers, saunas, steam rooms
- Heating pads and electric blankets
- Exercise
- Stress

Things Your Partner Should Avoid

- Ejaculation, including masturbation
- Tight underwear
- Tight pants
- Hot tubs, hot showers, saunas, steam rooms
- Heating pads and electric blankets
- Heavy physical activity

What You and Your Partner Should Do

- Avoid stress
- Increase vitamin C by 500 mg twice daily
- Increase B-Complex by 50 mg three times daily, B_6 by 100 mg daily
- Get at least eight hours of sleep a night for two nights in a row
- Avoid any use of alcohol, drugs, or tobacco
- Think about making love, not making babies

How Positive Emotions Can Help You Conceive: Nine Suggestions for a Happy, Healthy Pregnancy

One of the more interesting theories concerning fertility focuses on the benefits of positive emotions for couples trying to conceive. In much the same way that negative emotions can inhibit reproduction, positive thoughts and strong mental images of a happy, healthy pregnancy can increase your ability to conceive. Not only have several studies confirmed this idea, I have personally found this to be true. And I have also seen emotional health act as a deciding factor in some cases of unexplained infertility.

For this reason I strongly advise you to look forward to not only getting pregnant, but *being pregnant*. To achieve a positive state of mind, try the following suggestions in the months and weeks before your target conception date.

1. Enjoy your prepregnancy preparations. The time you spend getting ready to get pregnant should be joyful, even though you may be working very hard to achieve your goals. Feel positive about what you are doing and know in your heart that each step you take is bringing you that much closer to giving birth to a healthy, beautiful baby.

2. Feel positive about making changes. Don't dwell on negative feelings of deprivation, even if you have to give up lifelong habits, such as cigarettes or caffeine.

3. Relax about your pregnancy. Don't get uptight if you aren't accomplishing your goals right on schedule. Pregnancy preparation is not a race or a competition, just a method of helping you conceive a healthy child. It is something you can enjoy, and at your own pace.

4. Become dedicated to having a baby. Don't let the desire to have a baby run your life, but do feel your commitment deep inside you and feel good about that commitment.

5. Eliminate stress as much as possible. Don't worry about your pregnancy or your ability to conceive. Feel relaxed about not only getting pregnant, but being pregnant.

6. Think about the joys of parenthood. Concentrate on your happiness about being a parent, and believe that your child will be happy, healthy, and strong.

7. Feel your fertility. Several times a day close your eyes for a few moments and feel the power within you to create a wonderful, beautiful baby. Feel your body working for you and begin to imagine a child growing inside you.

8. Think about being in love—and not just about making babies. Never forget the role that love, and not just sex, has in conception. Focus on the love that you and your partner share.

9. Believe in yourself. If you embrace only one positive thought in the months before getting pregnant, let it be a belief in yourself and your ability to conceive and deliver a healthy baby.

Never forget the power you can have over your body and your pregnancy when you become a partner in your own health care. Believe that you can make a difference—and that what you do, say, think, and feel are as important as any doctor's diagnosis. Understand that sometimes what you feel in your heart can correctly contradict even the most learned medical opinion.

Most of all, believe in what you're doing and your ability to make positive things happen in your life, including pregnancy. You deserve the joy of parenthood. It can and will be yours. Good luck—and let us know if we can help you in any way!

Our website:
  GettingPregnant.net
Our e-mail:
  NLauersen@aol.com
  GettingPregnant@earthlink.net
Our office address:
  784 Park Avenue
  New York, NY 10021

Resources

Organizations

To learn more about protecting your fertility and expanding your child-bearing options, the following organizations can help.

American College of Obstetricians and Gynecologists
409 12th Street SW, PO Box 96920
Washington, DC 20090-6920
(202) 638-5577
www.acog.com

American Infertility Association
666 Fifth Avenue, Suite 278
New York, NY 10103
(212) 764-0802
www.Americaninfertility.org
(Note: The American Infertility Association [formerly the New York City chapter of Resolve] is, by far, one of the most important organizations and information sources for those experiencing fertility problems. Staffed with dedicated professionals to guide you every step of the way, they provide invaluable resources and information, including a database of fertility specialists around the nation.)

American Society of Andrology
74 Montgomery Street Suite 230
San Francisco, CA 94105
(415) 764-4823
www.godot.uriol.uic.edu~andrology.

American Society for Reproductive Medicine
1209 Montgomery Highway
Birmingham, AL 35216-2809
(205) 978-5000
www.asrm.org
(Check their website for a national listing of fertility experts.)

Endometriosis Association
8585 North 76th Place
Milwaukee, WI 53223
(800) 992-3636 (in United States)
(800) 426-2363 (in Canada)
www.IVF.com/endoassn.html

International Council on Infertility Information Dissemination
PO Box 6836
Arlington, VA 22206
(703) 379-9178
www.incid.org
(Here you will find a nationwide listing of fertility experts, testing facilities, and the latest information on treatment options and clinical trials.)

March of Dimes Birth Defects Foundation
1275 Marmaronek Avenue
White Plains, NY 10605
www.modimes.org

National Alliance to Prevent Birth Defects
www.birthdefectsprevent.org

Nine to Five—National Organization of Working Women
614 West Superior Avenue
Cleveland, OH 44113
(216) 566-9308

Repromedix Corp
10 Roessler Road, Suite A
Woburn, MA 01801
www.repromedix.com
(Information on immune system testing for chronic miscarriage, including where and how to obtain testing)

Resolve
1310 Broadway
Somerville, MA 02144
(617) 623-0744 (Helpline)
www.resolve.org

Society for Reproductive Endocrinology and Infertility
www.socrei.org/SREMAP.shtml
(Check their website for a listing of certified fertility experts nationwide.)

For Mail-Order Fertility Products, Including Medications, Custom Preparations, Ovulation Predictors, and Sex Selection Materials

Apthorp Pharmacy
2201 Broadway
New York City, NY 10024
Tel: (212) 877-3480
Fax: (212) 769-9095

Boghen Pharmacy
1080 Park Avenue
New York, NY 10128
(800) 842-6600

Clear Plan Easy Fertility Monitor
Unilever Corporation—Unipath Diagnostics
Free Brochure: (800) 931-1122
www.clearplan.com

Madison Pharmacy Wisconsin
1603 Monroe Street
PO Box 9641
Madison, WI 53715
(800) 558-7046

SELNAS—USA
For more information on how to obtain your personal sex selection cal-
endar
Call toll free: 877-NUBIRTH (682-4784)
Or on the Internet visit: *www.SELNASUSA.com*

Zetek Corporation—The Cue II
876 Ventura Street
Aurora, CO 80011
(303) 343-2122
www.zetek.com

Aromatherapy Products/Fragrances

Beauty by Tova (Tova Nights)
The Tova Corporation
Beverly Hills, CA 90210
(800) 852-9999 or the QVC Shopping Channel at (800) 345-1515
www.beautybytova.com

The Body Shop (lavender essential oils, vanilla)
(800) 263-9746
www.thebodyshop.com

Marilyn Miglin Products (pheromone)
112 East Oak Street
Chicago, IL
(800) 662-2871
www.marilyn-miglin.com
Or: Home Shopping Network Customer Service, (800) 284-3900

Perlier (Natural Vanilla products)
Home Shopping Network
(800) 284-3900

Fertility Experts

Baylor College of Medicine
Department of Obstetrics and Gynecology
1 Baylor Medical Plaza
Houston, TX 77054
(713) 798-7500

Alan Beers, M.D.
Reproductive Medicine Program
Finch University of Health Sciences—Chicago Medical School
3333 Green Baby Road
North Chicago, IL 60064
(847) 578-3233
www.repro-med.net
(Program specializes in chronic miscarriage, including immune-system testing and treatment.)

Brigham and Women's Hospital
IVF Program
75 Francis Street
Boston, MA 02115

Professor Ian Craft
London Fertility Center
Cozen's House
112A Harley Street
London, W1N1AF, England
011-44-71-224-0707

Alice Domar, Ph.D.
Mind-Body Center for Women's Health
Beth Israel Deaconess Medical Center
Boston, MA

Duke University Medical Center
Department of Obstetrics and Gynecology
Box 3527
Durham, NC 27404

Harry Fisch, M.D. (urology)
944 Park Avenue
New York, NY 10028
(212) 879-0800

Genetics and IVF Institute
Fairfax Hospital—Joseph Schulman, M.D.
3020 Javier Road
Fairfax, VA 22031

Mark Goldstein, M.D. (urology)
New York Weill-Cornell Center
525 East 68th Street
New York, NY 10021
(212) 746-5470

Steven Goldstein, M.D.
New York University Medical Center
317 East 45th Street
New York, NY 10016
(212) 263-7416

Jamie Griffo, M.D.
Chief of Reproductive Endocrinology
New York University Medical Center
317 East 45th Street, Floor 5
New York, NY 10016
(212) 263-7978

Hospital of the University of Pennsylvania
Department of Obstetrics and Gynecology
3400 Spruce Street, Suite 106
Philadelphia, PA 19104

The Johns Hopkins Hospital
Division of Reproductive Endocrinology
600 North Wolfe Street
Baltimore, MD 21205

Jones Institute for Reproduction
601 Colley Avenue
Norfolk, VA 23507
(757) 446-7100

Richard Marrs, M.D.
California Fertility Associates
1245 16th Street, Suite 220
Santa Monica, CA 90404

J. Victor Reyniak, M.D.
1107 Fifth Avenue
New York, NY 10128
(212) 410-4080

Zev Rosenwaks, M.D.
New York Weill-Cornell Center
Obstetrics and Gynecology Department
530 East 70th Street
New York, NY 10021
(212) 472-5003

Scott Rosoff, M.D.
741 Northfield Avenue, Suite 100
West Orange, NJ 07052
(201) 736-1200

Mark V. Sauer, M.D.
Chief of Endocrinology and Director of the Columbia Presbyterian
Center for Reproductive Medicine
161 Fort Washington Avenue, Suite 450
New York, NY 10032
(212) 305-3696

Jonathan Scher, M.D.
1126 Park Avenue
New York, NY 10021
(212) 427-7400
(Handles chronic miscarriage and high-risk pregnancy [OB/GYN].)

Richard Scott, M.D.
St. Barnabas Medical Center
94 Old Short Hills Road
Livingston, NJ 07039

Geoffrey Sher, M.D.
Pacific Fertility Center
2100 Webster Street, Suite 220
San Francisco, CA 94115
(415) 923-3344
or: Northern Nevada Fertility Clinic
350 West 6th Street
Reno, NV 89503

St. Barnabas Medical Center of New Jersey
Department of Reproductive Endocrinology
94 Old Short Hills Road
Livingston, NJ 07039

UMDNJ, New Jersey Medical School, Newark
Center for Reproductive Medicine, F342
150 Bergen Street
Newark, NJ 07103

University of Texas Health Science Center
Department of Reproductive Science
6431 Fannin, Suite 3204
Houston, TX 77030

University of Texas—SW Medical School
Division of Reproductive Endocrinology
Department of Obstetrics and Gynecology
Dallas, TX 07232

University of Wisconsin
Madison Fertility Clinic
600 Highland Avenue, H4/630 CSC
Madison, WI 53792

Vanderbilt University
Center for Fertility and Reproductive Research
IVF Program—D-3200 Medical Center North
Nashville, TN 37232

Michelle Warren, M.D.
Medical Director
Columbia Presbyterian Center for Menopause, Hormonal Disorders,
and Women's Health
16 East 60th Street
New York, NY 10022
(212) 326-8547

Yale University Medical School
Department of Obstetrics and Gynecology—IVF Program
333 Cedar Street
New Haven, CT 06510

Index